DATE DUE

AUG 0 7 2014			
MAY 3 1 2017			

Demco, Inc. 38-293

Radiologic Technology
at a Glance

Theresa S. Reid-Paul, MBA/HCM, R.T.(R)
Keiser University
Fort Lauderdale, Florida

DELMAR
CENGAGE Learning™

Australia Canada Mexico Singapore Spain United Kingdom United

DELMAR
CENGAGE Learning

Radiologic Technology at a Glance, **First Edition**

Theresa S. Reid-Paul, MBA/HCM, R.T.(R)

Vice President, Editorial: Dave Garza

Director of Learning Solutions: Matthew Kane

Senior Acquisitions Editor: Sherry Dickinson

Associate Acquisitions Editor: Christina Gifford

Managing Editor: Marah Bellegarde

Product Manager: Laura J. Wood

Editorial Assistant: Anthony Souza

Vice President, Marketing: Jennifer Ann Baker

Marketing Director: Wendy E. Mapstone

Associate Marketing Manager:
Jonathan Sheehan

Technology Project Manager: Ben Knapp

Technology Project Manager: Patricia Allen

Senior Director, Education Production:
Wendy A. Troeger

Production Manager: Andrew Crouth

Senior Content Project Manager:
Kara A. DiCaterino

Senior Art Director: David Arsenault

For product information and technology assistance, contact us at
Cengage Learning Customer & Sales Support, 1-800-354-9706.

For permission to use material from this text or product,
submit all requests online at **www.cengage.com/permissions**.
Further permissions questions can be e-mailed to
permissionrequest@cengage.com

The ARRT does not review, evaluate, or endorse publications. Permission to reproduce ARRT copyrighted materials within this publication should not be construed as an endorsement of the publication by the ARRT.

Library of Congress Control Number: 2011925448

ISBN 13: 978-1-4354-5405-7

ISBN 10: 1-4354-5405-7

Delmar

5 Maxwell Drive
Clifton Park, NY 12065-2919
USA

Cengage Learning is a leading provider of customized learning solutions with office locations around the globe, including Singapore, the United Kingdom, Australia, Mexico, Brazil, and Japan. Locate your local office at **international. cengage.com/region**

Cengage Learning products are represented in Canada by Nelson Education, Ltd.

To learn more about Delmar, visit **www.cengage.com/delmar**

Purchase any of our products at your local college store or at our preferred online store **www.cengagebrain.com**

Notice to the Reader

Publisher does not warrant or guarantee any of the products described herein or perform any independent analysis in connection with any of the product information contained herein. Publisher does not assume, and expressly disclaims, any obligation to obtain and include information other than that provided to it by the manufacturer. The reader is expressly warned to consider and adopt all safety precautions that might be indicated by the activities described herein and to avoid all potential hazards. By following the instructions contained herein, the reader willingly assumes all risks in connection with such instructions. The publisher makes no representations or warranties of any kind, including but not limited to, the warranties of fitness for particular purpose or merchantability, nor are any such representations implied with respect to the material set forth herein, and the publisher takes no responsibility with respect to such material. The publisher shall not be liable for any special, consequential, or exemplary damages resulting, in whole or part, from the readers' use of, or reliance upon, this material.

Printed in the United States of America
1 2 3 4 5 6 7 15 14 13 12 11

Table of Contents

Preface   ix

How to Use StudyWARE™   xiii

I Content Category
Professional Considerations and Patient Care 1

Chapter 1 – Imaging Modalities and Professional Organizations   **2**

Concept Thinking   2
Related Terms   6
Concept Thinking Questions   12
Practice Exercises   13
Matching   13
Retention of Material   14

Chapter 2 – Abbreviations and Word Parts   **15**

Concept Thinking   15
Abbreviations and Word Parts   16
Abbreviations   16
Prefixes   19
Root words   20
Suffixes   22
Concept Thinking Questions   23
Practice Exercises   23
Matching   24
Retention of Material   24

Chapter 3 – Medical and Legal Terms   **25**

Concept Thinking   25
Medical and Legal Terms   26
Concept Thinking Questions   39
Practice Exercises   40
Matching   40
Retention of Material   41

Chapter 4 – Infection Control   **42**

Concept Thinking   42
Related Terms   43
Concept Thinking Questions   59

Practice Exercises   59
Matching   60
Retention of Material   61

Chapter 5 – Pharmacology and Contrast Media   **62**

Concept Thinking   62
Related Terms   63
Concept Thinking Questions   79
Practice Exercises   79
Matching   80
Retention of Material   81

II   Content Category
Equipment Operation and Quality Control 83

Chapter 6 – Physics Terminology   84

Concept Thinking   84
Related Terms   85
Concept Thinking Questions   106
Practice Exercises   107
Matching   108
Retention of Material   108

Chapter 7 – Circuitry   **111**

Concept Thinking   111
Related Terms   112
Concept Thinking Questions   135
Practice Exercises   136
Matching   136
Retention of Material   137

Chapter 8 – X-ray Tube   **139**

Concept Thinking   139
Related Terms   140
Concept Thinking Questions   155
Practice Exercises   155
Matching   157
Retention of Material   158

Chapter 9 – Fluoroscopy   **159**

Concept Thinking   159
Related Terms   160
Concept Thinking Questions   174
Practice Exercises   175
Matching   176
Retention of Material   177

III Content Category
Image Production and Evaluation 179

Chapter 10 – Image Production **180**

Concept Thinking 180
Related Terms 181
Concept Thinking Questions 212
Practice Exercises 213
Matching 214
Retention of Material 214

Chapter 11 – Imaging Principles and Mathematical Equations **216**

Concept Thinking 216
Related Mathematical Equations 217
Concept Thinking Questions 228
Practice Exercises 229
Matching 230
Retention of Material 231

IV Content Category
Radiation Effects and Protective Measures 233

Chapter 12 – Radiation Biology **234**

Concept Thinking 234
Related Terms 235
Concept Thinking Questions 246
Practice Exercises 247
Matching 247
Retention of Material 248

Chapter 13 – Radiation Protection **249**

Concept Thinking 249
Related Terms 250
Concept Thinking Questions 262
Practice Exercises 263
Matching 263
Retention of Material 264

V Content Category
Anatomy and Imaging Procedures 265

Chapter 14 – Organ System Anatomy **266**

Concept Thinking 266
Organ Systems and Related Terms 267
Concept Thinking Questions 295
Practice Exercises 296
Matching 296
Retention of Material 297

Chapter 15 – Positioning Terms, Landmarks, and Lines   **298**

Concept Thinking   298
Abbreviations: Radiographic Examinations   299
Abbreviations: Projections and Positions   299
Common Vocabulary/Positioning Terms   301
Body Quadrants (Abdominopelvic)   304
Body Regions (Abdominopelvic)   304
Directional Terms   306
Directional X-ray Tube Terms   311
Bony Landmarks   314
Skull Topography   315
Skull Positioning Lines   316
Skull Morphology   318
Concept Thinking Questions   318
Practice Exercises   319
Matching   320
Retention of Material   320

Appendix A – ASRT Code of Ethics   **322**

Appendix B – Professional Organizations   **323**

Appendix C – ASRT Scope of Practice (Practice Standards for Medical Imaging and Radiation Therapy)   **331**

Appendix D – 2010 American Heart Association Guidelines for CPR and Emergency Cardiovascular Care: Lay Rescuer Adult Cardiopulmonary Resuscitation (CPR)   **333**

Appendix E – 381.026 Florida Patient's Bill of Rights and Responsibilities   **336**

Appendix F – Informed Consent   **341**

Appendix G – Steps for Contrast Administration (Venipuncture)   **342**

Appendix H – Incident Report Forum   **344**

Appendix I – Dosimetry Report   **345**

Answer Key   **346**

References   **375**

Index   **378**

Preface

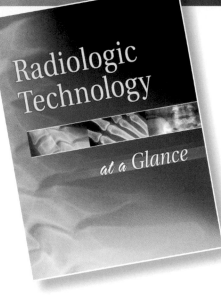

INTRODUCTION

The purpose of *Radiologic Technology at a Glance* is to provide learners with a straightforward overview of the radiologic profession. This book is intended to accompany learners throughout each course of study within their radiology program and serve as a guide to fully understanding the various aspects essential to the role of a registered radiologic technologist. Because retention of learned material is so important in preparing eligible candidates to achieve success on the American Registry of Radiologic Technologists (ARRT) national certification examination, this book also provides several test sections that incorporate exercises to strengthen memorization skills, develop critical thinking skills, and promote self-evaluation. In addition, this resource may prove valuable to novice professionals and to those needing a refresher of terms and concepts that relate to the field.

CONCEPTUAL APPROACH

After a decade of teaching students and observing their great ability to compartmentalize, I came to understand that a common recurring obstacle for students was the ability to retain previously learned material and integrate it into a continuum of information necessary for understanding the imaging profession as a whole. The biggest culprit hindering retention is what I refer to as an "informational gap," or a missing piece of information. An informational gap results in a break in the understanding of a particular concept, theory, or mathematical equation. The answer for helping students increase their level of retention became clear: Go backward rather than forward and identify the "informational gaps." Filling in these gaps with relevant "need-to-know" information and providing a transitional piece of information to bridge one aspect of the profession to another would promote the continuum of learning necessary for a full understanding of the imaging profession. Learning the role of radiologic technologist is not based on islands of information but an integration of all aspects of the imaging profession. This book came out of a strong desire to help students understand that the learning process first begins with establishing a solid foundation on which to build one conceptual objective at a time. My intent with this book is to provide students with a resource that encourages them to identify their strengths and weaknesses and fill any informational gaps they may uncover along the educational journey to become a registered radiologic technologist.

ORGANIZATION OF *RADIOLOGIC TECHNOLOGY AT A GLANCE*

This book is written in a manner that organizes information into five major content categories that are aligned with the ARRT national examination testing categories. These categories include: *Professional Considerations and Patient Care, Equipment Operations and Quality Control, Image Production and Evaluation, Radiation Biology and Radiation Protection,* and *Anatomy and Imaging Procedures.* Within each content category are chapters dedicated to defining specific imaging terminology relevant to the subject area. *Radiologic Technology at a Glance* is unique in its design, for each chapter is presented in a glossary format, providing a user-friendly approach to quickly locating specific radiology topics.

The book includes hundreds of figures and tables along with useful appendices that provide learners with visual images, data groupings, and reference materials correlated to the terminology, concepts, and mathematical equations presented. Each chapter begins with learning objectives and an introduction entitled *Concept Thinking*, where a brief overview of the chapter is provided along with insight on how best to gain knowledge of the subject matter. To allow the learner to locate terms easily, the defining terminology and concepts are listed in alphabetical order under *Related Terms.* Subentries and cross references to related terminology are provided where appropriate. At the end of each chapter is a review section composed of *Concept Thinking Questions, Practice Exercises, Matching,* and *Retention of Material.* The *Concept Thinking Questions* provide learners with an opportunity to test their understanding of a broad concept proposed within their course of study and summarized within the chapter. *Practice Exercises* challenge learners to seek a deeper level of understanding of the foundational concepts presented. The *Matching* section allows learners to assess their knowledge base utilizing word association. *Retention of Material* is the final testing section of each chapter where questions are purposefully reworded from the *Concept Thinking Questions* and the *Practice Exercises* to ensure the application of critical thinking skills while simultaneously reinforcing the retention of previously learned material.

Many useful appendices are provided along with answers to all end-of-chapter activities. Among other valuable documents, the appendices include the American Society of Radiologic Technologists *Code of Ethics* (Appendix A) and *Practice Standards for Medical Imaging and Radiation Therapy* (Appendix C), along with contact lists for professional imaging organizations (Appendix B).

FEATURES

Features of *Radiologic Technology At a Glance* include the following:
- A *first-of-its-kind resource designed specifically for radiographic technology programs* to promote review and retention of the most common terminology encountered in the imaging profession.

- *Learning objectives* that provide a framework for study and review of materials discussed in each chapter.
- An *easy-to-use, glossary-style format* that allows users to quickly locate relevant terms.
- A *full-color format* that enhances understanding of major concepts by presenting more than 200 detailed illustrations that provide visual support for key terms and concepts.
- *More than* 60 *tables* that detail important data and information related to major concepts.
- More than 650 *Practice Exercises and Critical Thinking Activities* that help students retain important concepts and terminology.
- A *comprehensive index* that allows users to quickly turn to information on a term or concept.

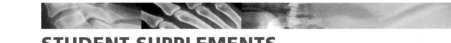

STUDENT SUPPLEMENTS

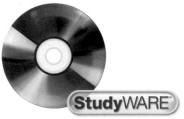

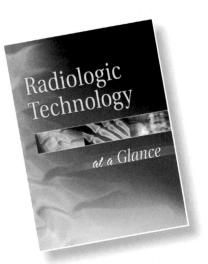

StudyWARE™ CD-ROM to accompany *Radiologic Technology at a Glance*

This interactive software accompanies the book and offers an exciting way to gain additional practice through exercises, game activities, and audio pronunciations for each chapter. See *"How to Use StudyWARE™"* on page xiii for details.

Also Available

StudyWARE™ CD-ROM stand-alone to accompany *Radiologic Technology at a Glance* (ISBN-13: 978-1-1115-3817-0) and *Book Only*: *Radiologic Technology at a Glance* (ISBN-13: 978-1-1113-2056-0).

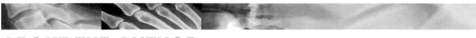

ABOUT THE AUTHOR

Theresa S. Reid-Paul, MBA/HCM, R.T.(R), has been involved in the radiologic profession for nearly 20 years and has served as a program director and regional program director for more than a decade. Her current role as educator involves managing programmatic accreditation processes within the Keiser University Collegiate System. She continues to serve as a radiography program accreditation site visitor.

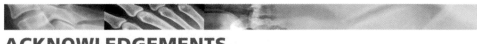

ACKNOWLEDGEMENTS

I would like to thank the many students I have had the pleasure to teach during the past twelve years, for they truly inspired the making of this book. I would like to express my sincere appreciation to the individuals and organizations that granted me permission to reproduce tables, images, illustrations, and photos. I extend my gratitude to Laura J. Wood, Product Manager, who supported me and guided me throughout this project, and to the reviewers who provided me with excellent feedback. A special thanks to Ms. Kathy Drotar, my friend and colleague, for her participation in the development of activities for the interactive software to accompany *Radiologic Technology at a Glance*. Finally, I would like to thank my loving husband, Edmund, whose unwavering encouragement kept me motivated and focused throughout this amazing journey, and my mother, Marion, who served as my personal cheerleader. I dedicate this book to my daughter, Keshia, stepson, Jordan, and brother, Kenny, so they may know that with desire, determination, and God's blessing, anything is possible at any age.

Reviewers

Lori Covington, M.S., R.T.(R)(M)
Radiology Technology
Program Director/Asst. Professor
San Diego Mesa College
San Diego, CA

Marie Hattabaugh, MAT, R.T.(R)(M)
Professor in the Radiography Program
Allied Health Department
Pensacola Junior College
Pensacola, FL

Rhonda Kern, MBA, R.T.(R)
Radiologic Technology Program
Coordinator
Southwestern Illinois College
Belleville, IL

Trina L. Koscielicki, M.Ed., R.T.(R)
Associate Professor and Director,
    Radiologic Technology Program
Department of Allied Health
Northern Kentucky University
Highland Heights, KY

William Nelson, MA, R.T.(R)
Professional Faculty
Washtenaw Community College
Ann Arbor, MI

Teal Sander, B.S., R.T.(R)(M)(CT)
LRT Instructor
Allied Health Department
Fort Hays State University
Hays, KS

How to Use StudyWARE™ to Accompany *Radiologic Technology At a Glance*

The StudyWARE™ software helps you learn terms and concepts in *Radiologic Technology at a Glance*. As you study each chapter in the text, be sure to explore the activities in the corresponding chapter in the software. Use StudyWARE™ as your own private tutor to help you learn the material in your textbook.

Getting started is easy. Install the software by inserting the CD-ROM into your computer's CD-ROM drive and following the on-screen instructions. When you open the software, enter your first and last name so the software can store your quiz results. Then choose a chapter from the menu to take a quiz or explore one of the activities.

Menus

You can access the menus from wherever you are in the program. The menus include quizzes and other activities organized by chapter.

Quizzes. Quizzes include multiple choice, true/false, matching, and fill-in-the-blank questions. You can take the quizzes in both practice mode and quiz mode. Use practice mode to improve your mastery of the material. You have multiple tries to get the answers correct. Instant feedback tells you whether you're right or wrong and helps you learn quickly by explaining why an answer is correct or incorrect. Use quiz mode when you are ready to test yourself and keep a record of your scores. In quiz mode, you have one try to get the answers right, but you can take each quiz as many times as you want.

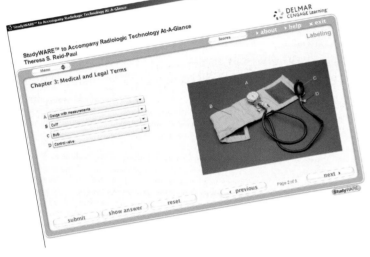

Scores. You can view your last scores for each quiz and print your results to hand in to your instructor.

Activities. Activities include image labeling, spelling bee, hangman, concentration, flash cards, and championship.

Animations. Animations help you visualize important concepts reviewed in the text, from ionizing radiation to infection control.

Audio Library. The StudyWARE™ Audio Library is a reference that includes audio pronunciations and definitions for over 2000 medical terms! Use the Audio Library to practice pronunciation and review definitions for medical terms. You can browse terms by content category or search by key word. Listen to pronunciations of the terms you select or listen to an entire list of terms.

I

Professional Considerations and Patient Care

CHAPTER 1

Imaging Modalities and Professional Organizations

OBJECTIVES

Upon completion of this chapter, the reader will be able to:

- Describe the role of the radiographer, radiologist assistant, and radiologist
- Define the role of the *American Registry of Radiologic Technologists (ARRT)*
- Differentiate between ARRT's primary pathway and postprimary pathway to certification
- Identify accrediting agencies related to the various specialized imaging modalities
- Define the role of The Joint Commission (TJC), formerly known as the Joint Commission, or JCAHO
- Distinguish between accreditation, certification, registration, and licensure
- Explain why continuing education is necessary for certified technologists

CONCEPT THINKING

Radiologic technology has been described as the merging of science and art. The science aspect of the profession involves a comprehensive understanding of human body composition and functional ability along with a knowledge base of radiation production, image formation, and radiation protection. The art aspect of the profession requires critical thinking skills to produce optimal images while taking into account internal and/or external variables that impact image quality. Imaging technology is ever-changing, requiring imaging professionals (radiologic technologists, radiologist assistants, and radiologists) to stay abreast of new and more effective methods for producing and viewing radiographic images. The American Registry of Radiologic Technologists (ARRT) mandates a minimum 24 category A or A+ continuing education credits completed every 2 years for technologists to renew and maintain national certification. State licensure (where applicable) is typically granted to individuals who possess national certification in a specialized imaging modality upon completion and submission of state licensure application and fees. Some states also require applicants to pass their state licensure examination. It is the responsibility of every registered technologist to abide by *ALARA principles* and the profession's *Code of Ethics (Refer to Appendix A – American Society of Radiologic Technologists (ASRT) Code of Ethics.)*

Specialized Imaging Modalities

The ARRT provides national certification examinations to eligible candidates (via primary pathways or postprimary pathways) seeking certification in a *specialized imaging modality*. All eligible candidates must have completed an accredited educational program recognized by the ARRT, successfully met all didactic and clinical ARRT competency requirements, and have followed the Rules of Ethics as stated in the ARRT *Standards of Ethics*. Once an eligible candidate has passed the voluntary national certification examination, the individual has the legal right to use the title of "Registered Technologist" in the abbreviated form of "R.T." behind their name along with the designated credentialing initial(s) representing the specialized imaging modality for which certification has been acquired. The exception to using "R.T." behind the certified technologist's name along with the initials indicating the specific discipline for which registration is held is the Radiologist Assistant. This title appears as "R.R.A," indicating "Registered Radiologist Assistant." However, certification achieved through the ARRT should be indicated with the abbreviation (ARRT) appearing after the credentialing initials representing the imaging modality discipline for which registration is held *(see Table 1–1).*

TABLE 1–1   Specialized Imaging Modalities

SPECIALIZED IMAGING MODALITY	CREDENTIALING INITIALS	PATHWAY	DEFINITION
Bone densitometry	BD	Postprimary	Imaging method that uses minimal radiation to determine bone mineral density (BMD) and aid in the diagnosis of osteoporosis. Procedure is recommended for individuals susceptible to bone loss and for postmenopausal women. Two common areas radiographically scanned for BMD measurements are the lumbar spine and the proximal femur.
Breast sonography	BS	Postprimary	Imaging method that uses high-frequency sound waves of >5 MHz via a transducer (probe) containing one or multiple crystals. Sound waves are reflected back from the internal structures of the breast to the transducer, where they are transformed into an electrical signal and sent to the scanning unit to be processed into a digital image for viewing on a TV monitor.

(Continued)

TABLE 1–1   **Specialized Imaging Modalities** *(Continued)*

SPECIALIZED IMAGING MODALITY	CREDENTIALING INITIALS	PATHWAY	DEFINITION
Cardiac-interventional radiography	CI	Postprimary	Specialized imaging modality that uses ionizing radiation for diagnostic cardiac studies, percutaneous coronary intervention, and therapeutic application.
Computed tomography referred to as (CT scan)	CT	Postprimary	Imaging method that requires the use of ionizing radiation and an array of detectors to image structures in thin slices. Data are collected and digitally manipulated to view images in various body planes on a computer monitor; three-dimensional (3-D) images can be produced.*
Magnetic resonance imaging	MRI	**Primary** Postprimary	Imaging method that uses a magnetic field strength of generally <2.0 Tesla and the manipulation of radiofrequency (RF) interactions with hydrogen nuclei of the body. Images are viewed on a computer monitor.*
Mammography	M	Postprimary	Imaging method specific to breasts that requires the use of ionizing radiation and image receptors (i.e., film, photostimulable phosphor plates [PSP] with computed radiography [CR], and solid-state detector plates with digital radiography [DR]).
Nuclear medicine technology	N	**Primary**	Imaging method that requires the patient to receive radiopharmaceuticals targeted to specific areas within the body. The gamma scintillation camera detects radioactivity of targeted areas depicting the presence or nonpresence of disease. Images can be viewed via film or computer monitor.
Quality management	QM	Postprimary	Specialized concentration of knowledge on various imaging systems (film, CR/DR, and picture archiving communication systems [PACS]), test instrumentation, and radiation protection. Data collection and analysis are continually performed with problem-solving techniques applied for producing optimal images and providing quality service to patients.
Radiography	R	**Primary**	Imaging method that requires the use of ionizing radiation and image receptors (i.e., film, photostimulable phosphor plates with CR, solid-state detector plates with DR, and an image intensifier with fluoroscopy).*

TABLE 1–1 **Specialized Imaging Modalities** *(Continued)*

SPECIALIZED IMAGING MODALITY	CREDENTIALING INITIALS	PATHWAY	DEFINITION
Radiologist assistant	RA	Postprimary	Radiologist assistant is a certified registered technologist with advance-level education who has taken and passed the national ARRT examination for an R.A. degree. The registered radiologist assistant works under the supervision of a radiologist to perform more complex radiographic procedures than those delineated within the scope of the RT.
Radiation therapy	T	**Primary**	Therapy used for malignant conditions and certain nonmalignant conditions in which greater levels (than required in diagnostic radiography) of ionizing radiation are used to effectively impact designated cells and tissues. In the treatment of cancer, cells dosage may be *fractionated (refer to Chapter 12: Radiation Biology)* to allow normal cells to recover while abnormal cells are destroyed.
Sonography	S	**Primary** Postprimary	Imaging method that uses high-frequency sound waves (1–17 MHz) via a transducer (probe) containing one or multiple specialized crystals. Sound waves are reflected back from the body's internal structures to the transducer, where they are transformed into an electrical signal and sent to the scanning unit to be processed into a digital image for viewing on a television monitor. Multidimensional images can be produced. Sonography has therapeutic application with frequencies in the kilohertz (kHz) range.
Vascular-interventional radiography	VI	Postprimary	Specialized imaging modality that uses ionizing radiation for diagnostic vascular-interventional procedures relevant to neurologic, genitourinary, gastrointestinal, peripheral, and thoracic categories.*
Vascular sonography	VS	Postprimary	Imaging method that uses high-frequency sound waves of <10 MHz via a transducer (probe) containing one or multiple crystals. Sound waves are reflected back from the body's internal structures to the transducer, where they are transformed into an electrical signal and sent to the scanning unit to be processed into a digital image for viewing on a TV monitor. Vascular structures are of interest.

Note: A medical-licensed, board-certified radiologist provides interpretation of images.

*Contrast media may be used to enhance visualization of internal structures.

© 2010 The American Registry of Radiologic Technologists

RELATED TERMS

accreditation – Accreditation is a voluntary peer-review process that an institution of higher education or a specialized program of study (which may or may not be located within an institution of higher education) undergoes to demonstrate compliance with set "*Standards*" developed by a specific accrediting agency. Meeting accrediting agency standards confirms that the level of education delivered is of the highest quality. Accrediting agencies recognized by the U.S. Department of Education and/or the Council of Higher Education Accreditation are categorized as follows:

- **National Institutional Accrediting Agencies** – National accrediting agencies are nonprofit organizations capable of accrediting institutions within the United States as well as institutions located outside the United States. There are numerous national institutional accrediting agencies located on the Council of Higher Education Accreditation website: http://www.chea.org.

- **Regional Institutional Accrediting Agencies** – Regional accrediting agencies are nonprofit organizations capable of accrediting institutions within specific regions of the United States.
  - Middle States Association of Colleges and Schools (Middle States Commission on Higher Education); http://www.msche.org
  - New England Association of Schools and Colleges (Commission on Institutions of Higher Education); http://www.neasc.org
  - North Central Association of Colleges and Schools (The Higher Learning Commission); http://www.ncahlc.org
  - Northwest Commission on Colleges and Universities; http://www.nwccu.org
  - Southern Association of Colleges and Schools (Commission on Colleges); http://www.sacscoc.org
  - Western Association of Schools and Colleges (Accrediting Commission for Community and Junior Colleges) and (Accrediting Commission for Senior Colleges and Universities); http://www.wascweb.org

- **specialized accrediting agencies** – Specialized accrediting agencies are nonprofit organizations that are capable of accrediting specialized programs of study (i.e., allied health programs, law, and engineering) in which unique standards specific to the profession have been met *(see Table 1–2).*

accreditation standards – Accreditation standards are a unique set of criteria developed by a particular accrediting agency for which an institution of higher education or a specialized program of study demonstrates compliance sufficiently to receive an award of accreditation.

- **award of accreditation** – Awards of accreditation vary greatly with each accrediting agency. Typical accreditation awards granted include periods ranging from 18 months to 8–10 years; annual reports or interim reports are required for continual monitoring and evaluation of the program of study or the institution. An accreditation award can be reduced and may even be

TABLE 1–2 **Programmatic Accreditation Agencies Recognized by the ARRT (in the United States)**

Recognized by the Council for Higher Education Accreditation (CHEA)

JRCERT	Joint Review Committee on Education in Radiologic Technology	http://www.jrcert.org
JRCNMT	Joint Review Committee on Educational Programs in Nuclear Medicine Technology	http://www.jrcnmt.org
JRC-DMS	Joint Review Committee on Education in Diagnostic Medical Sonography – under the Committee on Accreditation of Allied Health Education Programs (CAAHEP)	http://www.jrcdms.org

- The ARRT recognizes certain educational radiologic technology programs offered in postsecondary degree granting institutions that are accredited by one of the six regional institutional accrediting agencies *(see "accreditation").*
- The ARRT also recognizes certain educational radiology programs accredited outside the United States via:
  - Australian Institute of Radiography
  - Conjoint Accreditation Services of the Canadian Medical Association

© 2010 The American Registry of Radiologic Technologists

evoked if compliance with the established standards to which initial accreditation was awarded is not maintained.

ALARA principle – ALARA is a radiation protection mnemonic that stands for *"as low as reasonably achievable."* Radiographers follow the "ALARA principle" because it is their responsibility (as outlined in the radiologic technology profession's Code of Ethics) to use the least amount of radiation necessary to produce optimal images, thus keeping radiation exposure to the patient, technologist, and related health care workers minimal. Students in radiography programs are held to the same standard as registered technologists and must demonstrate appropriate radiation protection to patients and to themselves.

ARRT – The American Registry of Radiologic Technologists, often referred to as the ARRT, is a national organization that administers eligible candidates certification examinations in radiologic technology modalities such as radiography, cardiac-interventional radiography, vascular-interventional radiography, radiation therapy, nuclear medicine technology, magnetic resonance imaging, mammography, computed tomography, quality management, bone densitometry, sonography, vascular sonography, and breast sonography. The ARRT also provides a national certification examination for *eligible candidates* seeking certification as a radiologist assistant. The ARRT grants initial certification to candidates who successfully pass the ARRT credentialing examination. The ARRT also provides annual registration to certified technologists and radiologist assistants who adhere to the ARRT's *Standard of Ethics* and demonstrate continuing education as mandated by the ARRT *(see Table 1–3).*

TABLE 1–3   Examination and Certification Agencies/Organizations

ARDMS	American Registry of Diagnostic Medical Sonographers; http://www.ardms.org	■ Diagnostic medical sonography
		  • Abdomen
		  • Breast
		  • Fetal echocardiography
		  • Neurosonology
		  • Obstetrics and gynecology
		■ Diagnostic cardiac sonography
		  • Echocardiography
		    ■ Adult
		    ■ Fetal
		    ■ Pediatric
		■ Vascular sonography
		■ Registered physician vascular interpretation (exclusive to physicians)

ARRT	American Registry of Radiologic Technologists; http://www.arrt.org	■ Bone densitometry
		■ Computed tomography
		■ Mammography
		■ Nuclear medicine
		■ Quality management
		■ Radiation therapy
		■ Radiography
		■ Cardiac-interventional radiography
		■ Vascular-interventional radiography
		■ Radiologist assistant
		■ Sonography
		  • Breast sonography
		  • Vascular sonography

NMTCB	Nuclear Medicine Technology Certification Board; http://www.nmtcb.org	■ Nuclear medicine

Obtained via data from the American Registry for Diagnostic Medical Sonography, Inc. (http://www.ardms.org), the American Registry of Radiologic Technologists (http://www.arrt.org), and the Nuclear Medicine Technology Certification Board (http://www.nmtcb.org).

ARRT-eligible candidate – An ARRT-eligible candidate is an individual who meets the ethics, education, and examination requirements set forth by the ARRT and published in the *ARRT Rules and Regulations* and the *ARRT Standards of Ethics*.

ARRT National Certification Examination – The ARRT provides national certification examinations in various radiologic technology disciplines via computerized testing at designated test centers throughout the country. Candidates for an ARRT national examination must submit a completed application, endorsed by the candidate's educational program director (verification of completed programmatic requirements from an approved educational program). An application fee is also required by the ARRT for eligibility status consideration.

- ■ **ARRT primary pathway** – The ARRT offers eligible candidates a primary pathway to certification in the following five imaging disciplines: nuclear medicine technology, magnetic resonance imaging, radiography, radiation therapy, and sonography. The term "primary pathway" represents a direct area of study in one of the five imaging disciplines in which ARRT certification can be achieved upon the ARRT-eligible candidate passing the discipline-specific national examination.

- ■ **ARRT postprimary pathway** – The ARRT offers eligible candidates, i.e., those who are either ARRT-certified or certified by an ARRT-approved agency in one of the primary pathway imaging disciplines, an opportunity for additional certification in imaging disciplines that ARRT has approved as a progression of the supportive discipline in which initial certification was achieved. Postprimary certification candidates must meet all ARRT requirements for the imaging discipline in which they seek additional certification to be eligible to take the discipline-specific national examination.

ARRT rules and regulations – The ARRT has established specific rules and regulations regarding the necessary qualifications for individuals seeking either initial certification or annual registration within a designated discipline(s) of the radiologic technology profession.

ARRT standards of ethics – The ARRT has established *Standards of Ethics* comprising the ASRT "Code of Ethics" and "Rules of Ethics" for individuals seeking ARRT certification and for individuals who are ARRT-registered technologists. The *standards of ethics* serve as a guideline for professional conduct expected within the radiologic technology profession.

ASRT – The American Society of Radiologic Technologists (ASRT) is the largest professional worldwide organization for certified imaging professionals. The ASRT provides registered imaging professionals with a broad scope of knowledge reflecting current technological advancements within the imaging profession, along with providing an array of continuing education activities. The organization developed and promotes the profession's "Code of Ethics" and stresses the importance of delivering consistently high-quality patient care. The ASRT supports and encourages technologists to pursue life-long learning and professional advancement within the imaging profession. *(Refer to Appendix B: Professional Imaging Organizations.)*

certification – Certification is granted by the ARRT to an eligible candidate who has successfully met the ARRT requirements and received a passing score on the credentialing examination.

continuing education – Continuing education (CE) is mandated by the ARRT as a requirement for technologists to renew their certificate of registration. Individual states may also require technologists to submit documentation demonstrating

CE requirements for state licensure renewal have been met. The purpose of CE is to assist technologists in staying abreast of developing technologies and required technical skills evolving within the imaging profession as a means of providing improved patient care. CE activities may be classified as: Category A or A+ (approved by a *recognized continuing education evaluation mechanism (RCEEM)*) or Category B (not approved by a RCEEM). To fulfill the CE requirement for ARRT certification renewal, the technologist must either complete 24 category A or A+ CE credits (the maximum number of category-type credits accepted by the ARRT toward fulfillment of CE requirements is determined by the ARRT) within the biennium reporting cycle, or pass a primary or post primary examination in an additional discipline (other than discipline(s) for which they hold certification) for which they meet eligibility requirements. Academic courses pertinent to the profession and completed at an accredited educational institution may also be considered for CE credits by the ARRT.

- **biennium reporting cycle** – A biennium reporting cycle is a 2-year period, beginning on the first of day of the technologist's birth month and extending for 2 years, ending on the last day of the month before the technologist's birth month, during which CE requirements for certification renewal must be acquired.

credentials – Once an individual has completed the requirements for ARRT candidacy and has successfully passed a discipline-specific ARRT national examination, the individual is awarded initial certification as a "Registered Technologist" and may use R.T. (ARRT) after their name to confer credentials granted by the ARRT. The abbreviated radiologic technology discipline of study should also be indicated in parenthesis following R.T. *(see Table 1–1)*. The registered technologist may continue to use this title as long as certification is maintained with ARRT via compliance with annual registration requirements.

health care accreditation – Health care-accrediting agencies have established standards for evaluating and granting accreditation to various types of health care facilities *(see Table 1–4)*.

licensure – The majority of states within the country require individuals of the radiologic profession whose job duties involve performing imaging procedures on patients with the use of radiation or radioisotopes to be licensed in the state for which they are employed (in addition to holding ARRT national certification). State licensure requirements often vary from state to state; therefore, candidates seeking state licensure in more than one state should contact the individual State Licensing Agency for information regarding licensure qualifications, associated fees, and processing timeframes relevant to the state of interest.

radiologic technologist/radiographer – A radiologic technologist or radiographer's role in the health care profession is to use ionizing radiation to produce high-quality images (including both static and dynamic images) of the body's internal structures based upon knowledge of anatomy, physiology, pathology, patient care, radiation protection, and image production. A state-licensed, board-certified radiologist interprets these images for diagnostic or therapeutic purposes.

TABLE 1–4   Health Care Accreditation Agencies

ACHC	Accreditation Commission for Home Care, Inc.; http://www.achc.org	Evaluates and grants accreditation status to home health care agencies on the basis of compliance with accrediting agency standards.
CARF	Commission on Accreditation of Rehabilitation Facilities; http://www.carf.org	Evaluates and grants accreditation status to rehabilitation facilities on the basis of compliance with accrediting agency standards.
CCAC	Continuing Care Accreditation Commission (acquired by CARF); http://www.carf.org	Evaluates and grants accreditation status to senior care facilities on the basis of compliance with accrediting agency standards.
CHAP	Community Health Accreditation Program; http://www.chapinc.org	Evaluates and grants accreditation status to homecare businesses on the basis of ability to demonstrate adequate resources, quality management, and long-term viability.
TJC*	The Joint Commission (formerly referred to as Joint Commission on Accreditation of Healthcare Organizations or JCAHO); http://www.jointcommission.org	Evaluates and grants accreditation status to long-term care facilities, service providers, and hospitals on the basis of compliance with accrediting agency standards.

*Although there is no commonly used acronym for the Joint Commission, it is still commonly referred to by its previous name, JCAHO.

Obtained from data via the Accreditation Commission for Health Care, Inc. (http://www.achc.org); the Commission on Accreditation of Rehabilitation Facilities (http://www.carf.org); Community Health Accreditation Program (http://wwwchapinc.org); and The Joint Commission (http://www.jointcommission.org).

radiologic technology – Radiologic technology is a broad term used to describe numerous imaging disciplines *(also referred to as specialized imaging modalities or advanced imaging modalities)* offering high-quality images of the body's internal structures from different perspectives. A state-licensed, board-certified radiologist interprets these images for diagnostic and/or therapeutic purposes *(see Table 1–1)*.

radiologist – A radiologist is a physician who specializes in image interpretation of anatomical structures within the body that have been obtained through the various imaging modalities. This information is used in the diagnosis or treatment of patients. Educational requirements for a radiologist may vary slightly; however, typically 8 years of formal education in which a medical degree is awarded followed by 4 years of residency training and training in a subspecialty area are most common. For a radiologist to practice within the United States, he or she must possess:

- State medical license
- Board certification in radiology
- Hospital privileges

radiologist assistant – A radiologist assistant is an ARRT-certified technologist who has completed additional formal education in a nationally approved radiologist assistant program and passed the ARRT national examination for radiologist assistant. A registered radiologist assistant, R.R.A. (ARRT), provides an advanced level of patient care in diagnostic imaging under the supervision of a radiologist. Registered radiologist assistants may wish to include their radiography credentials in their professional title, listing their credentials as R.R.A.,R.T.(R)(ARRT).

registry – The term *registry* as it pertains to the radiologic profession is an ARRT national database listing of registered technologists who hold current ARRT certification and remain in compliance with ARRT credentialing requirements.

specialized imaging modality – Specialized imaging modality may be referred to as an advanced imaging modality or an imaging discipline. These terms relate to a specific branch of the radiologic technology profession. After initial certification as a registered technologist is granted by the ARRT, many technologists pursue additional education and/or hands-on training in a subspecialty area of the imaging profession. To gain postprimary certification in a specialized imaging modality *(see Table 1–1)*, the technologist must meet ARRT eligibility requirements for the advanced modality/discipline for which they wish to achieve certification and "pass" the national examination.

StudyWARE CONNECTION

After completing this chapter, take a practice quiz or play an interactive game on your StudyWARE™ CD-ROM that will help you learn the content discussed in this chapter.

CONCEPT THINKING QUESTIONS

1. Why is institutional and/or programmatic accreditation important, and to whom should it be important?

2. Is accreditation a voluntary or involuntary process?

3. What is the name of the accreditation agency that has specific educational standards for radiologic technology programs?

4. What is the name of the accreditation agency that has specific standards for hospitals and long-term care facilities?

5. What is the difference between the ARRT and the ASRT?

6. What qualifications are required by the ARRT for an individual to achieve eligibility status for the national examination in radiography?

7. Explain the difference between ARRT certification and ARRT registration.

8. Why is continuing education mandated as a requirement for renewal of ARRT certification?

9. List the five disciplines of radiologic technology for which the ARRT provides a *primary* pathway for certification.

10. Which radiologic technology discipline involves the use of radioisotopes?

PRACTICE EXERCISES

1. Explain what the term *radiologic technology* encompasses.

2. Distinguish between the role of a radiologic technologist and the role of a radiologic assistant.

3. Identify the accrediting agency that evaluates radiologic technology programs.

4. Identify the accrediting agency that evaluates hospitals and long-term care facilities.

5. List the organization that provides advanced certification in mammography, bone densitometry, and quality management.

6. What kind of an organization is the ASRT?

7. Explain the importance and value of accreditation standards.

8. List the six regional institutional accrediting agencies capable of accrediting institutions within specific regions of the United States.

9. Which specialized imaging modality requires high-frequency sound waves transformed into an electrical signal for processing into a digital image for viewing?

10. What does each credentialing title represent?

    A. R.T.(MR)(ARRT)

    B. R.T.(R)(ARRT)

    C. R.T.(T)(ARRT)

    D. R.R.A.(ARRT)

MATCHING

Match each term to the appropriate description.

registry	TJC	licensure
CE	accreditation	biennium
Tesla	transducer	category A credit
certification	ARRT	JRCERT
R.T.	radioisotopes	BMD
ASRT	quality management	fractionated

Description   **Term**

1. two-year period   _____

2. health care accrediting agency   _____

3. provides certification examinations _____

4. small doses of radiation over time   _____

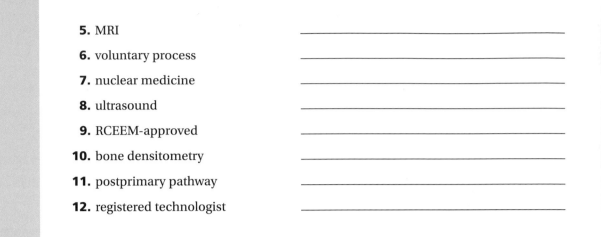

5. MRI _____

6. voluntary process _____

7. nuclear medicine _____

8. ultrasound _____

9. RCEEM-approved _____

10. bone densitometry _____

11. postprimary pathway _____

12. registered technologist _____

RETENTION OF MATERIAL

Retention requires practicing the use of previously learned material. Apply the knowledge you have learned regarding professional considerations and patient care to answer the following questions:

1. Define the following terms:

   A. accreditation

   B. certification

   C. registration

2. Explain how the following imaging modalities function:

   A. radiography

   B. computed tomography

   C. MRI

   D. nuclear medicine

   E. sonography

3. What does the mnemonic ALARA represent?

4. What is the role of a radiologist?

5. Differentiate between an ARRT primary pathway to certification and postprimary pathway to certification.

6. Why can't an individual take a postprimary pathway to certification initially?

7. List the two imaging disciplines that offer both a primary pathway and postprimary pathway to certification.

8. Is certification by the ARRT mandatory?

9. Which specialized imaging modality aids in the diagnosis of osteoporosis?

10. How can a patient know whether the technologist performing their procedure is qualified?

CHAPTER 2

Abbreviations and Word Parts

OBJECTIVES

Upon completion of this chapter, the reader will be able to:

- Identify common health care abbreviations encountered in the imaging profession
- Identify abbreviations regarding executive and administrative titles
- Differentiate between prefixes and suffixes
- Build medical words by combining prefixes, root words, and suffixes

CONCEPT THINKING

Building medical words consists primarily of combinations of word parts comprised of prefixes, root words, and suffixes. Remember that "pre" means before; therefore, all prefixes will come before a root word, whereas suffixes will be found after a root word. The root word is the foundation of the word, or the most basic meaning of the word. Adding a prefix to a root word typically means a more descriptive picture of the root word is provided. Descriptive word parts such as prefixes are similar to adjectives in that they provide clarifying information about the root word. As you change the prefix, you alter the meaning of the entire word. For example, the word *sthenic* refers to an average body habitus with slight muscularity and average strength, in which the thoracic and abdominal organs lie in a "normal" or expected position. When we add the prefix *hypo*, meaning lacking or insufficient in comparison to average, we can picture a body habitus thinner with less muscularity, in which the thoracic and abdominal organs lie lower and appear more vertical. Just as easily, we can change the prefix to *hyper*, meaning larger than average or excessive. This type of body habitus would demonstrate a broader, more muscular stature, with thoracic and abdominal organs appearing higher and more transverse. We can see that, by changing the prefix attached to the root word we have altered the word in such a way that three very different body habitus types can be visualized, even though the basic foundation of the word, *sthenic*, remained the same.

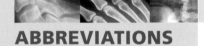

ABBREVIATIONS AND WORD PARTS
(Prefixes, Root Words, and Suffixes)

Building Words:

Abbreviations – letters indicating a medical word, phrase, or concept.

Prefixes *(precede root words)* – alter root words by providing specific additional information; usually in the form of adjectives.

Root Words *(main section or "body" of the word)* – provide the fundamental meaning of the word.

Suffixes *(follow root words)* – alter root words by providing specific additional information.

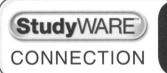

StudyWARE **CONNECTION** — *View the Word Parts animation on the StudyWARE™ CD-ROM for information about building words.*

ABBREVIATIONS

Letter or a grouping of letters indicating a medical word, phrase, or concept

$\overline{\textbf{a}}$	before
a.c.	before a meal
ADH	antidiuretic hormone
AF	atrial fibrillation
AIDS	acquired immune deficiency syndrome
ARDS	adult respiratory distress syndrome
ARS	acute radiation syndrome
ASAP	as soon as possible, immediately
b.i.d.	twice a day
b.i.n.	twice a night
BM	bowel movement
BP	blood pressure
bpm	beats per minute

Bx	biopsy
c̄	with
cath	catheter
CBC	complete blood cell count
CCU	critical care unit
CHF	congestive heart failure
c/o	complaints of
COPD	chronic obstructive pulmonary disease
CPR	cardiopulmonary resuscitation
CSF	cerebrospinal fluid
CV	cardiovascular
DNR	do not resuscitate
DOA	dead on arrival
DOB	date of birth
Dx	diagnosis
ECG	electrocardiogram *(sometimes referred to as* EKG*)*
ED	emergency department
EEG	electroencephalogram
ER	emergency room
FB	foreign body
FTT	failure to thrive
Fx	fracture
GI	gastrointestinal
GU	genitourinary
HIV	human immunodeficiency virus
Hx	history
ICU	intensive care unit
IM	intramuscular
IV	intravenous
lmp	last menstrual period
liq.	liquid
MI	myocardial infarction
MMR	measles, mumps, rubella
MVA	motor vehicle accident

Abbreviations (Continued)

NICU	neonatal intensive care unit
NKA	no known allergies
npo	nothing by mouth
NVD	nausea, vomiting, and diarrhea
O$_2$	oxygen
OR	operating room
p.c.	after meals
pH	hydrogen ion concentration; a measure of acidity
PPD	purified protein derivative; TB test
Pt.	patient
q.d.	every day
q.h.	every hour
q.i.d.	four times a day
RBC	red blood cell
RDS	respiratory distress syndrome *(infants)*
R/O	rule out
ROI	region of interest
ROM	range of motion
s̄	without
SOB	shortness of breath
STAT	immediately
TB	tuberculosis
TI	terminal ileum
t.i.d.	three times a day
TPR	temperature, pulse, respiration
Tx	treatment
WBC	white blood cell

Executive and/or Administrative Titles

CEO	Chief Executive Officer
CFO	Chief Financial Officer
CIO	Chief Information Officer
CNO	Chief Nursing Officer
RSO	Radiation Safety Officer

PREFIXES

Prefixes precede root words.

PREFIX	MEANING	EXAMPLE
a	without	anorexic – without appetite
ab	away from	abduct – move a limb away from the body (lateral)
ad	toward	adduct – move a limb closer to the body (medial)
ante	before	antecubital – in front of the elbow
anti	against	antibody – an immunoglobulin
bi	two	bilateral – both the left and right side
brachy	short	brachycephalic – short, broad skull
brady	slow	bradycardia – slow heartbeat
dys	difficult, painful	dysfunctional – inability to function normally
ecto	outside	ectopic – positioned outside the normal location
endo	within, inside	endoscope – optical instrument used for viewing structures within the body
epi	on, upon	epicondyle – bony projection on the superior part of a condyle
hemi	half	hemidiaphragm – only one side of the diaphragm
hyper	excessive	hyperactive – abnormally increased activity
hypo	insufficient, lacking	hypoxia – lack of oxygen
infra	below	infraorbital margin – inferior rim of the orbit
inter	between	interstitial – space between tissues
intra	within	intravenous – within the vein
iso	equal, balanced	isotonic – solutions with the same amount of solute
macro	large	macrophage – a large cell responsible for removing waste products from blood, lymph, and connective tissue as a means of protecting the body's immune system
micro	small	microcalcification – small or minute calcifications
olig	few, limited, little	oligospermia – limited quantity of spermatozoa in the semen
peri	around	pericardium – sac that surrounds the heart
poly	many	polyuria – frequent urination

Prefixes (Continued)

post	after	postoperative – after surgery
pre	before	precancerous – before becoming cancerous
retro	backwards, behind	retrograde – moving backwards, opposed to normal flow, against nature
scler	hard, hardening	sclerosis – condition in which tissues become hard
sub	below, under	sublingual – under the tongue
super	above	supercilliary ridge – ridge of bone above each orbit
supra	upon	supraorbital groove – depression or groove located on the frontal bone, above the eyebrow
tachy	fast, rapid	tachycardia – rapid heartbeat

ROOT WORDS

Root words are also known as combining forms and provide the fundamental meaning of the medical term. Root words appear as the first part of the medical term unless a prefix is added to the root word. Root words typically combine with suffixes by way of a connecting vowel.

COMBINING FORM	MEANING	EXAMPLE
acr/o	extremities	acrocyanosis – blue discoloration of the extremities
aden/o	gland	adenitis – inflamed lymph node or gland
angi/o	vessel	angiography – imaging study of vessels
arthro/o	joint	arthroscopy – visual examination of a joint with the aid of an endoscope
cardi/o	heart	cardiomegaly – enlarged heart
cerebr/o	brain	cerebrospinal – pertaining to the brain and spinal cord
chol/e	bile	cholangiography – radiographic procedure in which a positive contrast media is used to visualize the biliary system
chondr/o	cartilage	chondroma – a benign tumor found in cartilage
cost/o	rib	costovertebral joint – joint located between thoracic vertebrae and the head of the rib
cyan/o	blue	cyanosis – condition in which skin turns blue due to lack of oxygen

cyt/o	cell	cytoplasm – cellular material composed of fluid and organelles; located between the cell membrane and the nucleus (cyt or -cyte)
derm/o	skin	dermatitis – inflammation of the skin
enter/o	intestines	enterolith – a calculus or stone located within the intestines
erythr/o	red	erythrocyte – red blood cell
gastr/o	stomach	gastritis – inflammation of the stomach lining
hem/o	blood	hemoptysis – coughing or spitting up blood
hemat/o	blood	hematocrit – a centrifuged blood sample
hepat/o	liver	hepatorrhea – flow of bile from the liver
heter/o	different	heterogeneous – unlike parts
hist/o	tissues	histology – the study of tissues
homeo	same, stable	homeostasis – stable internal environment
hydr/o	water, hydrogen	hydrotherapy – therapy involving the use water
hyster/o	uterus	hysterectomy – surgical removal of the uterus
leuk/o	white	leukocyte – white blood cell
lip/o	fat	liposuction – to remove fat via a vacuum suction
lith/o	calculus, stone	lithotripsy – destruction of calculi (stones)
lymph/o	clear body fluid	lymphocyte – a leukocyte responsible for immune responses
myel/o	spinal cord, bone marrow	myelogram – radiographic image depicting the subarachnoid space of the spinal cord
necr/o	death	necrosis – condition in which cells or tissues die
nephr/o	kidney	nephrolith – kidney stone (calculus)
neur/o	nerves	neurotransmitter – chemical that permits transmission of information between neurons, or between neurons and other cell types
oste/o	bone	osteoporosis – thinning of bone
path/o	disease	pathogenesis – the cause or origin of a disease
phleb	vein	phlebostenosis – condition resulting in narrowing of veins
pneum/o	air	pneumothorax – air in the pleural cavity
pyel/o	renal pelvis	pyelogram – radiographic study of renal pelvis of kidneys, ureters, and bladder (often referred to as IVP or IVU)
thorac/o	chest, thorax	thoracocentesis – surgical procedure involving a needle puncture through the chest into the pleural cavity to remove fluid or retrieve tissue sample.

SUFFIXES

Suffixes follow root words.

SUFFIX	MEANING	EXAMPLE
-algia	pain, suffering	cephalalgia – headache, head pain
-ectomy	excision, removal	appendectomy – removal of the appendix
-dipsia	thirst	oligodipsia – having little thirst
-gram/ graphy	image	myelogram
-ia	condition	insomnia – inability to sleep
-ism	disease of a specific cause	autism – mental disorder characterized by withdrawal, isolation, and lack of interaction
-itis	inflammation of	arthritis – inflammation of the joints
-megaly	enlargement	acromegaly – enlarged extremities
-ologist	specialist	cardiologist – physician who specializes in conditions of the heart
-ology	study of	biology – study of living organisms
-oma	tumor (benign or malignant)	sarcoma – malignant tumor arising in connective tissue, i.e., bone, fat, muscle, cartilage, or lymph
-osis	condition of	mononucleosis – abnormal increase of leukocytes in the blood
-ostomy	surgical opening	colostomy – surgical opening in which the colon is brought to the surface of the abdomen either temporarily or permanently
-otomy	surgical incision	phlebotomy – incision of vein for purpose of blood collection
-penia	lack of, deficient	leukopenia – decrease of white blood cells
-phagia	swallow	dysphagia – difficulty swallowing
-phasia	speech	dysphasia – difficulty speaking
-plegia	paralysis	quadriplegia – condition in which extremities and torso are paralyzed due to injury of the spinal cord
-pnea	breath, respiration	apnea – without breath
-rrhage	burst open	hemorrhage – loss of blood due to rupture
-rrhea	flow	diarrhea – frequent watery discharge of feces
-scope	imaging instrument	endoscope – imaging instrument used to aid in the visualization of structures within the body
-uria	urine	pyuria – white blood cells in the urine; symptomatic of a urinary tract infection

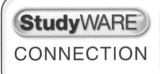

After completing this chapter, review the Flashcards or play an interactive game on your StudyWARE™ CD-ROM that will help you learn the content in this chapter.

CONCEPT THINKING QUESTIONS

1. What prefix and root word combined would mean a body habitus without strength? _____

2. List two prefixes or suffixes that mean difficult or painful.
_____ and _____

3. What three lowercase letters of the alphabet stand alone, appear with a score mark above them, and are abbreviations to the following terms?

    A. with _____

    B. without _____

    C. before _____

PRACTICE EXERCISES

Build a word from the list of prefixes, root words, and suffixes that has the same meaning as the definition provided:

poly-	-pnea	dys-
-ectomy	cardi/o	-dipsia
-ia	thorac/o	cyt/o
-oma	cyan/o	pneu-
a-	erythr/o	leuk/o
brady-	-uria	tachy-
appendic/o	nephr/o	-osis

Definition   **Build A Word**

1. White blood cells   _____

2. Blue condition   _____

3. Difficulty urinating   _____

4. Slow heartbeat   _____

5. Without respiration   _____

6. Removal of appendix   _____

7. Tumor of the kidney   _____

8. Air in pleural cavity (thorax) _____

9. Excessive thirst _____

10. Rapid respiration _____

MATCHING

Match each term to the appropriate body description.

a. hypersthenic   **b. asthenic**   **c. hyposthenic**   **d. sthenic**

1. The abdominal organs are situated higher and more transverse *(horizontal)* than the average body type.

2. The abdominal organs are situated so as to occupy the abdominal cavity with an even distribution of contents; neither appearing too transverse nor too vertical.

3. The abdominal organs are situated very close to the spine, appear almost vertical, and descend lower in the abdominopelvic cavity than the other three body types.

4. The abdominal organs are situated in close proximity to the spine and appear more vertical than the average body type.

RETENTION OF MATERIAL

Retention requires practicing the use of previously learned material. Try writing a **prefix** for each term.

1. inside _____

2. outside _____

3. above _____

4. below _____

5. between _____

Now, try writing a **suffix** for each term.

6. condition _____

7. tumor _____

8. inflammation _____

9. surgical incision _____

10. removal _____

CHAPTER 3

Medical and Legal Terms

OBJECTIVES

Upon completion of this chapter, the reader will be able to:

- Explain what is meant by "*professional conduct*"
- Identify appropriate body mechanics involved with lifting, moving, and transferring a patient
- Describe the role of the radiographer in dealing with cultural diversity
- Identify *subjective* and *objective* data in patient assessment
- List the criteria necessary for obtaining an appropriate patient history
- Differentiate between a *felony* and a *misdemeanor*
- Identify the four vital signs and their acceptable ranges

CONCEPT THINKING

Medical terms and legal terms are languages unto themselves. Although each is very different in scope and practice, they do share some commonalities when it comes to patient care. In caring for a patient, one must have an expected level of medical knowledge and technical skills to be able to offer quality care to patients. It is not enough to have the desire to provide medical care to the public, but rather there must be qualifying standards established through laws and/or governing agencies/ organizations that mandate the quality of health care to ensure public safety. The term "health care" encompasses a broad range of medical professions, which is why *Practice Standards* are so valuable in their design to define the role and scope of specific branches of the medical profession. *Practice Standards* also identify professional responsibilities unique to various medical disciplines. Professional health care organizations are known to provide guidelines specifying minimum expectations for professional conduct and ethical behavior as it relates to a particular branch of the medical professions. The American Registry of Radiologic Technologists (ARRT) provides this type of guide for eligible candidates seeking ARRT certification and for registered technologists who have previously held or currently hold ARRT certification; this guide is referred to as the profession's *Standards of Ethics*. It is important to remember that, even when adhering to professional *Practice Standards* and/or *Standards of Ethics*, unforeseen incidents may still arise affecting the health and well-being of the patient and/or the health care provider. To reduce the chances of unfortunate incidents occurring, imaging professionals must abide by professional *Practice Standards*, comply with state and federal regulations (as they pertain to the profession), and demonstrate ethical conduct/judgment as specified in the profession's *Standards of Ethics*. All persons who become a member of the health care profession are to provide quality standard care to the public regardless of gender, race, religious beliefs, socioeconomic status, mental status, and form of illness/injury.

MEDICAL AND LEGAL TERMS

advanced health care directive (AHCD) – An advanced health care directive (AHCD) is a legal document declaring the wishes of individuals regarding their own health care and/or treatment in the event they are unable to convey their choices and/or decisions for well-being.

■ **health care proxy decision maker/surrogate** – The health care proxy decision maker or designated surrogate is the appointed individual stated on the AHCD that has legal authority to make health care decisions on behalf of the individual who appointed them.

ambulatory – Ambulatory describes an individual who is able to walk or move freely.

ARRT Rules of Ethics – The American Registry of Radiologic Technologists (ARRT) provides rules of ethical behavior termed "Rules of Ethics" as part of their *Standards of Ethics*. These rules mandate the professional conduct of Registered Technologists, Registered Radiologic Assistants, and individuals seeking ARRT certification. The ARRT has the authority to impose *sanctions* to individuals (candidates seeking ARRT certification, Registered Technologists, and Registered Radiologic Assistants) determined by the ARRT Ethics Committee and/or the ARRT Board of Trustees to have breached the ARRT Rules of Ethics.

ASRT Code of Ethics – The American Society of Radiologic Technologists (ASRT), in conjunction with the American Registry of Radiologic Technologists (ARRT), developed a "Code of Ethics" outlining minimum expectations of professional conduct and ethical behavior specific to the radiologic imaging profession. The "Code of Ethics" and the "Rules of Ethics" comprise the ARRT *Standards of Ethics. (Refer to Appendix A – ARRT "Code of Ethics.")*

ASRT – The Practice Standards for Medical Imaging and Radiation Therapy – The *Practice Standards* for medical imaging and radiation therapy clearly state the role and scope of knowledge, technical skills, patient care, and ethical conduct required of a practicing radiologic technologist in the health care profession. *(Refer to Appendix C, – ASRT Scope of Practice.)*

authorization – Legal authorization or permission is required for health care providers to provide care or treatment to patients. Authorization is also required for the disclosure of private patient information to be released to a third party.

- **health care power of attorney** – To appoint an individual with a "health care power of attorney" is to legally grant authorization for health care decisions to be made on your behalf by the appointee.

- **informed consent** – *(see definition in Chapter 5)*

- **legal guardian** – A legal guardian is a person who has the legal authority to make health care, business, or financial decisions for someone who is unable to make decisions for him or herself. Typically, parents of children younger than 18 years of age are considered legal guardians and can make decisions on their child's behalf.

autonomy – Autonomy refers to individuals who are able to function independently and make decisions for themselves regarding their course of treatment.

beneficence – Beneficence describes a kind act, an act that promotes a positive effect without consideration to self.

body mechanics – Body mechanics for health care personnel refers to use of correct body positioning when lifting, moving, and transferring patients.

- **good body mechanics** – Good body mechanics refers to proper posture and body alignment for lifting, moving, and transferring patients *(see Table 3–1)*. The practice of good body mechanics helps reduce the occurrence of back injuries, which are known to be the number one cause of job-related injuries among health care personnel.

blood pressure reading – To obtain a blood pressure reading, a sphygmomanometer and a stethoscope are required. The *systolic* reading or top number (i.e., <120 mmHg) indicates the contraction phase of left ventricle of the heart, whereas the *diastolic* reading or bottom number (i.e., <80 mmHg) indicates the relaxation phase of the left ventricle of the heart.

- **sphygmomanometer** – A sphygmomanometer is a medical device used to obtain blood pressure readings. It consists of an inflatable cuff that fits over an individual's bicep (area above the elbow) and tightens around the upper arm as air inflates within the cuff. The pressure gauge provides a meter for monitoring the blood pressure rate as the cuff is slowly deflated.

- **stethoscope** – A stethoscope is a medical device designed to allow an individual to hear sounds naturally occurring in the body, such as heart beat, respiration, and digestive activity.

body temperature reading – Normal body temperature is an individual's internal core temperature during normal daily activity. To obtain an individual's body temperature, a thermometer is required. Temperature readings can be achieved via the following types of thermometers: oral thermometer, rectal thermometer, and electronic thermometer. Readings can be obtained at any one of the following five body point locations.

TABLE 3–1 Good Body Mechanics

BEST PRACTICE RULE	RATIONALE
Establish a good base of support.	A good base of support constitutes a person standing with approximately 6–10 inches of space between the feet, with body weight evenly distributed. Feet should be parallel to one another and at right angles to the lower (tibia-fibula) legs.
Be aware of the body's center of gravity; the weight of the body is centered at this point. The center of gravity should be positioned directly over the base of support when lifting a heavy object.	The center of gravity for a standing person is in the pelvic region, at approximately the level of the second sacral segment.
Keep the chest up and slightly forward with waist extended.	This position will allow good lung expansion when lifting a heavy object.
Keep the head held erect with the chin in as to avoid curvature in the neck.	This position allows for proper alignment of the entire spine and avoids undue pressure placed on the upper (proximal) portion of the spine.
Keep the knees slightly bent when lifting an object.	This position allows the knees to absorb any strain from lifting and avoids undue pressure placed on the spine.
Keep the buttocks tucked in and abdomen up and in.	This position allows for the center of gravity to be involved with the lifting process and avoids undue pressure being placed on the spine.
If lifting or moving a patient, first inform them of the move.	Informing the patient of the move will allow them to assist in the move (if they are able), which will reduce the amount of exertion required from the health care provider(s).
Align the patient's body before lifting, moving, or transferring.	Aligning the patient's body (i.e., shoulders, hips, feet) will allow for ease of movement.

Based on data from: Beebe, R., Scadden, J., & Funk, D. (2010) *Fundamentals of basic emergency care* (3rd ed.). Clifton Park, NY: Delmar Cengage Learning and the Institute for Caregiver Education, Good Body Mechanics/Employee Safety: A Skills Update. Retrieved February 25, 2010, from http://www.caregivereducation.org/products/sample_inservice.pdf.

■ **axillary** – An axillary temperature reading is achieved by placing the thermometer bulb directly under the axilla (the arm pit), with the arm placed close to the body to hold the thermometer in place for approximately 5–10 minutes. The normal body temperature range for an axillary reading is generally 0.3°–0.4° lower than an oral temperature reading. It should be noted that the axillary temperature reading is considered the least accurate of the five methods mentioned for obtaining body temperature.

■ **oral** – An oral temperature reading is achieved by placing the oral thermometer bulb directly under the tongue for up to 3 minutes. Times will vary depending on the type of oral thermometer being used; electronic versions used in health care facilities generally only require a few seconds, whereas the standard glass type thermometer requires a longer time to produce an accurate reading. Normal body temperature range for an oral reading is considered 97.8°–99.1°F.

- ■ **rectal** – A rectal reading is achieved by placing the rectal thermometer bulb in the rectum for approximately 2.5–5 minutes. Normal body temperature range for a rectal reading is generally 0.5°–0.7° higher than an oral temperature reading.

- ■ **temporal artery (TA)** – A temporal artery reading, or TA reading, is obtained by placing a swiping electronic device across the forehead where the temporal artery lies close to surface of the skin. The sweeping motion provides for a quick and accurate reading. TA readings closely resemble rectal readings, which tend to run 0.5°–0.7° higher than oral temperature readings.

- ■ **tympanic** – A tympanic reading is achieved by placing an electronic thermometer within the ear for approximately 3 seconds. Tympanic readings closely resemble rectal readings, which tend to run 0.5°–0.7° higher than oral temperature readings.

cardiopulmonary resuscitation (CPR) – Cardiopulmonary resuscitation, more often referred to as CPR, is a physical act performed in an emergency situation on an individual who has stopped breathing and whose heart has stopped beating. The life-saving act of CPR involves a series of chest compressions and rescue breaths performed in a cyclic manner in an attempt to keep the individual alive while waiting for medical help to arrive. *(Refer to Appendix D or http://www.americanheart.org for the 2010 American Heart Association Guidelines for Cardiopulmonary Resuscitation and Emergency Cardiovascular Care.)*

> **Note**   *The American Registry of Radiologic Technologists (ARRT) requires candidates seeking ARRT certification to demonstrate CPR competency as one of the six general patient care components mandated by the ARRT for national certification examination eligibility. (Refer to Appendix D.)*

communication – Communication is a transmission of information between two individuals, which can be accomplished via speaking, writing, sign language, body language, and through the aid of electronic devices. The majority of communication that takes place in a medical environment focuses on verbal and written communication. As stated in the *Patient's Bill of Rights*, "the patient has the right to and is encouraged to obtain from physicians and other direct caregivers relevant, current, and understandable information concerning diagnosis, treatment, and prognosis." It should be noted that patients who are minors, legally incompetent, or lack decision-making capabilities may have a legal guardian, designated surrogate, or proxy decision-maker communicate and make decisions on their behalf regarding the type of care or treatment to be received.

- ■ **verbal** – Verbal communication to the patient may include but is not limited to: questions regarding patient history, explanation of procedure/s to be performed, directions for patients to follow before and during the procedure, and/or instructions for follow-up care.

- ■ **written** – Written communication regarding the patient may include but is not limited to *Patient's Bill of Rights*, preparatory directions for the procedure/s to be performed, a consent form explaining the procedure and any possible side effects, and instructions for follow-up care.

compassion – Compassion is the ability to understand another person's pain or suffering without feeling emotional.

competence – Competence is a required standard that has been met. When a health care worker is designated as competent, the public can feel secure in knowing the person has demonstrated competency as it relates to the position they hold in the health care profession. Often a demonstration of competency regarding health care professionals involves passing a national certification examination and/or a state licensure examination.

compliance – Compliance refers to meeting established standards or requirements or abiding by set rules or regulations.

conviction – A conviction is a legal term used by the court to declare an individual guilty of committing a crime.

criminal background check – A state or national criminal background check is a report many employers require of prospective employees and educational institutions require of prospective students. This type of report requires a signed authorization form from the individual for an investigative search to be conducted of their past history and reveals any criminal activity or legal misconduct to the potential employer or to the educational institution. An arrest and/or conviction resulting in a felony, misdemeanor, or sex crime would be disclosed in the report unless the individual's legal records have been expunged (removed or sealed). Criminal background reports are deemed confidential because of personal identifying information contained within the report and are not to be used for purposes other than the intent stated on the disclosure form. In addition to state and federal laws, The Joint Commission has established requirements for performing criminal background checks in which individuals subject to receiving a criminal background check are identified. *(The Joint Commission, 2008)*

> Staff, students, and volunteers who work in the same capacity as staff who provide care, treatment, and services would be expected to have criminal background checks, verified when required by law and regulation and organization policy.
>
> ———————————————————————
>
> Source: The Joint Commission. (2008). Requirements for Criminal Background Checks. Retrieved June 29, 2010, from http://www.jointcommission.org.

cultural diversity – Cultural diversity is a broad term used to describe a population or group of people in which a variety of ethnic, racial, religious beliefs, morals, values, traditions, socioeconomic circumstances, and gender coexists.

defendant – In a court of law the defendant may be an individual, group, or company accused of committing an unlawful act and therefore must answer to the court regarding the charge.

dependent – A dependent is an individual who is unable to act independently and on their own behalf either financially, legally, physically, or mentally.

diagnosis – Diagnosis refers to the recognition of an illness, disorder, or disease by a physician.

DNR code – DNR is the code for "do not resuscitate." This code is placed in the patient's chart so health care personnel caring for the patient are aware that an attempt to restart the patient's heart or respiration is not desired should the patient experience cardiac or respiratory arrest. Terminally ill patients or individuals with legal authority to act on behalf of the patient may choose to have a DNR code placed in the patient's chart. A DNR order is recognized as a legal document in the United States but is not recognized worldwide.

doctrine – A doctrine is an accepted rule, theory, or concept used to clarify a particular action, event, or policy.

drug screening/testing – A drug screening is a medical laboratory test performed to detect the presence of medications and/or illegal drugs within the human body. A person must voluntarily provide a urine or blood sample (other bodily fluids or hair follicles can be used) for testing purposes; however, many health care facilities along with other institutions and organizations require prospective employees, trainees, and volunteers to undergo a drug screening as part of the application process. Drug screening results are usually available within 24–48 hours after the test and are only released to individuals named on the authorization form.

■ **10-panel drug test** – The 10-panel drug test is a common drug screening test designed to detect the presence of any of the following drugs:

- amphetamines/methamphetamines
- barbiturates
- benzodiazepines
- cocaine
- marijuana
- methadone
- methaqualone
- opiates
- phencyclidine
- propoxyphene

empathy – Empathy is the ability for a person to identify with another person's set of circumstances. Often, emotions are involved with empathy.

ethics, ethical – Ethics and/or ethical behavior refers to adapting our moral belief (knowing right from wrong) to make appropriate professional decisions and judgments expected within the scope of practice for a given profession.

fidelity – Fidelity implies a commitment to the truth, a demonstration of loyalty, or devotion.

felony – A felony is a crime that is considered serious in nature and may or may not involve a violent act. There are various classifications of felonies with degrees of punitive actions, including incarceration. Registered technologists seeking renewal of their registration and candidates seeking ARRT certification are required to disclose a felony conviction or charge resulting in a plea of guilty, plea of nolo contendere (no contest), withheld or deferred adjudication, suspended or stay of sentence, pretrial diversion, and military court-martial to the ARRT. Excluded in the reporting process are speeding and parking violations unrelated to drug or alcohol use. The ARRT conducts a review process for applicants reporting a felony charge or conviction when renewing their registration and for candidates reporting a felony charge or conviction when applying for the national certification examination.

flight-or-fight response – The "flight-or-fight response" is a physiological response to fear, danger, or stress. Under such conditions, the human body releases hormones (adrenaline and cortisol), after which a surge of energy becomes available to either run away (flight) from what is perceived as a threatening situation or to stay and fight.

fraud – Fraud is the act of deception, i.e., to intentionally mislead an individual to believe or to act on a belief that is not true.

health care – Health care is a very broad term that encompasses a variety of medical disciplines, methods for care and treatment, and avenues for promoting, maintaining, or improving the overall health and well-being of the public.

health care team – A health care team consists of health care members with specialized knowledge and technical skills that work collaboratively to provide the best possible plan of care for the patient.

Heimlich maneuver – The Heimlich maneuver is a life-saving procedure named after Dr. Henry Jay Heimlich, the person who is credited for developing it. The procedure involves a series of upward abdominal thrusts underneath the diaphragm of a choking victim. The abdominal thrusts force air from the lungs upward and out the mouth in an attempt to dislodge any material that could be causing an airway obstruction *(see Figure 3–1).*

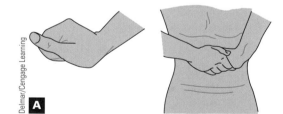

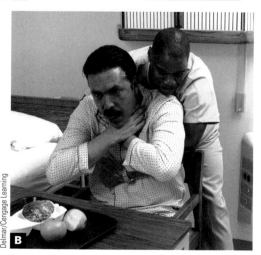

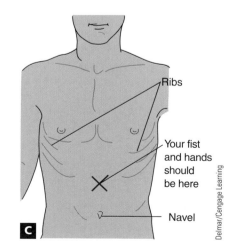

FIGURE 3–1. Performing the Heimlich maneuver.
1. Stand behind the person and lean him forward slightly.
2. Clench your fist with one hand, keeping the thumb straight *(A)*.
3. Place your arms around the person and grasp your fist with your other hand near the top of the stomach and just below the center of the rib cage *(B)*.
4. Thrust forcefully, inward and upward, with the thumb side of your fist just above the navel *(C)*.

HIPAA – Health Insurance Portability and Accountability Act of 1996 – In 1996, Congress enacted a federal law known as the *Health Insurance Portability Act* to provide national compliance standards for health care providers and insurance companies to abide by regarding the disclosure and transmission of patients, identifiable health information. Under HIPAA law, a patient's identifiable health care information or medical record is protected and secured from public access.

- **confidentiality** – To maintain confidentiality is to not disclose patient information to others outside the circle of health care personnel involved in the care and treatment of the patient.

- **privacy** – Privacy is a respect of personal and confidential information contained within a patient's medical chart and/or medical record. Health care personnel typically have limited access to full disclosure of patient information, with privileges to specific information deemed relevant (within the role and scope of *Professional Practice Standards*) to the care and/or treatment of the patient.

hospice – A hospice facility is a place that provides care for terminally ill patients, making their lives as comfortable as possible as life nears an end.

incident report – An incident report is a document used by a health care facility or by an employer in the event of an accident occurring on the premises. The document details the event (date and time of occurrence, how the event occurred, and individuals involved in the accident) and any actions the facility or employer took during and following the event. The incident report should be filled out immediately following the accident to ensure accuracy of details, and it should be kept on file for future reference should the incident become a legal matter. *(Refer to Appendix H.)*

law – A law (as considered in this text) is a rule enacted by state or federal legislature requiring compliance of a community. Noncompliance to a law can result in civil and/or criminal charges against the individual.

- **Americans with Disabilities Act** – The Americans with Disabilities Act of 1990 (ADA) was amended in 2008, passed by Congress, and signed into law by President George W. Bush. The ADA Amendments Act became effective January 1, 2009, in which a broader definition of "disability" was established in order to provide better protection from employer discrimination to persons with a disability.

- **The CARE Bill** – The CARE Bill is a piece of federal legislation that was first introduced to Congress in 2000 as the *"Consumer Assurance of Radiologic Excellence" bill*; however, since that time, the name has changed to the *"Consistency, Accuracy, Responsibility, and Excellence in Medical Imaging and Radiation Therapy" bill*. Still referred to as the CARE bill, the name change was made in an attempt to more accurately reflect the broader scope of imaging professions for which standardized education and credentialing is deemed necessary to assure public safety. The CARE bill is intended to amend the current Consumer-Patient Radiation Health and Safety Act of 1981.

- **The Good Samaritan Law** – Good Samaritan Laws are laws enacted on a state-by-state basis and are designed to legally protect citizens who voluntarily and in good faith come to the aid of a stranger in need of emergency medical care. The Good Samaritan Law is intended to protect the citizen should their actions result in unintentional injury or damage to the assisted individual.

legislature – Legislature is a group of elected individuals that have the authority to create, revise, and enact laws that govern the citizens they represent.

malice – Malice is the desire for someone to feel pain or to experience harm.

malpractice – Malpractice is negligence that occurs in a medical or professional setting.

medical record – A medical record is a legal document that contains pertinent, confidential patient information regarding care, treatment, and the patient's response throughout the duration of the care provided.

misdemeanor – A misdemeanor is a crime considered less serious than a felony and results in a lesser degree of punitive action. Often misdemeanor offenses result in a fine imposed by the court.

mission statement – A mission statement is a statement declaring an organization's focus or purpose. A company mission statement is designed to provide its employees with an overall goal that all work toward in effort to maintain or achieve the vision for the company's existence. Many companies, organizations, and institutions make their mission statement known to the public. Mission statements are reviewed periodically and updated as deemed necessary to accurately depict the purpose of a growing, evolving organization *(see Box 3–1)*.

BOX 3–1   ASRT Mission Statement

The mission of the American Society of Radiologic Technologists is to advance the medical imaging and radiation therapy profession and to enhance the quality of patient care.

© 2010 American Society of Radiologic Technologists. Reprinted with permission.

---

morals/morality – Morality refers to what we have been taught to be right and wrong. To have morals or morality is to be able to recognize right from wrong and then choose to do the right thing not because you have to, but because it is the right thing to do.

patient assessment data collection – When obtaining a patient history, collecting objective data and subjective data is important to developing an overall picture of what factors may be contributing to the patient's illness and/or injury.

- **objective data** – Objective data are factual data.
  - Observing the patient, e.g., coughing, spitting up blood, fainting, vomiting

- **subjective data** – Subjective data are determined by emotions and feelings.
  - Patient statement of "feeling sick," "feeling tired," or "feeling out of sorts"

patient chart – A patient's chart houses relevant information regarding care the patient receives while in the medical facility. The chart typically accompanies the patient to and from any medical department within the facility in which they receive care. Each department the patient receives care in is responsible for documenting or *charting* the type of care that was provided along with any information deemed important in the treatment and response of the patient. All examinations and/or medical procedures ordered by a physician should be clearly indicated in the patient's chart and initialed, stamped, or stickered upon completion of the examination/procedure by the appropriate health care provider. Should the examination/medical procedure not be able to be performed, the appropriate health care provider is responsible for notifying the department head overseeing the patient's care (or the ordering physician) and documenting in the patient's chart the reason for not performing the examination/procedure.

- ■ **charting** – Charting refers to relevant information regarding the care of the patient being documented within the patient's medical chart. Documented information should be accurate, thorough, and legible, and it should clearly delineate subjective and objective data.

patient history – Obtaining a "good patient history" is essential to establishing a foundation to provide appropriate patient care. A good patient history begins with an interview process initiated by the health care provider to determine the patient's chief complaint and/or multiple complaints contributing to their lack of wellness. That information will be entered into the patient's medical chart. On the basis of the information collected, the primary physician or attending physician may order radiologic examinations to gain further insight into the patient's illness or injury. Specific to the imaging profession is an additional patient history conducted by the radiologic technologist to provide the radiologist with additional information to assist in image interpretation. This detailed patient history consists of seven questions, known as the "*Sacred Seven*," which are designed to provide the radiologist with pertinent patient information correlated to the radiographic procedure/examination ordered.

- ■ **Sacred Seven** – The "Sacred Seven" comprise a series of seven (7) patient care questions specific to the imaging profession.

  - **aggravating and alleviating factors** – Aggravating factors are factors that have a negative impact on the pain, injury, or illness, causing an increase in symptoms or severity. Alleviating factors are factors that have a positive impact on the pain, injury, or illness, causing a decrease in symptoms or severity.

  - **associated manifestations** – Associated manifestations apply to any other accompanying complaints the patient may have. This information is important in determining if a relationship exists between the accompanying complaints and the patient's chief complaint.

  - **chronology** – Chronology is a determined timeframe that spans the onset of pain, injury, or illness to the present time of the imaging procedure in terms of *duration*, *frequency*, and *symptoms*.

  - **localization** – Localization is the process of establishing the exact point of pain, injury, or illness.

  - **onset** – Onset is marking the first moment the pain, injury, or illness manifested and detailing possible circumstances or events that might have led to the occurrence.

- **quality** – Quality is a description by the patient as to how the pain feels (e.g., hot, itchy, burning, stabbing, sharp, dull, pressure, radiating, throbbing, wavelike, constant ache). The radiologic technologist would indicate apparent symptoms if present (e.g., coughing, sweating, bleeding, spitting, vomiting, diarrhea, lesions, dizziness) as acute (sudden onset) or chronic (during a long period of time).

- **severity** – Severity refers to the degree of pain or illness the patient is experiencing. Oftentimes a rating scale can be used to determine the "severity" of pain. For example, one might ask the patient on a scale of 1–10, with 10 being the most severe pain, "What rating number would you equate to the level of pain you are experiencing?"

Patient's Bill of Rights – The American Hospital Association first adopted the Patient Bill of Rights in 1973 and revised the doctrine on October 21, 1992. The bill states the rights patients are entitled to and can exercise in the course of their own care and treatment. For patients who are unable to exercise their rights, a legal guardian, health care proxy decision maker, or designated surrogate can make health care decisions on their behalf. Many states and health care institutions have tailored the bill through language modification to better serve their community in understanding the rights they are entitled to as a patient. *(Refer to Appendix E – 2010 Patient's Bill of Rights.)*

patient type – Patient type refers to a classification of patients by age, degree of injury or illness, mental capacity, or degree of impairment. Such categories are devised to assist health care providers in providing the best possible care or treatment (as stated by a specific protocol) to patient types that present unique circumstances or needs. Such patient types include but are not limited to pediatric, adolescent, adult, geriatric, trauma, mentally altered, comatose, vision impaired, and hearing impaired.

- **elective booking** – Elective booking is a term used to describe a female patient scheduling an appointment for a radiographic procedure on the basis of her menstrual cycle. The first 10 days after the onset of menstruation is considered the safest time (decreased chance of pregnancy) for a female of childbearing age to have a radiographic procedure performed.

plaintiff – In a court of law, the plaintiff is an individual (typically the patient) who has initiated a lawsuit against another individual, group, or company that may be responsible for the performance of an unlawful act that resulting in some form of personal damage, injury, or harm.

pregnancy – To safeguard against accidental radiation exposure to a developing fetus, imaging departments provide women of childbearing age a specific questionnaire in which the possibility of pregnancy is addressed. Oftentimes a signed consent form from the patient is required before the radiologic procedure can be performed. Since the first 10 days after the onset of patient's menstrual cycle is considered the safest time for radiographic procedures, the patient may choose *elective booking*. For female patients who are pregnant, the physician (along with patient/family) will determine whether the procedure's benefits outweigh its risks. If a determination to proceed with the imaging procedure is made, then the radiologic technologist will adhere to the ALARA principles employed for all patients in which protective shielding (unless relevant anatomy will be obscured) and tight collimation are used to reduce radiation exposure.

prognosis – Prognosis refers to an expected outcome as it relates to an illness, disorder, or disease diagnosed by a physician. A therapeutic plan may be discussed in the prognosis of an illness, disorder, or disease.

reprimand – In the health care profession, a reprimand is a warning given to an individual from someone of higher authority for an inappropriate action considered to be unprofessional.

sanction – A sanction is a disciplinary action imposed on an individual who breaches a policy, rule, protocol, or law.

state regulations – State regulations are rules imposed by individual states addressing expected behaviors. Failure to abide by a state regulation will prompt the state to sanction the individual.

tort – A tort is a civil wrongdoing resulting in injury or harm to an individual (patient) or to their property attributable to a lack of care by the caregiver. Torts can be classified into two main categories, *intentional misconduct* and *unintentional misconduct*, often referred to as negligence.

■ **intentional misconduct** – Intentional misconduct is an action taken by an individual with the purpose or intent to cause harm to another.

• **assault** – Assault is a legal term meaning to threaten someone or to imply harm may occur.

• **battery** – Battery is a legal term meaning to bring physical harm to an individual or to make unwanted physical contact with another individual.

• **defamation** – Defamation is to make false statements about an individual, i.e., to intentionally malign someone's character. Defamation can occur through written form (libel) or verbal form (slander) and requires witness by a third party.

• **false imprisonment** – False imprisonment as it pertains to the health care profession is to restrict a patient's movements against their will. The use of *restraints* on a patient requires written orders by a physician and is not to be misconstrued with protective measures taken by health care workers for the safety of the patient, such as raising the side rails on a stretcher.

• **restraints (immobilization methods)** – There are various types of immobilization methods and/or restraints used in the health care profession, particularly within general radiography. Because unwanted motion can produce undesirable radiographic images, the technologist may need to use Velcro straps, sandbags, or other simple immobilization methods to limit a patient's movement during an imaging procedure. However, this action should only be taken after a thorough explanation to the patient of the procedure and the need for immobilization has occurred. Special restraints for pediatric, geriatric, combative, and trauma patients are also available to protect the patient from unwanted motion that could result in injury or excessive radiation exposure. These types of immobilization methods may be more sophisticated and should be in place for the duration of the procedure or until the physician has removed the restraint order.

■ **unintentional misconduct** – Unintentional misconduct is an action taken by an individual with no intent to cause harm to another.

- **negligence** – Negligence is the term used to describe injury or harm inflicted on a patient as a result of a breach of duty regarding expected care. Expected care in the medical profession often refers to *Professional Practice Standards*, which serve as a guide to identify the role and scope (duties) for health care personnel within various branches of the health care profession. In order to declare negligence, four factors must be determined.

  - **breach of duty** – A breach of duty is a failure on the part of the caregiver to carry out an expected duty or level of standard care as determined in the role and scope of the profession's *Practice Standards* or as stated in the medical facility's standing protocol.

  - **causation** – Causation refers to a direct effect resulting from the wrongful action.

  - **damage** – Damage can be described as harm, injury, or a loss of value to the individual or to their property.

  - **duty** – The duty or duties of the individual providing care must be identified as part of an expected standard of care.

- **negligence doctrines** – There are two main negligence doctrines that are commonly referred to regarding the claim of negligence within the medical profession.

  - **res ipsa laquitur** – The Latin phrase *res ipsa laquitur*, meaning *"the thing speaks for itself,"* is a legal term used to describe a resulting action as true, clear, and undebatable, i.e., there could be no other conclusion.

  - **respondeat superior** – The Latin phrase Respondeat Superior, meaning *"let the superior respond"* or *"let the master speak for the servant,"* is a legal term used to imply that responsibility for a wrongful action taken by an employee should reside with a higher authority such as an employer or medical facility.

values – Values are a set of beliefs an individual or organization deems important to achieving success.

veracity – Veracity is a term used to denote sincerity, honesty, and/or truthfulness about someone or something.

vital signs – Vital signs are monitoring points by which the body's functional ability can be assessed. There are four main vital signs routinely assessed to determine a patient's overall well being. The normal vital sign range for the average healthy adult (at rest) is provided separately under each vital sign-monitoring category.

(MedlinePlus Medical Encyclopedia, U.S. Library of Medicine, National Institutes of Health, 2009. Retrieved February 25, 2010, from http://www.nlm.nih.gov/medlineplus)

- ■ **blood pressure** – Blood pressure rate is a measurement of the force of blood against the walls of the arteries as the heart pumps blood through the circulatory system. The systolic reading is a recording of the blood flow force as the ventricles of the heart contract, whereas the diastolic reading is a recording of the blood flow force while the ventricles of the heart are at rest. A blood pressure rate of less than 120 mmHg systolic and less than 80 mmHg diastolic is considered the normal blood pressure range for the average healthy adult *(see blood pressure reading)*.

- ■ **pulse** – Pulse rate or heart rate is a measurement of the heart's ability to beat or pump blood through the circulatory system. A pulse rate of 60–80 beats per minute (bpm) is considered within the normal pulse range for the average healthy adult.

- ■ **respiration** – Respiration rate is a measurement of the body's ability to move air (oxygen) into the lungs and move carbon dioxide out of the lungs. This gas exchange occurs via inhalation and exhalation. A respiration rate of 12–18 breaths per minute is considered within the normal respiration range for the average healthy adult.

- ■ **temperature** – Normal body temperature is considered the temperature in which homeostasis exists between heat produced within the body and heat exerted by the body. An oral body temperature reading of 97.8°–99.1°F is considered within the normal body temperature range for the average healthy adult, with 98.6°F being the average *(see body temperature reading)*.

vulnerable – Vulnerable means to be open to and unprotected from potential harm.

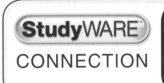

StudyWARE
CONNECTION

After completing this chapter, complete the image labeling exercises or play another interactive game on your StudyWARE™ CD-ROM that will help you learn the content in this chapter.

CONCEPT THINKING QUESTIONS

1. Describe what a tort is and list the two main classifications of torts.

2. Differentiate between intentional misconduct and unintentional misconduct.

3. Identify the four vital signs and explain what each represents.

4. Explain what is meant by subjective patient data and objective patient data.

5. Differentiate between an assault and a battery.

6. Explain how the *Health Insurance Portability and Accountability Act (HIPAA)* protects a patient.

7. Differentiate between a felony and a misdemeanor.

8. Discuss what are considered the normal ranges for each of the four vital signs.

9. Explain the difference between morals, values, and ethics.

10. Discuss reasons for having an advanced health care directive.

PRACTICE EXERCISES

1. List the "*Sacred Seven*" regarding a patient history.

2. Devise a case study depicting a patient who has fallen while receiving medical care in a health care facility. Apply the knowledge that you have of medical and legal terms to build a case in support of the plaintiff and then to build a case in support of the defendant.

3. Explain what the systolic and diastolic numbers represents in a blood pressure reading.

4. Describe how a patient might appear whose respiration is at 25 breaths per minute.

5. Provide an example of how the negligence doctrine *respondeat superior* might be used.

6. Describe a medical situation that would demonstrate veracity and one that would demonstrate malice.

7. Explain the type of information contained within the ARRT *Standard of Ethics*.

8. Provide an example of when the *Good Samaritan Law* might be used in a court of law.

9. List recommended practices for maintaining good body mechanics.

10. Explain what type of imaging procedures would require a signed consent form.

MATCHING

Match each term to the appropriate description.

negligence	warning	102°F
open	female patient scheduling	prognosis
deception	98.6°F	slander
70 bpm	ADA Amendments Act	mmHg
12–20 breaths/min	medical record	intentional misconduct
defendant	compliance	DNR code

Description	Term
1. law	_____
2. fraud	_____

   3. reprimand   _____

   4. pulse rate   _____

   5. vulnerable   _____

   6. fever   _____

   7. mercury   _____

   8. unintentional misconduct   _____

   9. established standards   _____

  10. false imprisonment   _____

  11. confidential patient information   _____

  12. elective booking   _____

RETENTION OF MATERIAL

Retention requires practicing the use of previously learned material. Apply the medical and legal knowledge you have gained throughout your studies to answer the following questions.

   1. What is the purpose of obtaining a good patient history?

   2. What should a mission statement tell you about an organization?

   3. Why should a technologist be familiar with the normal ranges for vital signs?

   4. Explain ways in which a patient could be considered vulnerable when receiving care or treatment in a hospital or medical facility.

   5. Describe the purpose of completing an incident report.

   6. Give examples of simple to sophisticated restraints (immobilization methods) that are commonly found in a radiology/imaging department.

   7. Explain the difference between "diagnosis" and "prognosis."

   8. Give three examples of intentional misconduct an RT could be accused of.

   9. Give an example of unintentional misconduct an RT could be accused of.

  10. List the four factors that must be present to determine whether negligence has occurred.

     _____ and _____

     _____ and _____

  11. Give an example of a medical incident that could occur involving an RT in which the legal doctrine *res ipsa laquitur* could be used.

  12. Give an example of a medical incident that could occur involving an RT in which the legal doctrine *respondeat superior* could be used.

CHAPTER 4

Infection Control

OBJECTIVES

Upon completion of this chapter, the reader will be able to:

- Differentiate between medical asepsis and surgical asepsis
- Explain the technique for hand washing
- Discuss isolation classifications
- Discuss the cycle of infection
- List four types of pathogens
- Identify various types of personal protective equipment (PPE)
- Differentiate between direct and indirect contact

CONCEPT THINKING

Infection control combines a common sense approach along with CDC (Centers for Disease Control and Prevention) guidelines on practices and protocols designed to assist health care workers to reduce the spread of infectious pathogens from one individual to another as they care for patients with various illnesses, diseases, and injuries. The most common practice for reducing the spread of infection in a health care setting is for caretakers to wash their hands before and after care is given to a patient. *Standard Precautions* are infection control guidelines and practices published by the CDC to assist health care workers to reduce the spread of pathogens within a health care setting. Hand washing is the easiest practice and the best way to minimize the spread of microorganisms from one individual to another. Hand washing is a common practice we learn as children. However, busy adults with limited time can become neglectful of a routine practice that doesn't demand full attention. The frequency and duration of hand washing can and does affect our health significantly, causing everything we touch to be a potential vehicle for the transmission of infectious pathogens. We tell children not to put objects in their mouths because "they have germs." We cover our mouths when we cough or sneeze to prevent airborne droplets from spreading. We wash off any utensil that has fallen to the floor before we put it back in our mouth. We rinse off vegetables and fruits before we eat them, and of course we wash our hands after using the rest room. On a very basic level, we understand that direct contact (touch) and indirect contact (inanimate objects) carry germs (pathogens) from one place to another and from one individual to another. Further development of the germ-spreading concept would lead us to the conclusion that the risk for spreading infection would increase in areas where interaction between the sick and injured and the nonsick (health care providers, family, and visitors) would be prevalent, such as hospitals and health care settings.

Infection control pertains to limiting the spread of pathogenic microorganisms that cause disease by understanding *transmission modes* and the *cycle of infection*. The World Health Organization (WHO) provides health care facilities with guidelines regarding standard infection control precautions. (WHO: *Interim Infection Control Guideline for Health Care Facilities*; May 2007. Retrieved March 1, 2010, from http://www.wpro.who.int.

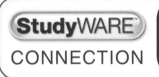

StudyWARE CONNECTION *View the Infection Control animation on your StudyWARE™ CD-ROM for more information.*

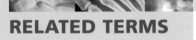

RELATED TERMS

antibiotic – An antibiotic is a form of medication prescribed by a physician to rid a patient of infection brought on by harmful bacteria.

antibody, antibodies – Antibodies are specialized proteins produced by plasma cells within the body. Antibodies serve to provide a line of defense against antigens (bacteria and viruses) that could be harmful to the body.

antiseptic – An antiseptic is a substance (e.g., ethanol, propanol, hydrogen peroxide, or iodine) applied to the skin (living tissue) to reduce the spread of microorganisms.

asepsis – Asepsis means being without infection *(prefix "a" means without; root word "septic" means infection).*

■ **medical asepsis** – Medical asepsis is an infection control practice used to reduce the presence of microorganisms.

■ **surgical asepsis** – Surgical asepsis is an infection control practice used to eliminate the presence of microorganisms (i.e., during surgical procedures).

autoclave – An autoclave is a device used to sterilize instruments through the use of steam and pressure.

FIGURE 4–1. Containers for contaminated items are identified with a biohazard label. The symbol is black with an orange or red background.

Delmar/Cengage Learning.

biohazard – Biohazard refers to any substance or material that poses a health threat to humans, animals, or the environment. Containers for contaminated items are identified with a biohazard label. The biohazard symbol is black with an orange or a red background *(see Figure 4–1)*.

biospill – A biospill is any fluid or substance that is not contained and poses a health threat to humans, animals, or the environment.

bodily fluids – Bodily fluids are fluids that can be found within the human body. They include bile, blood, blood plasma, chyme, interstitial fluid, lymph, pleural fluid, saliva, sebum, sputum, sweat, tears, and gender-specific fluids such as female vaginal secretions, breast milk (produced after childbirth), and male semen.

communicable disease – A communicable disease is a disease that can be transmitted from one individual to another via direct and/or indirect contact.

contaminate, contamination – Contaminate or contamination is to have the presence of an infectious agent, or the risk of an infectious agent spread from one individual to another via direct and/or indirect contact.

disease – A medical disorder or condition in which normal body function and/or body structure is disrupted either temporarily or permanently is referred to as a disease. Signs or symptoms of a disease can manifest quickly or may go unnoticed for a period of time. The underlying cause of a disease may or may not be detectable, and the disease itself may or may not be treatable.

disinfectant – A disinfectant is a chemical used to inhibit the spread of microorganisms surviving on nonliving surfaces. Common disinfectants in the health care setting include alcohols (e.g., ethanol, isopropanol), aldehydes (e.g., glutaraldehyde), halogens (e.g., hypochlorite bleach), and phenolics.

hand washing – Hand washing should be performed before and after contact with a patient. The following steps are basic guidelines to follow to ensure appropriate hand washing is accomplished. The process takes approximately 1 minute to complete. The CDC website (http://www.cdc.gov) provides hand-washing technique guidelines.

- Remove jewelry (e.g., rings, bracelets, watches).
- Wet hands under warm running water (do not touch the faucet again).
- Use antibacterial soap and rub together to create friction for at least 15 seconds.
- Wash palms of hands, between fingers, under the fingernails, tips of the fingers, and the backs of hands.
- Rinse hands thoroughly and dry with a towel or paper towel.
- Turn off faucet with the use of a clean, dry towel or paper towel to avoid contamination of the hands.

health organizations

- **CDC** – Centers for Disease Control and Prevention; http://www.cdc.gov
- **DOH** – Department of Health (individual state web addresses vary)
- **HHS** – U.S. Department of Health and Human Services; http://www.hhs.gov
- **OSHA** – U.S. Department of Labor's Occupational Safety and Health Administration; http://www.OSHA.gov
- **WHO** – World Health Organization; http://www.who.int

host – A host is a living organism that provides nourishment for another living organism.

idiopathic – Idiopathic refers to a disease of unknown origin.

immune, immunity – To be immune or have immunity is to be protected from the effects of pathogenic microorganisms or harmful agents. Immunity can occur through a natural body response or through an acquired response from a vaccine.

immunization – Immunization is the process of introducing the body to a dead or weakened strain of an infectious disease to stimulate the body's immune system to create antibodies for defending the body against acquiring the actual disease.

immunization record – An immunization record is a medical record depicting the dates of immunizations *(inoculations)* the patient has received.

infection – An infection is the reproduction and spread of infectious pathogens within the body.

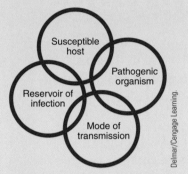

FIGURE 4–2. The cycle of infection.

▪ **cycle of infection** – The cycle of infection is a series of events that runs in a continuum. If the cycle of infection is broken, the transmission of infection can no longer continue. The cycle consists of a susceptible host, pathogenic organism, means of transmission, and a reservoir of infection *(see Figure 4–2).*

    • **susceptible host** – A susceptible host can be the human body, an animal, or an environment in which pathogenic organisms can thrive.

    • **pathogenic organism** – Pathogenic organisms include bacteria, fungi, protozoan parasites, and viruses.

    • **means of transmission** – The mode of transmission for pathogenic organisms can occur through direct or indirect contact.

    • **reservoir of infection** – A reservoir of infection is a place in which pathogenic organisms can exist and be easily transmitted to an individual when a means of transmission is established. This reservoir can be a living organism (humans, animals, and vectors), an inanimate object (fomites), or an environment conducive to sustaining life.

▪ **iatrogenic infection** – An iatrogenic infection is an infection that a patient acquires directly as the result of treatment provided by a physician or prescribed therapy.

▪ **nosocomial infection** – A nosocomial infection can also be referred to as a health care-associated infection (HAI). This type of infection arises after the patient has entered the health care setting. The most common nosocomial infection a patient acquires when hospitalized is a urinary tract infection (UTI).

inoculation – An inoculation is a vaccine injected into the body for the purpose of creating immunity to a specific disease.

isolation – Isolation refers to separating an individual from others as a means of either protecting the individual or protecting others from receiving infectious agents or potentially harmful microorganisms. Before a patient is placed in an isolation area, the health care team must determine what type of isolation is required to best minimize the spread of infectious pathogens. This is accomplished by evaluating the mode of transmission of the identified pathogen(s). The three main modes of transmission for infectious agents include contact (direct and/or indirect contact), airborne, and droplet. Health care workers are required to adhere to the appropriate precautions designated for the mode of transmission identified.

- ■ **contact precautions** – Contact precautions require health care workers to protect themselves by donning gloves and gowns (and masks if deemed necessary) when anticipating direct and/or indirect contact with an infected patient. Contact precautions require a private room for the patient with all necessary protective clothing located outside the room for health care workers to apply prior to entering the room. Diseases that require contact precautions include but are not limited to MRSA (*Staphylococcus aureus*), VRE (vancomycin-resistant enterococcus), C-diff (*Clostridium difficile* colitis), impetigo, scabies, *Varicella* (chickenpox), hepatitis A, and certain wounds such as abscesses or decubiti *(see Figure 4–3)*.

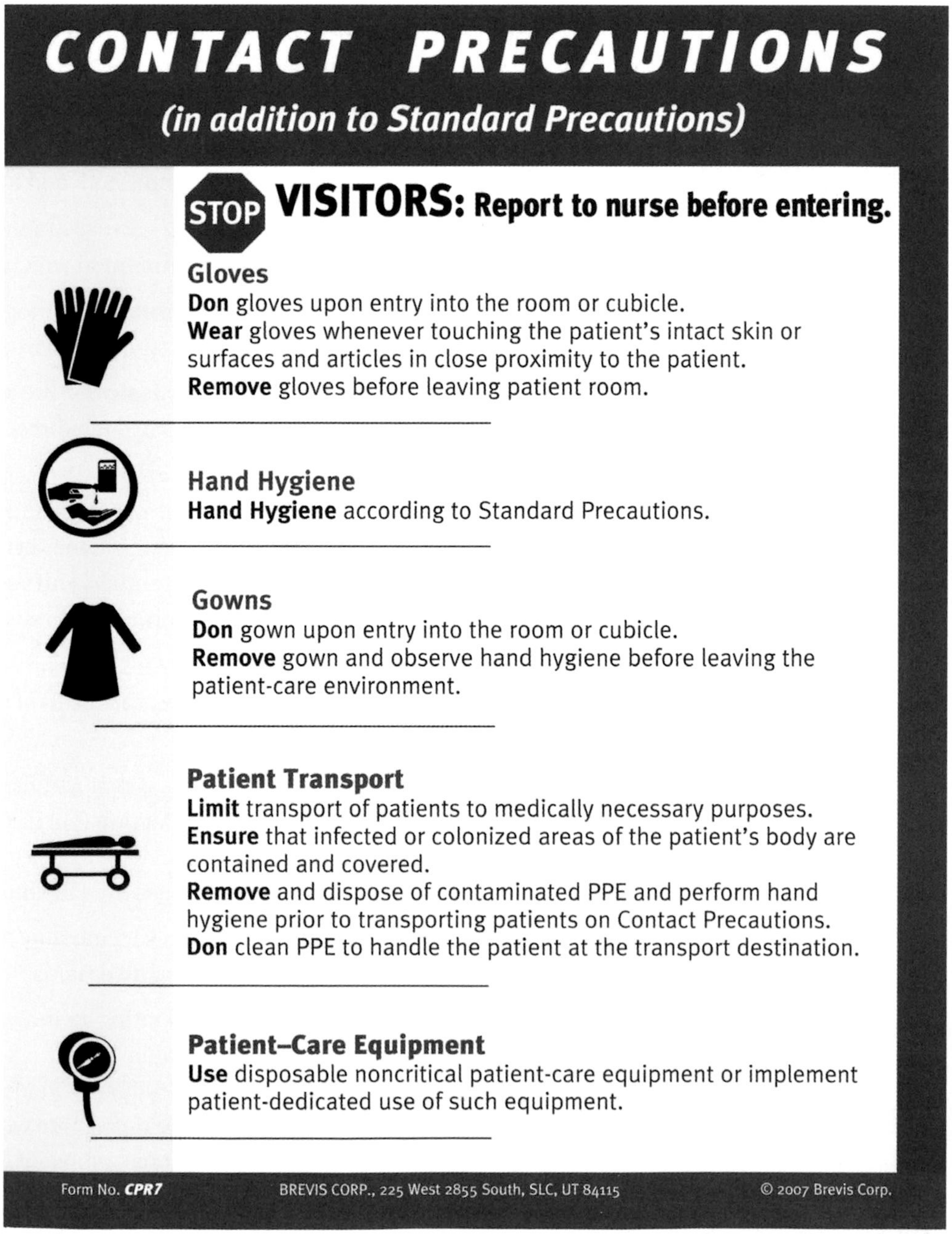

CONTACT PRECAUTIONS
(in addition to Standard Precautions)

STOP VISITORS: Report to nurse before entering.

Gloves
Don gloves upon entry into the room or cubicle.
Wear gloves whenever touching the patient's intact skin or surfaces and articles in close proximity to the patient.
Remove gloves before leaving patient room.

Hand Hygiene
Hand Hygiene according to Standard Precautions.

Gowns
Don gown upon entry into the room or cubicle.
Remove gown and observe hand hygiene before leaving the patient-care environment.

Patient Transport
Limit transport of patients to medically necessary purposes.
Ensure that infected or colonized areas of the patient's body are contained and covered.
Remove and dispose of contaminated PPE and perform hand hygiene prior to transporting patients on Contact Precautions.
Don clean PPE to handle the patient at the transport destination.

Patient–Care Equipment
Use disposable noncritical patient-care equipment or implement patient-dedicated use of such equipment.

Form No. **CPR7**   BREVIS CORP., 225 West 2855 South, SLC, UT 84115   © 2007 Brevis Corp.

FIGURE 4–3. Contact precautions poster.

■ **airborne precautions** – Airborne precautions require health care workers to protect themselves when caring for infected patients by wearing special masks or using respirators such as the N95 respirator, which is specifically designed to prevent the inhalation of small or evaporated airborne droplets. Airborne precautions require a private *negative pressure* room in which the air within the patient's room is not permitted access beyond the room. This precautionary measure is taken to keep the infectious agent contained and away from uninfected individuals who may be in close proximity to the patient's room. The airflow within the patient's room is typically directed through a filtration system with HEPA (high-efficiency particulate air) filters that may or may not lead to the exterior of the medical facility. Diseases that require airborne precautions include but are not limited to TB (tuberculosis) *Varicella* (chickenpox), and rubeola (measles) *(see Figure 4–4)*.

AIRBORNE PRECAUTIONS
(in addition to Standard Precautions)

VISITORS: Report to nurse before entering.

Use Airborne Precautions as recommended for patients known or suspected to be infected with infectious agents transmitted person-to-person by the airborne route (e.g., M. tuberculosis, measles, chickenpox, disseminated herpes zoster).

Patient placement

Place patients in an **AIIR** (Airborne Infection Isolation Room).
Monitor air pressure daily with visual indicators (e.g., flutter strips).

Keep door closed when not required for entry and exit.

In ambulatory settings instruct patients with a known or suspected airborne infection to wear a surgical mask and observe Respiratory Hygiene/Cough Etiquette. Once in an AIIR, the mask may be removed.

Patient transport

Limit transport and movement of patients to **medically-necessary purposes.**

If transport or movement outside an AIIR is necessary, instruct patients to **wear a surgical mask**, if possible, and observe Respiratory Hygiene/Cough Etiquette.

Hand Hygiene

Hand Hygiene according to Standard Precautions.

Personal Protective Equipment (PPE)

Wear a fit-tested NIOSH-approved **N95** or higher level respirator for respiratory protection when entering the room of a patient when the following diseases are suspected or confirmed: Listed on back.

APR   ©2007 Brevis Corporation www.brevis.com

Reprinted with permission from Brevis Corporation (www.brevis.com).

FIGURE 4–4. Airborne precautions poster.

■ **droplet precautions** – Droplets tend to be large particles (>5 μm) secreted from an individual's respiratory tract (nose and mouth) and expelled into the air via coughing, sneezing, talking, or spitting. These particles tend to travel short distances (<6 feet from the patient) as the result of their large size and can easily spread disease if infectious pathogens are present and come in contact with the mucous membranes of a healthy individual. Diseases spread by droplet include but are not limited to common cold, influenza, mumps, and rubella *(see Figure 4-5).*

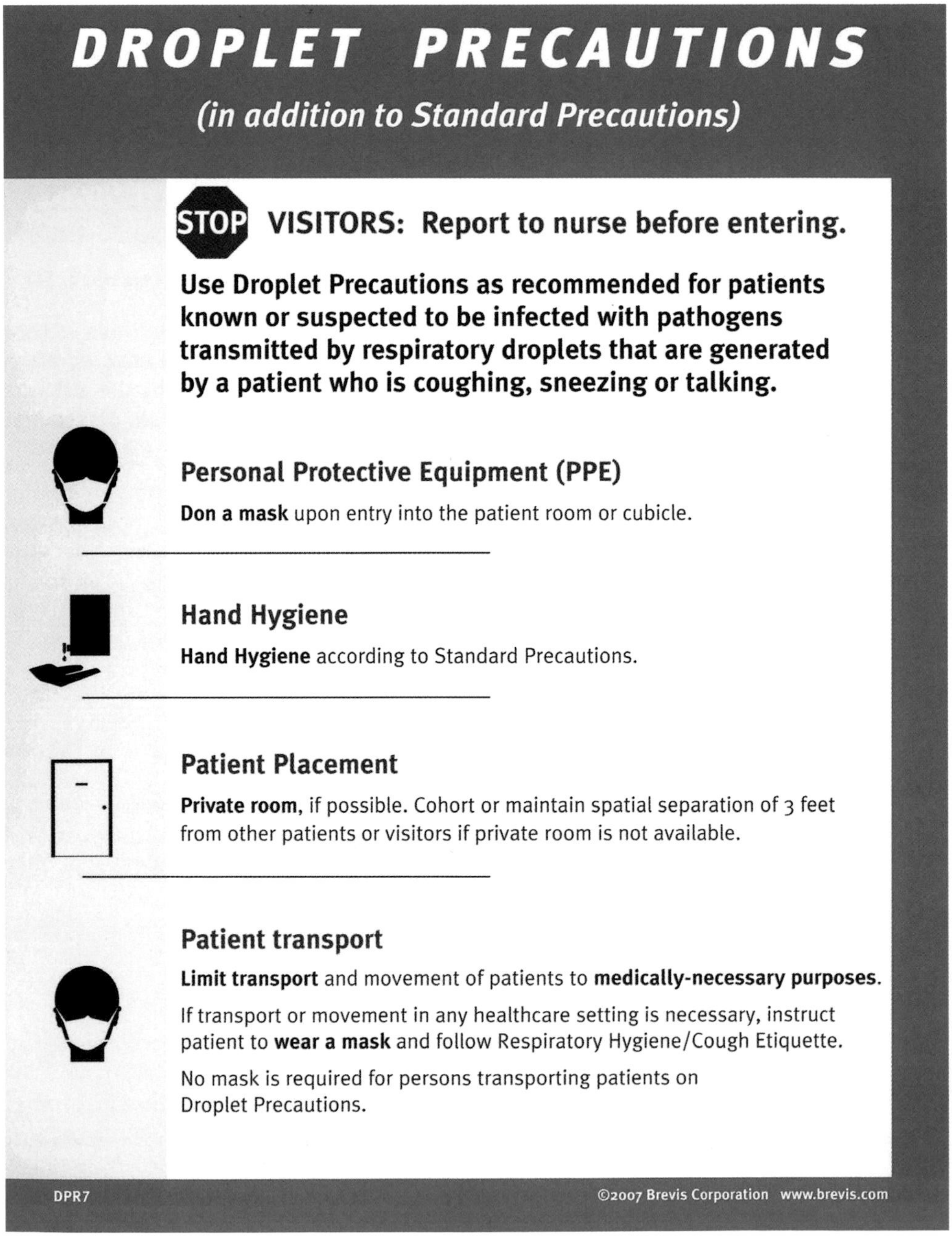

DROPLET PRECAUTIONS

(in addition to Standard Precautions)

 STOP **VISITORS: Report to nurse before entering.**

Use Droplet Precautions as recommended for patients known or suspected to be infected with pathogens transmitted by respiratory droplets that are generated by a patient who is coughing, sneezing or talking.

 Personal Protective Equipment (PPE)

Don a mask upon entry into the patient room or cubicle.

Hand Hygiene

Hand Hygiene according to Standard Precautions.

Patient Placement

Private room, if possible. Cohort or maintain spatial separation of 3 feet from other patients or visitors if private room is not available.

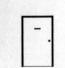 **Patient transport**

Limit transport and movement of patients to **medically-necessary purposes**.

If transport or movement in any healthcare setting is necessary, instruct patient to **wear a mask** and follow Respiratory Hygiene/Cough Etiquette.

No mask is required for persons transporting patients on Droplet Precautions.

DPR7   ©2007 Brevis Corporation   www.brevis.com

FIGURE 4–5. Droplet precautions poster.

microorganism – A microorganism is considered to be the smallest living organism *(prefix "micro" means small; root word "organism" means living body)*. To see a microorganism, one would need the aid of a microscope.

MSDS – MSDS (Material Safety Data Sheets) are information sheets on specific chemicals and substances that are used within the health care facility and educational institutions with dedicated laboratories for health care training. These data sheets are important to the employer, employees, trainees, and emergency personnel in providing valuable information on how best to handle workplace substances regarding storage, temperature, ventilation, skin contact, spills, and other occurrences that could pose potential health risks. MSDS sheets should be readily available to health care workers and trainees in case of a chemical emergency.

needle – Needles are used to draw blood and administer drugs to patients via the following three routes: intravenous, intramuscular, and subcutaneous. Needles are identified by their length and diameter (gauge). The average length of a needle ranges between 0.25 inch and 5 inches with a diameter typically between 14 and 28 gauge. The smaller the needle gauge, the larger the needle diameter. Needles are made of stainless steel with a beveled edge to help with insertion and distribution of solution. Although needles may vary in length and gauge, the three main sections of a needle remain constant: the hub, the cannula, and the bevel. Needles should always be disposed of appropriately after use to avoid accidental injury *(see Figure 4-6)*.

■ **bevel** – The bevel of the needle refers to the angle of the tip of the needle. The bevel varies slightly in length as it is designed to accommodate the three routes of drug administration.

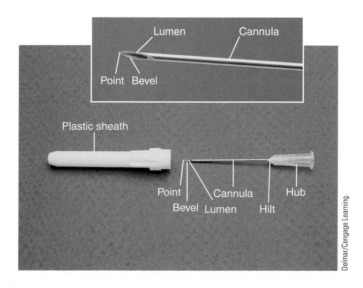

FIGURE 4–6. Needle with bevel, cannula, and hub.

Delmar/Cengage Learning.

■■ **cannula** – The cannula is the long slender shaft of the needle, and it can vary in length between 0.25 inch and 5 inches.

■■ **hub** – The hub is the connecting area that joins the needle to the syringe.

needleless devices – Needleless devices are devices specially designed to protect health care workers from exposure to needlestick injuries. These devices are made to either retract the sharp needle back into the syringe or to provide a protective housing the needle can be projected forward into. Various types of needleless devices and systems can be viewed at http://www.OSHA.gov.

needle recapping – Recapping a needle refers to the attempt to place the removed cap, originally covering the needle tip, back over the used needle. This practice is considered dangerous to health care workers and should be avoided because of the high risk of needlestick injuries. All used needles should be disposed of in a "sharps container," which is puncture resistant, usually red in color, and clearly labeled with the *biohazard symbol*.

needlestick injury – A needlestick injury is an accidental injury to a health care worker in which a contaminated needle (i.e., with a patient's blood) has broken the surface of the health care worker's skin, allowing the transmission of microorganisms.

parasite – A parasite is an organism that depends on a host to sustain its life.

pathogen – A pathogen is a microorganism capable of producing a disease. There are four main types of pathogens: bacteria, fungi, protozoan parasites, and viruses.

■■ **bacteria** – Bacteria are single-celled microorganisms that can function independently or as a parasite to a host. Bacteria have no nuclei and are classified according to their morphology *(shape and structure)*: spheric (cocci), comma-shaped (vibrios), rod-shaped (bacilli), and spiral (spirochetes). Common bacteria include but are not limited to:

  • chlamydia, *Escherichia. coli (E. coli)*, meningitis, pneumonia, scarlet fever, streptococcus (strep throat), syphilis, tetanus, tuberculosis, and typhoid fever

■■ **fungi** – Fungi are living organisms that have their own unique classification because they cannot be classified as animal or plant. Growth conditions determine whether the fungi will manifest as a single-cell yeast or as a mold (filamentous hypha). Fungi can be helpful to the human body, like penicillin and yeast, or deadly to the human body, like the *death cap* mushroom. Common ailments manifesting from fungi include but are not limited to:

  • athlete's foot, ringworm, and tinea nigra

■■ **protozoan parasites** – Protozoan parasites are one-celled organisms that have their own unique classification because they are considered neither animal nor plant. They are larger than bacteria and are classified by their method of movement: amoeboid locomotion, cilia, or flagella. Common protozoan parasites include but are not limited to:

  • giardiasis (giardia infection), hookworm infection, intestinal roundworms, malaria, pinworm infection, scabies, and toxoplasmosis

■ **viruses** – A virus is a parasite in need of a host to survive. A virus particle *(virion)* will invade a cell and alter cell function by depositing its own genetic information in the form of DNA or RNA. The effect the virus has on the host can vary depending on the type of virus and the type of cells involved. Common viruses include but are not limited to:

- common cold (rhinovirus), herpes simplex, human immunodeficiency virus (HIV), human papilloma virus, influenza, mononucleosis (Epstein-Barr virus), mumps, rubella, and smallpox.

personal protective equipment (PPE) – *Personal protective equipment* encompasses numerous types of clothing and accessories designed to protect health care workers (and patients) from contact with potentially infectious agents and infectious agents, as well as reduce the risk of spreading infectious agents from one individual to another within a health care facility.

■ **facemask** – A facemask (or mask) is to be used by either the health care worker or the patient when attempting to prevent inhalation of airborne contaminants. Facemasks can be secured by a tie or by elastic bands that fit over and behind the ears. The two main types of facemasks are the *surgical mask* and the *isolation mask (see Figure 4-7).*

■ **face shield** – A face shield is a transparent protective barrier that covers the health care worker's face (forehead to chin) from any splashing fluids that may be encountered during invasive procedures or when patient interaction dictates such protection. Face shields are flexible enough to wrap around the face without causing discomfort and can be held in place by ties or elastic bands that fit over and behind the ears. For radiation protection purposes, face shields with a lead equivalent material are available to those participating in procedures that require fluoroscopy *(see Figure 4-7).*

■ **gloves** – Disposable gloves are considered part of *Standard Precautions* and should be used by health care workers in direct or indirect contact with patients. Disposable gloves come in various sizes to accommodate all health care workers. Disposable gloves may be made of latex, vinyl, or nitrate and include powdered or nonpowdered types. The powdered glove type helps

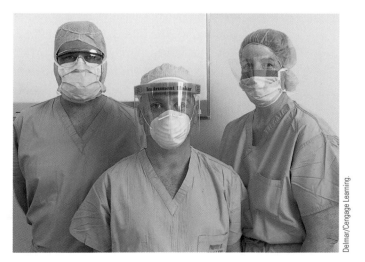

FIGURE 4–7. Surgical masks and protective eyewear, including face shields.

to prevent the hand from sticking to the inside surface of the glove where sweat can create a tight bond. Most medical facilities use latex-free gloves as the result of reported incidents of health care workers experiencing adverse (allergic) reactions to latex. Surgical technique requires individuals who will be in contact with the sterile field to don disposable sterile gloves to reduce the risk of infection to the patient. There are strict aseptic guidelines for how to appropriately perform the closed or open glove technique to avoid contamination of the sterile field. For radiation protection purposes, lead gloves are available to those participating in procedures that require fluoroscopy *(see Figures 4-8 and 4-9).*

- **goggles** – Goggles are a form of protective eyewear providing health care workers with a transparent barrier between their eyes and any splashing fluids. Goggles should fit snuggly around the eyes, leaving no gaps for fluid entry, and they should possess an anti-fog coating to prevent fog build up. Goggles should be designed to permit comfort without obstructing peripheral vision. For radiation protection purposes, goggles with a lead equivalent material are available to those participating in procedures that require fluoroscopy.

- **gowns** – The two types of disposable gowns health care workers commonly use are the isolation gown and the surgical gown. Isolation gowns are to be worn by health care workers to protect themselves from contact with a patient's bodily fluids. These gowns are readily available to health care workers and are required as part of isolation precautions. Gowns are designed to cover the complete torso from neck to knee and the upper extremities down to include the wrists. Surgical gowns are donned for procedures requiring sterile technique. There are strict aseptic guidelines for how to appropriately put on a surgical gown (both for self-gowning and gowning another individual) to avoid contamination of the sterile field *(see Figure 4-10).*

- **hair cap** – A hair cap is a protective head covering in which the health care worker's hair is concealed, preventing strands of hair from floating into the sterile field and contaminating the microorganism-free environment.

- **particulate respirators** – Particulate respirators are a type of specialized face mask that covers the nose and mouth and prevents inhalation of airborne infectious agents. Particulate respirators are ranked according to their level of filtration. The minimum level of filtration for particulate respirators is 95%. The N95 respirator filters 95% of airborne inhalants and is approved by the National Institute for Occupational Safety and Health (NIOSH), a branch of the CDC. The N95 respirator has been cleared by the Food and Drug Administration (FDA) as a surgical mask. A user-seal check (sometimes referred to as a "fit-check") is a method for testing air leakage gaps around the face where the respirator should fit securely. There should be no gaps between the face and the particulate respirator *(see Figure 4-11).*

proliferate – Proliferate is to reproduce, multiply, or grow in number.

protective/reverse isolation – Protective isolation is often referred to as reverse isolation because the susceptible person is the patient rather than the health care worker. Patients in protective isolation often have a weakened immune system, which tends to increase their risk for infection.

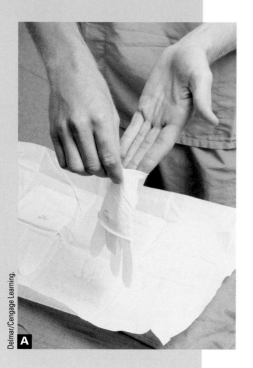

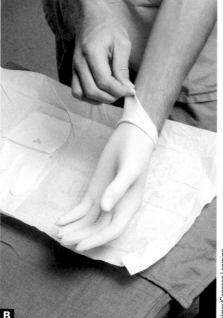

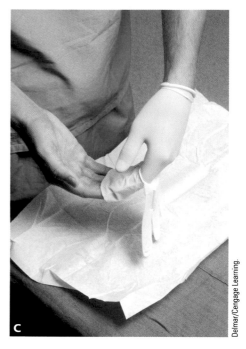

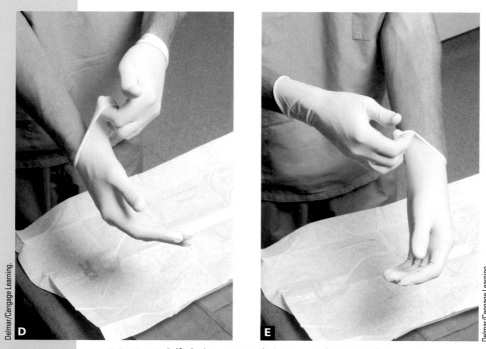

FIGURE 4–8. Self-gloving, open technique. *A.* and *B.* Open the inner glove wrapper and don the first glove, leaving the cuff rolled down. *C.* Slide the fingers of the partially gloved hand into the outer side of the opposite glove cuff. *D.* Gently unroll the cuff and slide the hand into the glove. *E.* Using the gloved hand, unroll the cuff of the first glove.

Delmar/Cengage Learning.

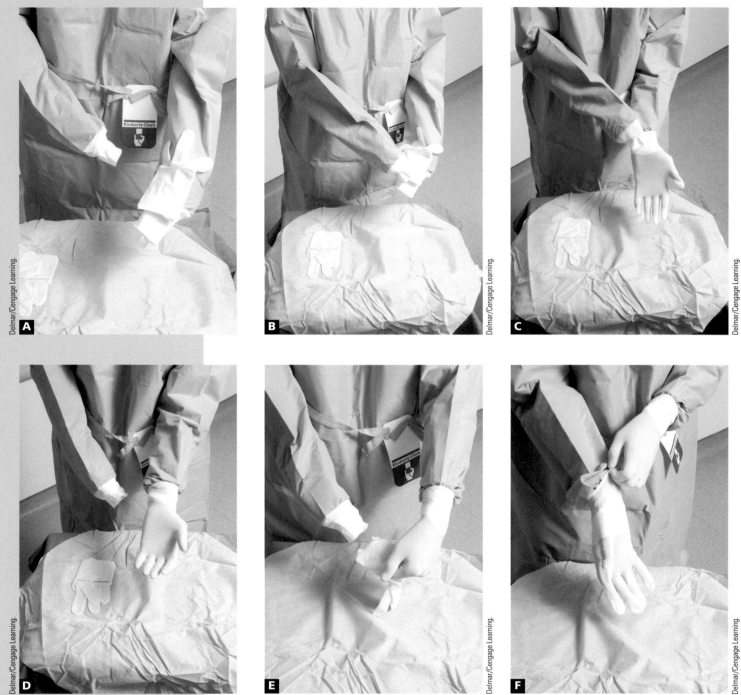

FIGURE 4–9. Self-gloving, closed technique. *A.* Position the first glove palm to palm, thumb to thumb over the cuff of the gown. *B.* Working through the gown sleeve, grasp the cuff of the glove and bring it over the open cuff of the sleeve. *C.* and *D.* Unroll the glove cuff so that it covers the sleeve cuff of the gown. *E.* and *F.* Repeat with the opposite hand using the same technique.

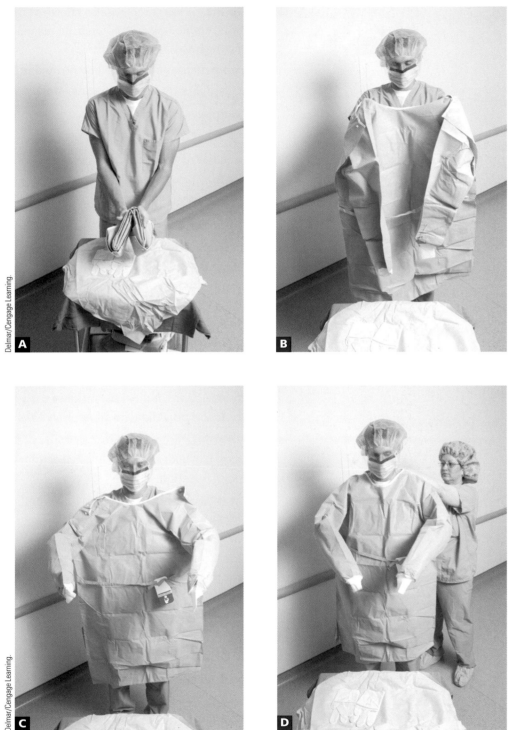

FIGURE 4–10. Self gowning. *A.* Pick up gown and move it away from the table. It is folded so that the outside faces away. *B.* Holding the gown at the shoulders, identify the arm openings and unfold the gown. *C.* Guide each arm through the gown sleeves. Do not bring your hands through the outside cuffs of the gown. *D.* The circulator helps pull the gown over the shoulders and ties it.

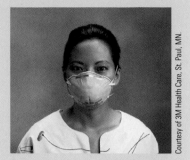

FIGURE 4–11. Particulate respirator.

Courtesy of 3M Health Care, St. Paul, MN.

skin prep kit – A skin prep kit, also known as a sterile pack, contains a commercially prepared sterile tray with compartments to house items that may be needed during the invasive procedure.

Skin prep items may include but are not limited to:

■ glass tubes (3–4) for collecting bodily fluids for testing purposes

■ gauze pads for maintaining a moisture-free environment

■ local anesthetic provided to patient to temporarily lessen the sensation of pain

■ needles of various gauge sizes

■ sterile drapes for maintaining a sterile field

■ syringes for administering drugs, contrast media, and collecting bodily fluid samples

standard precautions – *Standard Precautions* are a set of infection control guidelines and practices published by the CDC to assist health care workers to reduce the spread of pathogens within the health care setting as they provide patient care. Health care professionals should assume that all patients are potentially infectious and that contamination can result from contact with a patient's bodily fluids (e.g., secretions, excretions, blood, feces), open skin sores, soiled items, and fomites with which the patient has had direct contact. As a means of preventing the spread of infection, health care workers follow a strict hand-washing regimen and use disposable gloves, fluid-resistant gowns, masks, face shields, and goggles as deemed necessary for providing the appropriate level of patient care *(see Figure 4–12).*

sterile – Sterile or aseptic means free from microorganisms. Surgical instruments and surgical fields must be kept free of microorganisms to prevent the onset and spread of infection.

■ **sterilization** – Sterilization is the removal of all living microorganisms. In the medical field, sterilization typically refers to the surgical instruments or sterile field that must be initiated and maintained during all invasive procedures. The most common method of sterilization involving invasive instrumentation is the autoclave, which uses steam under pressure to remove any and all living organisms. Other methods include dry heat, chemicals, and gases. Sterile fields must be set up before the introduction of sterile instruments and sterile kits.

sterile field – A sterile field is a clean area free of microorganisms. A sterile field is required for surgical procedures to reduce the risk of infection to the patient.

sterile technique – Sterile technique is the process used to ensure a microorganism-free environment is established and maintained during invasive procedures. Each step listed has specific CDC guidelines (www.cdc.gov) that should be studied in depth before initiating sterile technique.

■ hand-washing technique for sterile technique *(surgical scrub)*

■ use of sterile clothing *(i.e., facemask, gloves, goggles, gown, and hair cap)*

■ preparation of work area to establish a sterile environment *(sterile field)*

■ sterile kits or packages introduced to work area appropriately and handled only by individuals adhering to sterile technique

■ preparation of patient *(skin prep kit)*

STANDARD PRECAUTIONS

Assume that every person is potentially infected or colonized with an organism that could be transmitted in the healthcare setting.

Hand Hygiene

Avoid unnecessary touching of surfaces in close proximity to the patient.

When hands are visibly dirty, contaminated with proteinaceous material, or visibly soiled with blood or body fluids, wash hands with soap and water.

If hands are not visibly soiled, or after removing visible material with soap and water, decontaminate hands with an alcohol-based hand rub. Alternatively, hands may be washed with an antimicrobial soap and water.

Perform hand hygiene:
> Before having direct contact with patients.
> After contact with blood, body fluids or excretions, mucous membranes, nonintact skin, or wound dressings.
> After contact with a patient's intact skin (e.g., when taking a pulse or blood pressure or lifting a patient).
> If hands will be moving from a contaminated-body site to a clean-body site during patient care.
> After contact with inanimate objects (including medical equipment) in the immediate vicinity of the patient.
> After removing gloves.

Personal protective equipment (PPE)

Wear PPE when the nature of the anticipated patient interaction indicates that contact with blood or body fluids may occur.

Before leaving the patient's room or cubicle, remove and discard PPE.

Gloves

Wear gloves when contact with blood or other potentially infectious materials, mucous membranes, nonintact skin, or potentially contaminated intact skin (e.g., of a patient incontinent of stool or urine) could occur.

Remove gloves after contact with a patient and/or the surrounding environment using proper technique to prevent hand contamination. Do not wear the same pair of gloves for the care of more than one patient.

Change gloves during patient care if the hands will move from a contaminated body-site (e.g., perineal area) to a clean body-site (e.g., face).

Gowns

Wear a gown to protect skin and prevent soiling or contamination of clothing during procedures and patient-care activities when contact with blood, body fluids, secretions, or excretions is anticipated.

Wear a gown for direct patient contact if the patient has uncontained secretions or excretions.

Remove gown and perform hand hygiene before leaving the patient's environment.

Mouth, nose, eye protection

Use PPE to protect the mucous membranes of the eyes, nose and mouth during procedures and patient-care activities that are likely to generate splashes or sprays of blood, body fluids, secretions and excretions.

During aerosol-generating procedures wear one of the following: a face shield that fully covers the front and sides of the face, a mask with attached shield, or a mask and goggles.

Respiratory Hygiene/Cough Etiquette

Educate healthcare personnel to contain respiratory secretions to prevent droplet and fomite transmission of respiratory pathogens, especially during seasonal outbreaks of viral respiratory tract infections.

Offer masks to coughing patients and other symptomatic persons (e.g., persons who accompany ill patients) upon entry into the facility.

Patient-care equipment and instruments/devices

Wear PPE (e.g., gloves, gown), according to the level of anticipated contamination, when handling patient-care equipment and instruments/devices that are visibly soiled or may have been in contact with blood or body fluids.

Care of the environment

Include multi-use electronic equipment in policies and procedures for preventing contamination and for cleaning and disinfection, especially those items that are used by patients, those used during delivery of patient care, and mobile devices that are moved in and out of patient rooms frequently (e.g., daily).

Textiles and laundry

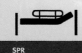

Handle used textiles and fabrics with minimum agitation to avoid contamination of air, surfaces and persons.

FIGURE 4–12. Standard precautions poster.

superbug – A "superbug" is a strain of bacteria resistant to antibiotics.

surgical scrub – A surgical scrub is a regimented hand-washing practice used by health care personnel involved with invasive procedures requiring sterile technique. There are two methods for performing a surgical scrub: the *numbered stroke method* and the *timed scrub method*. The estimated length of time for either procedure is between 3 and 5 minutes. However, many health care facilities have a standing protocol requiring a longer surgical scrub time.

■ **numbered stroke method** – This method involves counting a predetermined amount of brush strokes with a nailbrush for each finger, anterior hand (palm side), posterior hand (knuckle side), and lower arm beginning slightly above the elbow.

■ **timed scrub method** – The timed scrub method is very similar to the numbered stroke method except that, instead of counting brush strokes, the surgical scrub is performed for a predetermined amount of time as dictated by facility protocol.

toxin – A toxin is a substance produced by a living organism that is considered poisonous to the human body. The following websites provide further information on toxins:

■ Food and Drug Administration (FDA); http://www.fda.gov

■ Centers for Disease Control and Prevention (CDC); http://www.cdc.gov

■ United States Department of Agriculture (USDA); http://www.usda.gov

■ National Institutes of Health (NIH); http://www.nih.gov

transmission mode – Transmission mode refers to the method by which pathogens can be spread to a healthy individual.

■ **direct contact** – Touch between two individuals constitutes direct contact.

■ **indirect contact** – Indirect contact is the transmission of microorganisms by means other than direct contact, such as airborne, airborne droplets, vehicles (fomites), and vectors.

  • **airborne** – Airborne transmission involves extremely small dust particles or small evaporated airborne droplets.

  • **airborne droplets** – Airborne droplets tend to be large particles (>5 μm) secreted from an individual's respiratory tract (nose and mouth) and expelled into the air via coughing, sneezing, talking, or spitting. These particles tend to travel short distances (<6 feet from the patient) because of their large size.

  • **vector** – A vector is a living animal or insect capable of transmitting infectious microorganisms to individuals. Common vectors are ticks, mosquitoes, and fleas.

  • **vehicle** – A vehicle is an inanimate object (fomite) or material (food, water, transfusion blood) that permits the transmission of infectious microorganisms.

- **fomite** – A fomite is an inanimate object (e.g. faucet handle, glass, examination table, wall bucky, lead shields) that serves as a vehicle for transmission of infectious microorganisms.

vaccine – A vaccine is a dead or weakened strain of disease used to stimulate the body's immune system to create antibodies for defending the body against acquiring the actual disease.

vaccination – A vaccination or inoculation is an injection of a dead or weakened strain of disease given to an individual to cause their immune system to become resistant to the disease.

StudyWARE™ CONNECTION

After completing this chapter, complete the quiz questions or play an interactive game on your StudyWARE™ CD-ROM that will help you learn the content in this chapter.

CONCEPT THINKING QUESTIONS

1. What are *Standard Precautions* and how do they apply to a health care setting?
2. Differentiate between a pathogen and nonpathogen organism.
3. Identify the four types of pathogens.
4. Identify two common characteristics for each type of pathogen.
5. Name two ways in which a communicable disease can spread.
6. What is the name of the organization that provides infection control guidelines for health care workers?
7. Ringworm would be considered what type of pathogen?
8. What are toxins and are they lethal to the body?
9. Why does the hand-washing technique require friction?
10. Why is acquiring a "superbug" of great concern?

PRACTICE EXERCISES

1. Draw a diagram of the cycle of infection.
2. Provide examples for each link in the cycle of infection.
3. Discuss methods for breaking the cycle of infection.
4. Write the steps in sequential order for performing the *hand-washing technique*.
5. Differentiate between the two types of surgical scrub techniques.

6. Differentiate between medical asepsis and surgical asepsis.

7. Identify the classifications of bacteria by their morphology.

8. What conditions make for a suitable environment for proliferation of pathogens?

9. Explain what a "user-seal check" or "fit-check" is and its importance.

10. Explain what a *virion* is and how it affects the host cell.

11. When should a health care worker don gloves when caring for patient?

12. What conditions require a patient to be placed in protective isolation?

MATCHING

Match each term to the appropriate description.

disinfectant	antiseptic	indirect contact
cannula	direct contact	MSDS
kills viruses	N95	kills bacteria
autoclave	organism	HAI
idiopathic	vector	fomite
strep throat	sterile	pathogens

Description	Term
1. life	_____
2. antibiotic	_____
3. bleach	_____
4. chemical information	_____
5. kissing	_____
6. respirator	_____
7. unknown origin	_____
8. UTI	_____
9. mosquito	_____
10. free of microorganisms	_____
11. drinking glass	_____
12. infectious agents	_____

RETENTION OF MATERIAL

Retention requires practicing the use of previously learned material. Apply the knowledge you have of infection control to answer the following questions.

1. What is the purpose of using a "skin prep kit"?

2. Identify the three types of imaging procedures typically performed in a radiology department that require sterile technique.

   _____

   _____

   _____

3. The following diseases *(mumps, measles, rubella, and smallpox)* should be classified by which type of infectious pathogen?

4. The following diseases *(syphilis, strep throat, pneumonia, and meningitis)* should be classified by which type of infectious pathogen?

5. Explain the type of information expected to be found on a material safety data sheet (MSDS).

6. List the various types of personal protective equipment (PPE) and indicate when a health care worker would use each.

7. Identify three main types of isolation categories recognized for their mode of transmission.

8. List three communicable diseases for each mode of disease transmission.

9. Identify four types of environments (reservoirs) that can sustain the life of a pathogen.

10. List fluids found within the human body that constitute "bodily fluids."

CHAPTER 5

Pharmacology and Contrast Media

OBJECTIVES

Upon completion of this chapter, the reader will be able to:

- Identify medications common to the imaging profession
- Discuss types of contrast media and their usage
- Explain the scheduling protocol for imaging procedures with and without contrast
- Describe indications and contraindications for contrast media
- Differentiate between mild, moderate, and severe contrast media reactions
- Explain the difference between a bolus injection and a drip infusion
- Discuss the "five rights" of drug administration
- Discuss the role of informed consent and invasive procedures
- Discuss routes of drug administration and venipuncture protocol

CONCEPT THINKING

Radiologic technologists (RTs) are required to have a knowledge base of drug administration not only for procedures involving contrast media but for common medications that can impact functional ability of the body's organ systems. Because the body can have an adverse reaction to contrast media and certain medications, the RT must obtain a thorough patient history by the use of probing questions regarding allergies and possible allergic reactions to food and drugs. The RT must be able to recognize mild to severe contrast reactions and respond immediately and appropriately to the patients needs. Just as important to the technologist is recognizing the indications and contraindications for specific imaging procedures, thus avoiding the initiation of a procedure that could be potentially harmful to a patient. It is not within the RT's scope of practice to make decisions regarding performance or nonperformance of a physician-ordered examination. It is, however, the technologist's responsibility to report pertinent patient information to the radiologist so all medical factors can be considered in the decision to continue or discontinue with an imaging procedure. The premise for using contrast media is to make anatomical structures within the body that are normally not visible on an image become visible. This is accomplished by altering the atomic number of tissues with similar radiographic densities to create visible distinctions between comparable tissues for the purpose of evaluating structural integrity and organ function. Examples of human tissues and related atomic numbers can be seen under the term *human tissue*. As a member of the health care team, the RT is expected to know the normal ranges of all four vital signs and the procedures involved in obtaining accurate readings, thus gaining the skills necessary to assist in a medical emergency.

RELATED TERMS

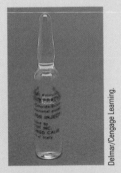

FIGURE 5–1. Ampule.

Delmar/Cengage Learning.

allergic reaction – An allergic reaction is a systemic reaction to an allergen introduced into the body; symptoms can appear mild to severe and can cause great distress and in rare instances even death. Allergic reactions can occur from food, drugs, insect bites, inhalants, and direct contact.

ampule – An ampule is a sealed container of small stature, usually made of glass, that holds a single dose of medication *(see Figure 5–1)*.

arterial system – The arterial system functions to distribute oxygenated blood from the heart to the body's organ systems via vessels of various size. The oxygenated blood moves from the largest vessels (closest to the heart), referred to as *arteries*, to smaller vessels, known as *arterioles*, to the smallest vessels (and furthest from the heart) of the arterial system, the *capillaries (see Figure 5–2)*.

cathartic or laxative – A cathartic or laxative is a solution/substance taken to cleanse the large bowel. Certain radiographic procedures require the large bowel to be to be empty (no fecal material) to optimize the imaging of anatomical structures required of the radiographic procedure. The most common types of laxative recommended for radiographic procedures of the large bowel are saline laxatives (magnesium citrate and magnesium sulfate); irritant laxatives (castor oil) are rarely used today.

central venous catheter – A central venous catheter is a tube inserted into a patient's circulatory system to provide an open line for continuous access during an extended period of time for the purpose of drug administration/ therapy, dialysis, blood transfusion, blood drawings, parenteral nutrition, and monitoring heart function/pressures. Types of central venous catheters include:

■ **CV (central venous) lines** – A *CV line* is a catheter inserted into a vein located within the neck, upper arm, or groin and positioned into the superior vena cava for short-term use in drug administration/therapy, blood drawings, blood transfusions, and monitoring heart function/pressures. The *Groshong*, *Hickman*, and *Raaf* are tunneled CV lines, requiring two incisions to allow the catheter to travel under the skin (tunnel) to the desired vein, allowing the

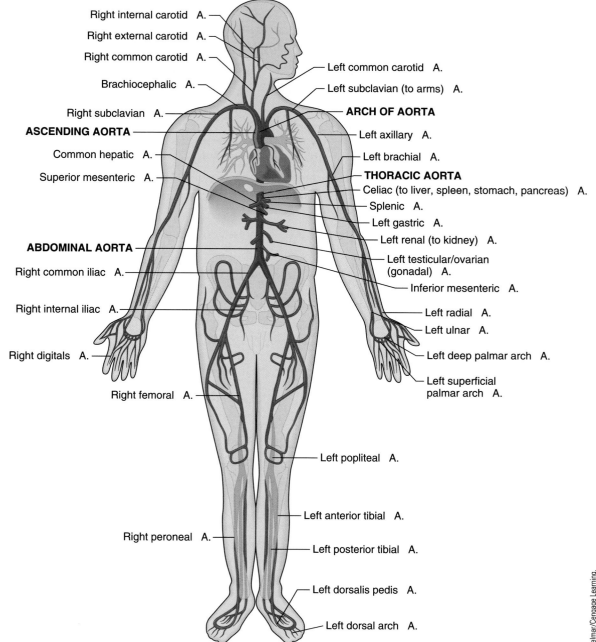

Right internal carotid A.
Right external carotid A.
Right common carotid A.
Left common carotid A.
Brachiocephalic A.
Left subclavian (to arms) A.
Right subclavian A.
ARCH OF AORTA
ASCENDING AORTA
Left axillary A.
Common hepatic A.
Left brachial A.
Superior mesenteric A.
THORACIC AORTA
Celiac (to liver, spleen, stomach, pancreas) A.
Splenic A.
Left gastric A.
Left renal (to kidney) A.
ABDOMINAL AORTA
Left testicular/ovarian (gonadal) A.
Right common iliac A.
Inferior mesenteric A.
Right internal iliac A.
Left radial A.
Left ulnar A.
Right digitals A.
Left deep palmar arch A.
Left superficial palmar arch A.
Right femoral A.
Left popliteal A.
Left anterior tibial A.
Right peroneal A.
Left posterior tibial A.
Left dorsalis pedis A.
Left dorsal arch A.

Delmar/Cengage Learning.

FIGURE 5–2. Diagram of arterial distribution.

external ends of the catheter to be accessible on the surface of the skin midway between the axilla and the sternum (*see Figure 5–3*).

- **Groshong** – The *Groshong* catheter has a single or double lumen and is inserted under the skin of the chest wall skin and tunneled to a specific vein (usually the subclavian vein), where it is advanced into the superior vena cava for long-term use in drug administration and blood drawings.

- **Hickman** – The *Hickman* catheter has a single lumen and is inserted under the skin of the chest wall skin and tunneled to a specific vein (usually the subclavian vein), where it is advanced into the superior vena cava for long-term use in providing drug administration/therapy and parenteral nutrition.

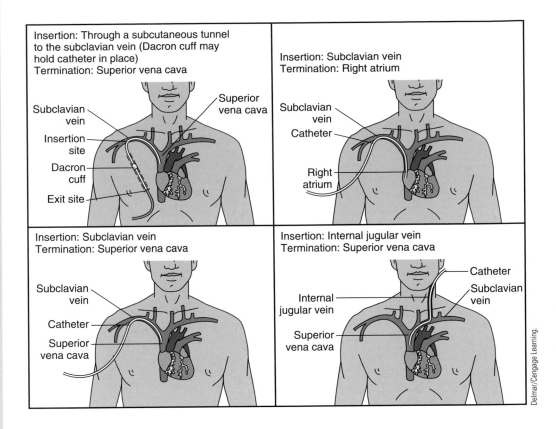

FIGURE 5–3. CV catheters.

- **PICC Line (peripherally inserted central catheter)** – A PICC line is a small catheter inserted into a vein located within the anterior part of the elbow and advanced into the superior vena cava for short-term use in drug administration/therapy and blood drawings.

- **Port-a-Cath** – A *Port-a-Cath* or venous access port is an infusion port implanted under the skin of the upper arm or chest designed for long-term use in drug administration, blood transfusions, and/or blood drawings from the superior vena cava. Other names of venous access ports include the *Infusa-Port* and *Mediport*.

- **Raaf** – The *Raaf* catheter has a large double lumen and is inserted under the skin of the chest wall and tunneled to a specific vein (usually the subclavian vein), where it is advanced into the superior vena cava for long-term use in providing dialysis.

- **Swan-Ganz catheter** – The *Swan-Ganz* catheter may have one lumen or several lumens. This catheter contains a small electrode at the distal end along with a balloon tip to secure the catheter's position (balloon inflation). Once the tip is advanced from the subclavian vein, internal vein, external vein, or femoral vein into the right atrium of the heart, cardiac function/pressures can be monitored.

contrast contraindications – Contrast contraindications are indicators that a contrast agent should not be used on a patient because of the likelihood that an adverse reaction or negative outcome would manifest (*see Table 5–1*).

TABLE 5–1   Contraindications for Contrast Media

CONTRAINDICATIONS FOR BARIUM CONTRAST MEDIA	CONTRAINDICATIONS FOR IODINATED CONTRAST MEDIA
Presurgical patients	Hypersensitivity to iodinated contrast, severe allergies (e.g., shellfish or nut allergy)
Suspected perforation (organ, intestines)	Diabetes, hepatic disease, renal disease, renal failure, anuria (absence of urine)
Suspected large bowel obstruction	Congestive heart failure, sickle-cell anemia
	Pheochromocytoma (adrenal gland tumor), multiple myeloma (malignant condition of bone marrow)
	Patient on glucophage. An examination can still be performed; however, glucophage should be withheld for 48 hours before the contrast procedure and for 48 hours after the contrast procedure.

Data from Bontrager, K. L. (2010). *Radiographic positioning and related anatomy* (7th ed.). St. Louis, MO: Mosby Elsevier; Greathouse, J. S. (2006). *Radiographic positioning & procedures: A comprehensive approach.* Clifton Park, NY: Delmar Cengage Learning; and Ballinger, P. W., & Frank, E. D. (2003) *Merrill's atlas of radiographic positions and radiologic procedures* (10th ed.). St. Louis, MO: Mosby Elsevier.

contrast media – A contrast media or contrast agent is a substance that, when introduced into the human body, will either increase tissue/organ density (higher atomic number) or decrease tissue/organ density (lower atomic number). Contrast agents are used in imaging procedures to enhance visualization of anatomic structures. There are two main types of contrast media: positive contrast agents (radio-opaque) and negative contrast agents (radiolucent).

■ **negative contrast/radiolucent** – A negative contrast agent, or radiolucent contrast agent, has a lower atomic number than the tissue to which it will be introduced. A negative contrast agent is used to create a noticeable difference in similar tissue by decreasing the tissue/organ density. Examples of negative contrast agents include air, oxygen (O_2), carbon dioxide (CO_2), and nitrous oxide.

■ **positive contrast/radio-opaque** – A positive contrast agent or radio-opaque contrast agent has a higher atomic number than the tissue to which it is introduced. A positive contrast agent is used to create a noticeable difference in similar tissue by increasing the tissue/organ density. Examples of positive contrast agents include barium sulfide ($BaSO_4$) and iodinated (water-soluble and fat soluble) contrast agents. Barium sulfate is the contrast agent of choice for studies of the digestive system (alimentary canal-pharynx, esophagus, stomach, small intestines, large intestines, rectum, and anus), whereas iodinated contrast media (ionic and nonionic contrast agents) are primarily used for radiographic examinations of the urinary system (kidney function, ureters, bladder, and urethra).

• **fat-soluble iodinated contrast media** – Nonwater-soluble contrast agents are oil-based iodine contrast agents made from fatty acids that do not dissolve in water and are not easily absorbed by the body.

- **ionic contrast media** – Ionic contrast agents contain a complex molecular arrangement of iodine and other compounds, resulting in a contrast agent with high osmolality. Although ionic contrast agents are more cost efficient than nonionic contrast media, the likelihood of adverse reactions is greater.

- **nonionic contrast media** – Nonionic contrast agents are two to three times greater in cost than ionic contrast agents, and although they still contain an iodine compound, the molecular arrangement produces a low-osmolality contrast agent with less adverse reactions.

- **water-soluble iodinated contrast media** – Water-soluble iodinated contrast agents contain the element iodine with an atomic number of 53, which serves as a good radio-opaque material for contrast studies in which an increase in tissue/organ density is desired. Water-soluble iodinated contrasts agents easily dissolve in water, are less viscous than fat-soluble iodinated contrast agents, are used more frequently than fat-soluble contrast agents, are easily absorbed, and leave no residual evidence in the body.

contrast reactions – Contrast reactions are adverse reactions patients experience upon the administration of a contrast agent. Contrast reactions can range from mild to severe, and in rare instances cause shock and even death. Health care professionals who administer drugs or assist with drug administration are required to be trained to recognize symptoms of adverse reactions and respond appropriately to the patient's needs.

- **mild reactions** – Mild reactions to a contrast agent include anxiety, urticaria (hives), itching, swelling (eyelids, lips, and face), sweating, sneezing, coughing, flushing, dizziness, shaking, chills, nausea, vomiting, pallor (loss of skin color, pale), and experiencing a metallic taste in the mouth. These symptoms usually begin to dissipate within minutes of the contrast injection. If, however, these symptoms increase in intensity or frequency, they should be considered moderate or severe adverse reactions and warrant immediate medical attention.

- **moderate reactions** – Moderate reactions to a contrast agent include bradycardia (slow heart rate), tachycardia (rapid heart rate), asthmatic symptoms, dyspnea (difficulty breathing), wheezing, broncospasms, swelling of the tongue, laryngeal edema, hypotension (decrease in blood pressure), hypertension (increase in blood pressure), and progression of intensity and/or frequency of mild reactions. Moderate reactions warrant immediate medical attention.

- **severe reactions** – Severe reactions to a contrast agent include a progression of mild or moderate reactions, extreme hypotension (dramatic decrease in blood pressure) unconsciousness, cyanosis (turning blue), convulsions, shock, arrhythmia (irregular heart beat), acute renal failure, respiratory arrest, and cardiopulmonary arrest (heart ceases beating). Severe reactions warrant immediate medical attention.

crash cart – A crash cart, also known as an emergency response cart, is a mobile cart that houses drugs, equipment, and supplies that may be needed in a medical emergency. Crash carts must be easily accessible to medical care personnel in the event a patient experiences an emergency medical crisis (*see Figure 5–4*).

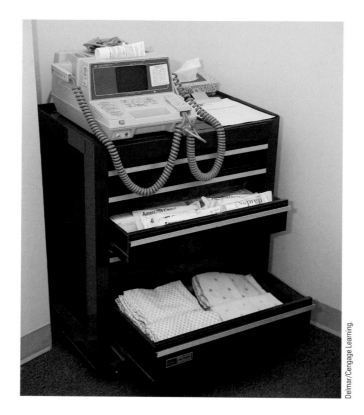

Delmar/Cengage Learning.

FIGURE 5–4. Crash cart with defibrillator.

BOX 5–1 Crash Cart Items

IV tubing

Disposable gloves *(recommended latex-free)*

Face masks

Disposable needles

Disposable syringes

Tourniquet

Hypoallergenic tape

Gauze pads

Cotton balls

Alcohol wipes

CPR equipment *(defibrillator and monitor)*

Portable oxygen with O_2 masks and cannulas

Ambu bags *(adult and pediatric)*

Emergency drugs

Suction equipment and tubing

Blood pressure apparatus

Tongue blades

ET tubes

Injectable saline

Data from Adler, A. M., & Carlton, R. R. (2007). *Introduction to radiologic sciences and patient care* (4th ed.). St. Louis, MO: Saunders Elsevier; and Ehrlich, R. A., McCloskey, E. D., and Daly, J. A. (2004). *Patient care in radiography* (6th ed.). St. Louis, MO: Mosby Elsevier.

defibrillator – A defibrillator is a medical device used in a medical emergency in which an individual's heart ceases to beat. The defibrillator induces an electrical shock, prompting the heart to resume a normal rhythm *(see Figure 5-4)*.

diuretic – A diuretic is a substance that causes the body to increase urine excretion.

drip infusion – A drip infusion, or intravenous (IV) infusion, is a slow distribution of a solution into a patient's vein via IV tubing and needle insertion. An infusion pump is often utilized to provide consistent distribution of a specified quantity of solution over a determined period of time.

drug – A drug is a chemical substance that has a biological effect on the body. Drugs may be classified as legal or illegal. This text will only address legal drugs approved by the United States Food and Drug Administration (FDA) and those used within the medical profession for the purpose of diagnosing, preventing, or treating illness and disease. There are three drug classifications or drug names: the *chemical name*, the *generic name*, and the *trade name (see Table 5-2)*.

- **chemical name** – The chemical name of a drug is derived from its molecular arrangement and is seldom used because of its complexity.

- **generic name** – The generic name of a drug is similar to the chemical name without the molecular arrangement included. As mandated by the FDA, generic drugs must be bioequivalent to their trade name counterpart. Generic drugs are typically less expensive than the trade name drug.

- **trade name** – The trade name (also referred to as brand name or proprietary name) of a drug is a name given by the manufacturer.

endotracheal tube – An endotracheal (ET) tube can be used for various respiratory conditions. The purpose of the ET tube is to provide oxygen to the lungs when normal respiratory function is hindered. The ET tube is typically inserted through the mouth or nose, advanced through the trachea, and positioned slightly superior (vertebral level T4-T5) to the carina, the point at which the trachea bifurcates into the right and left primary bronchi. ET tube placement requires a chest radiograph to confirm proper placement. This procedure is often performed in an emergency situation and is commonly referred to as an *intubation*.

extravasation – Extravasation or infiltration is a condition in which a drug, contrast agent, or IV solution is mistakenly injected into the surrounding tissues of a vein (as opposed to directly into the vein) or when a solution leaks out of the vein into the surrounding tissues. This condition can cause severe pain at the injection site and requires immediate medical attention to reduce the chance of a hematoma developing. If extravasation occurs, the technologist should immediately remove the injection needle and apply light pressure and warm compresses to the puncture site.

TABLE 5–2 Example of One Drug's Three Classifications

CHEMICAL NAME	GENERIC NAME	TRADE NAME
N-(4-hydroxyphenyl) acetamide	Acetaminophen	Tylenol

Data from: http://www.merck.com (2010)

"Five rights" of drug administration – The "five rights" of drug administration are five safety rules for RTs to follow in ensuring patient safety when administering a drug *(see Table 5–3).*

TABLE 5–3   **"Five Rights" of Drug Administration**

RULE	ACTIONS
Right patient	Ensure the "right" patient by checking three patient identifiers: ■ patient's identification arm band or bracelet ■ patient's medical record number (MR #) ■ patient's date of birth (DOB)
Right drug	Ensure the "right" drug for administration: ■ Check the label on the container 3 times • when removing from shelf • when removed from container • immediately prior to administering ■ Check expiration date ■ Prepare drug administration independently
Right amount	Ensure the "right" amount of the drug for administration: ■ form of drug (tablet, liquid, powder, etc.) ■ correct dosage (unit of measurement)
Right route	Ensure the "right" route of drug administration: • oral • parenteral • sublingual • topical
Right time	Ensure the "right" time for drug administration*:

Abbreviation	Meaning
a.c.	Before a meal
p.c.	After a meal
o.m.	Each morning
o.n.	Each night
q.d.	Every day
b.i.d.	Two times a day
t.i.d.	Three times a day
q.i.d.	Four times a day
p.r.n	When needed

*The abbreviations listed are common times for drug administration but do not reflect all possible times for drug administration.

Data from Adler, A. M., & Carlton, R. R. (2007) *Introduction to radiologic sciences and patient care* (4th ed). St, Louis, MO: Saunders Elsevier; and Venes, D. (ed). (2011). *Taber's cylclopedic medical dictionary* (21st ed). Philadelphia, PA: F. A. Davis.

flush, flushing – A flush or flushing is a cleansing process for peripheral intermittent IV catheters. A flush solution (typically heparin and/or saline) is injected through the IV line to remove any residual drugs and to discourage blood coagulation forming in the line or at the infusion site. The flush keeps the established venous line accessible and clear for subsequent drug administration.

Foley catheter – A Foley catheter is a retention catheter (stays securely in place via an inflated balloon) inserted through the urethra and into the bladder for the purpose of urine drainage. Urine collects in the drainage bag, which is to be positioned below the level of the bladder to avoid back flow of urine into the bladder, potentially causing a urinary tract infection. The drainage bag is emptied at scheduled intervals, and urine output is often charted for assessing kidney function *(see Figure 5-5)*.

glucagon – Glucagon is a hormone secreted by the pancreas, causing an increase in blood glucose levels.

glucophage – Glucophage is a common medication taken by patients for the treatment of noninsulin-dependent diabetes mellitus. It is important for RTs to ask patients scheduled for a contrast study involving iodinated contrast media if they are taking the drug glucophage; the combination of this drug and iodinated contrast could cause renal failure. Imaging departments may vary their protocol regarding patients taking glucophage; however, the common safety precaution routine is to instruct patients to discontinue the use of glucophage 48 hours before the scheduled iodinated contrast procedure and wait 48 hours after the procedure before resuming glucophage use.

human tissue – The human body is composed of different types of tissue, each having a different atomic number and therefore having a varying degree of radiation absorption. It is this variation of radiation absorption that permits a noticeable distinction between tissue types on a radiographic image. Contrast agents are used to enhance visual differences within an organ system of similar tissues, making anatomic structures more detectable on a radiographic image *(see Table 5-4 and Table 5-5)*.

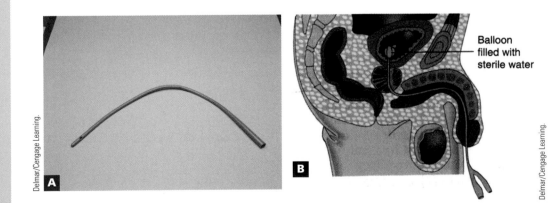

Balloon filled with sterile water

FIGURE 5–5. Urinary catheters. *A.* Straight catheter. *B.* Foley catheter.

Delmar/Cengage Learning.

TABLE 5–4   Human Tissues and Effective Atomic Number

HUMAN TISSUE	ATOMIC NUMBER (Z#)
Lung	7.4
Fat, muscle, and organs	Range of 6 to13
Bone	13.8
■ calcium	20

Note: The greater the atomic number of a tissue (bone), the more radiation absorption, resulting in a structure that will appear light on a visible image. The lower the atomic number of a tissue (lung), the less radiation absorption, resulting in a structure that will appear dark on a visible image.

Data from IUPAC–*Periodic Table of the Elements*; Adler, A. M., & Carlton, R. R. (2007). *Introduction to radiologic sciences and patient care* (4th ed.). St, Louis, MO: Saunders Elsevier; and Bushong, S. C. (2008). *Radiologic science for technologists; physics, biology, and protection* (9th ed.). St. Louis, MO: Mosby.

TABLE 5–5   Contrast Media and Related Atomic Number

CONTRAST MEDIUM	ATOMIC NUMBER (Z#)
Oxygen (negative contrast)	8
Iodine (positive contrast)	53
Barium (positive contrast)	56

Data from IUPAC–*Periodic Table of the Elements*; Adler, A. M., & Carlton, R. R. (2007). *Introduction to radiologic sciences and patient care* (4th ed.). St, Louis, MO: Saunders Elsevier; and Bushong, S. C. (2008). *Radiologic science for technologists; physics, biology, and protection* (9th ed.). St. Louis, MO: Mosby.

hypodermic needle – A hypodermic needle is a disposable needle with a beveled edge and a hollow lumen to allow fluid to flow through it; it is used for extracting bodily fluid or for drug administration. Hypodermic needles come in various lengths and gauge sizes. Needle gauges include a large diameter lumen such as a 7-gauge to a small 33-gauge lumen. The typical needle gauge range used with radiologic procedures is 16–25 gauge *(see Figure 5–6)*.

■ **needle types** – Various needles commonly used for radiologic procedures include:

- **butterfly needle** – The butterfly needle has two flaps or wings to securely hold the needle in place and maintain an open venous line during the radiologic procedure.

- **over-the-needle catheter** – The over-the-needle catheter allows for an open venous line to be maintained during the radiologic procedure in the event that drug administration is required.

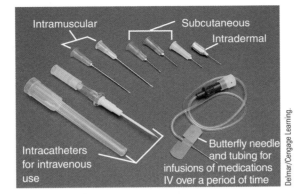

FIGURE 5–6. Hypodermic needles: butterfly needle; over-the-needle catheter; and straight-through the needle.

- **straight-through the needle** – The straight-through the needle allows for easy drug administration but is not used for maintaining an open venous line during radiologic procedures.

infiltrate – See *extravasation*.

informed consent – An informed consent is a document provided by a health care facility to a patient in which the procedure or treatment being considered is explained and any associated risks are disclosed. Invasive procedures require an informed consent be signed by the patient (or legal guardian in the case of a minor) in order for the procedure/treatment to legally be performed. *(Refer to Appendix F – Consent Form.)*

inject/injection – An injection refers to a solution introduced to the body via a hypodermic needle and disposable syringe.

- **bolus injection** – A bolus injection is an injection of a specified amount of solution drawn into a disposable syringe and dispersed into the patient's body at one time. Bolus injections are common for the administration of contrast agents into veins.

- **intrathecal injection** – An intrathecal injection is an injection of a solution directly into the subarachnoid space of the spinal canal, as required in myelography of the cervical, thoracic, and lumbar spine. The most common puncture site for a cervical myelogram is C1-C2, whereas the most common puncture site for the lumbar myelogram is L3-L4. Thoracic myelography is not commonly performed.

- **intravascular injection** – An intravascular injection is an injection of a solution into the vascular system, which is composed of both arterial and venous blood vessels.

IV push – An IV push is a bolus IV injection of a solution given rapidly at one time.

miscibility – Miscibility refers to how well two or more liquids blend together. Miscibility regarding contrast media refers to how well a contrast agent mixes with fluids of the body.

nasoenteric tube – A nasoenteric tube *(NE tube)* is a tube placed through the nose and positioned into the stomach where peristalsis advances the tube into the small intestines. NE tubes are used for drainage or decompression, in which gas and fluid are removed from the small intestines, or for radiographic imaging purposes in which a contrast medium is introduced into the small intestines. Common types of NE tubes include the single lumen *Cantor tube* and *Harris tube* and the double lumen *Miller-Abbott tube (see Figure 5–7)*.

nasogastric tube – A nasogastric tube *(NG tube)* is a tube placed through the nose and positioned into the stomach for the purpose of providing nutrients (feeding) to the patient or for drainage and/or decompression in which gas and fluid are removed from the stomach. NG tubes are also used for radiographic imaging purposes in which a contrast medium is introduced directly into the stomach. Common types of NG tubes include the *Dobbhoff feeding tube*, the single lumen *Levin tube*, and the double lumen *Salem-Sump tube (see Figure 5–7)*.

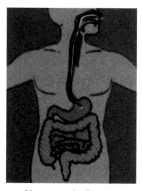

Nasogastric Route

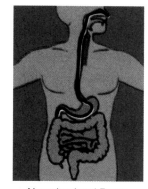

Nasoduodenal Route

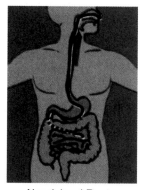

Nasojejunal Route

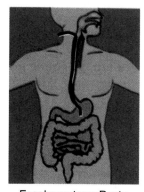

Esophagostomy Route

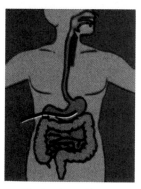

Gastrostomy Route

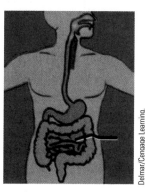

Jejunostomy Route

Delmar/Cengage Learning.

FIGURE 5–7. Various enteral feeding routes.

osmolarity – The concentration or number of particles (solute) within a specific solvent. The ratio of solute (particles) to solvent (water) per kilogram of solvent is referred to as osmolarity. Osmolarity affects the osmosis process in which water molecules move across a semipermeable membrane from an area of low solute particle concentration to an area of high solute particle concentration to create balance. This movement helps the body to maintain homeostasis.

■ **high osmolarity** – High osmolarity refers to a solution that contains a high concentration of solute particles and a low concentration of solvent molecules.

■ **low osmolarity** – Low osmolarity refers to a solution that contains a low concentration of solute particles and a high concentration of solvent molecules.

osmosis – Osmosis is the process of water moving across a semipermeable membrane (e.g., cell membrane) from an area of greater concentration to an area of lower concentration *(see Figure 5–8).*

oxygen administration – Oxygen (O_2) administration must be prescribed by a physician. Oxygen can be administered to a patient in several ways and is categorized by the amount (liters per minute [LPM] or concentration percentages) of oxygen distribution required (low-flow delivery systems, high-flow delivery systems, and enclosure delivery systems). Low-flow oxygen systems typically involve the use of a nasal cannula, transtracheal catheter, or oxygen mask. High-flow systems include the use of an air-entrainment mask or an air-entrainment nebulizer. Enclosure delivery systems are generally used for pediatric patients and include the oxygen tent (for children) and the oxyhood (for infants).

patient history – Obtaining a good patient history is essential to establishing a foundation for providing appropriate patient care. A good patient history begins with an interview process initiated by the health care provider to determine the patient's chief complaint and/or multiple complaints contributing to their lack of wellness. For radiographic procedures involving the use of contrast media, probing questions relevant to current medications the patient is taking, known allergies, and the possibility of experiencing an adverse reaction to contrast agents must be explored. This information will be entered into the patient's medical chart and relayed to the radiologist. On the basis of the information provided to the radiologist, a decision to continue or discontinue with the radiologic contrast examination will be determined. *(Refer to Chapter 3: Medical and Legal Terms, Patient History; the "Sacred Seven.")*

pharmaceutical – Pharmaceutical refers to the manufacturing, distribution, and sales of drugs approved by the FDA for medical purposes.

Initial stage

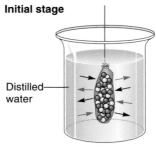

Distilled water

(A) Initially, the sausage casing contains a solution of gelatin, salt, and sucrose. The casing is permeable to water and salt molecules only. Because the concentration of water molecules is greater outside the casing, water molecules will diffuse into the casing. The opposite situation exists for the salt.

● Gelatin   ○ Salt   ● Sucrose

10-12 hours later

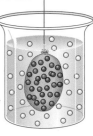

(B) The sausage casing swells due to the net movement of water molecules inward. However, the volume of distilled water in the beaker remains constant.

FIGURE 5–8. Osmosis.

prescription – A prescription (often referred to as a *script*) is a written physician order for a pharmacy to provide a prescribed medication to a patient. Dosage instructions and possible side effects of the medication are provided to the patient along with the medication.

radiolucent – Radiolucent describes a material that easily allows x-ray photons to transmit through it with little or no x-ray absorption. Radiolucent objects or negative contrast agents do not absorb x-ray photons. Therefore, the result is a decrease in tissue/organ density and an increase in radiographic density (darkness) on the visible image.

radio-opaque – Radio-opaque describes a material that does not allow x-ray photons to transmit through it, due to x-ray absorption. Radio-opaque objects or positive contrast agents absorb x-ray photons. Therefore, the result is an increase in tissue/organ density and a decrease in radiographic density (whiteness) on the visible image.

routes of drug administration – There are several routes for drug administration to the body. These routes include the oral route, the parenteral route, the sublingual route, and the topical route *(see Table 5–6 and Figure 5–9).*

syringe – A syringe is a plastic disposable container used for drug administration and for aspirating fluids and gases from the body. Although syringes vary in size and shape, they share three common features: a *plunger*, a *barrel*, and a *tip (see Figure 5–10).*

- **barrel** – The barrel houses the drug to be dispersed and shows units of measure on the outside for determining precise dosage.

- **plunger** – The plunger is a sliding piece of plastic that moves backward and forward within the barrel to remove air and permit suction.

- **tip** – The tip attaches to the needle or to IV tubing.

tourniquet – A tourniquet is an elastic band that is applied to an extremity to control blood flow. A tourniquet is often used for venipuncture procedures to dilate the veins, making them more pronounced; this helps to access the vein easily when performing IV injections.

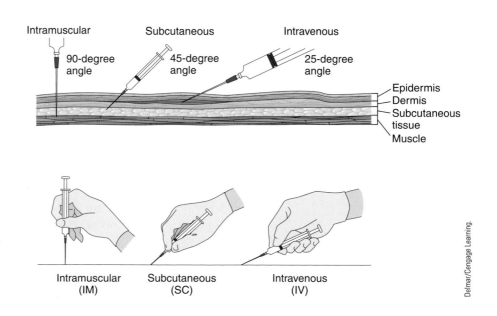

FIGURE 5–9. Needle placement for injections (angles).

Delmar/Cengage Learning.

TABLE 5–6 Routes of Drug Administration

TYPE OF ROUTE	DEFINITION OF DRUG ADMINISTRATION ROUTE
Oral route	Drug administered by mouth and digested
Parenteral route	A route involving an injection or a route excluding the alimentary canal. The four most common parenteral routes are: ■ **intramuscular injection** – Injection into the muscle at a 90° angle ■ **intrathecal injection** – Injection into the subarachnoid space of the spinal canal; for cervical puncture, C1-C2; for lumbar puncture, L3-L4 ■ **intravenous injection** – Injection into the vein at an approximate 25° angle ■ **subcutaneous injection** – Injection below the skin at a 45° angle
Sublingual route	Drug administered under the tongue and dissolved
Topical route	Drug administered on top of the skin and absorbed

Data from Adler, A. M., & Carlton, R. R. (2007). *Introduction to radiologic sciences and patient care* (4th ed.). St. Louis, MO: Saunders Elsevier; and Bontrager, K. L. (2010). *Radiographic positioning and related anatomy* (7th ed.). St. Louis, MO: Mosby Elsevier.

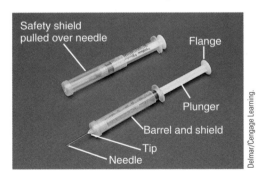

FIGURE 5–10. A syringe with all three components labeled (plunger, barrel, and tip).

vasoconstrictor – A vasoconstrictor is a drug that causes the body's blood vessels to constrict and become narrow, hindering blood flow and causing an increase in blood pressure. Common vasoconstrictors include epinephrine, antihistamines, and decongestants. Epinephrine is the drug most commonly given to patients experiencing anaphylactic shock in a medical emergency.

vasodilator – A vasodilator is a drug that causes the body's blood vessels to dilate and become larger, permitting greater blood flow and causing a decrease in blood pressure. Common types of vasodilators include angiotensin-converting enzyme inhibitors, alpha-blockers, and nitrates. Nitroglycerin is a common nitrate vasodilator prescribed to patients with angina pectoris (chest pain caused by a narrowing of the coronary arteries) to lessen the workload on the heart and allow oxygenated blood to flow with ease to the heart.

venipuncture – Venipuncture is the process of accessing a vein for the purpose of drug administration or for the purpose of withdrawing blood. *(Refer to Appendix G – Venipuncture Protocol.)*

venous system – The venous system functions to return deoxygenated blood to the heart via vessels of various sizes. The deoxygenated blood moves from the smallest vessels (furthest from the heart), referred to as *venous capillaries*, to larger vessels, known as *venules*, to the largest vessels (closest to the heart) of the venous system, the *veins*. *(See Figure 5–11; Refer to Chapter 15: Cardiovascular System.)*

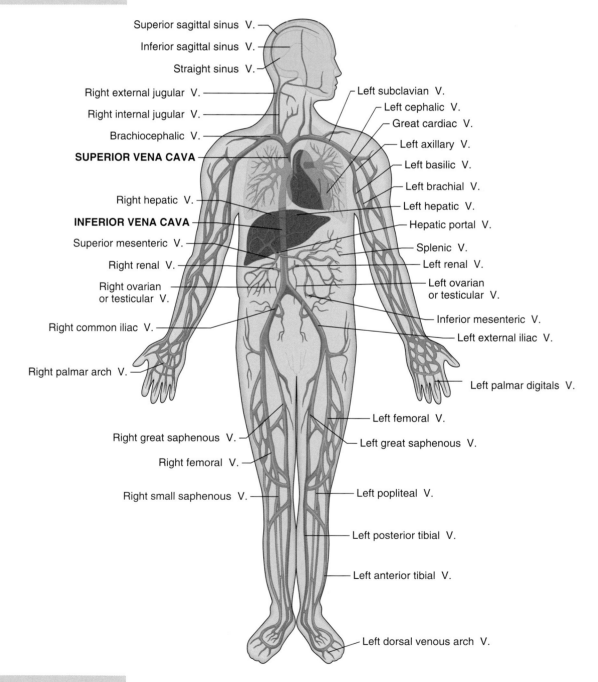

Superior sagittal sinus V.
Inferior sagittal sinus V.
Straight sinus V.
Right external jugular V.
Right internal jugular V.
Brachiocephalic V.
SUPERIOR VENA CAVA
Right hepatic V.
INFERIOR VENA CAVA
Superior mesenteric V.
Right renal V.
Right ovarian or testicular V.
Right common iliac V.
Right palmar arch V.
Right great saphenous V.
Right femoral V.
Right small saphenous V.

Left subclavian V.
Left cephalic V.
Great cardiac V.
Left axillary V.
Left basilic V.
Left brachial V.
Left hepatic V.
Hepatic portal V.
Splenic V.
Left renal V.
Left ovarian or testicular V.
Inferior mesenteric V.
Left external iliac V.
Left palmar digitals V.
Left femoral V.
Left great saphenous V.
Left popliteal V.
Left posterior tibial V.
Left anterior tibial V.
Left dorsal venous arch V.

FIGURE 5–11. Venous distribution.

Delmar/Cengage Learning

vial – A vial is a sealed container, usually made of glass, that holds more than one dose of a medication.

viscosity – Viscosity refers to the amount of resistance a solution encounters in its ability to flow. Solutions of low viscosity flow easily with little required force or pressure, whereas solutions of high viscosity are slow to flow and require increased force or pressure. High-viscosity solutions such as iodinated contrast agents should be warmed to body temperature to reduce viscosity and lessen the force required for administering the IV injection.

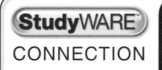

StudyWARE™ CONNECTION

After completing this chapter, complete the Spelling Bee or play another interactive game on your StudyWARE CD-ROM that will help you learn the content in this chapter.

CONCEPT THINKING QUESTIONS

1. What are the *"five rights"* regarding drug administration?

2. Differentiate between ionic and nonionic contrast media.

3. Define an IV push.

4. Identify two mild adverse reactions to contrast media.

5. Identify two severe adverse reactions to contrast media.

6. Name the three parts of a disposable syringe.

7. List the four common routes for drug administration.

8. What is the difference between an ampule and a vial?

9. Differentiate between low–viscosity and high–viscosity solutions.

10. What purpose does a tourniquet serve?

PRACTICE EXERCISES

1. Identify at least 10 items that are commonly found on a crash cart.

2. Provide examples of good patient history questions posed to a patient who is scheduled for a radiographic procedure involving contrast media.

3. Discuss the importance of obtaining a signed informed consent regarding invasive radiographic procedures.

4. Write the steps in sequential order for performing *venipuncture*.

5. Differentiate between positive and negative contrast agents and explain how they appear radiographically with regard to density.

6. Differentiate between an IV injection and an intrathecal injection.

7. Identify the three classifications of drugs.

8. Explain the correlation between the atomic number of human tissue and its ability to absorb radiation.

9. Explain the relationship between "tissue density" and "radiographic density."

10. Discuss the impact nitroglycerin has on the vessels of heart.

11. Differentiate between a vasodilator and a vasoconstrictor.

12. Describe osmolarity and the role it plays regarding ionic and nonionic contrast media.

MATCHING

Match each term to the appropriate description.

barium sulfate	air	viscosity
cannula	radiolucent	air-entrainment nebulizer
sacred seven	epinephrine	radio-opaque material
sublingual	mask	intrathecal
osmosis	LPM	Levin tube
Groshong	Harris tube	nitroglycerin

Description	Term
1. high-flow O_2 delivery system	_____
2. under the tongue	_____
3. NG tube	_____
4. a positive contrast agent	_____
5. CV catheter	_____
6. vasodilator	_____
7. a negative contrast agent	_____
8. NE tube	_____
9. vasoconstrictor	_____
10. patient history	_____
11. resistance to flow	_____
12. absorption of photons	_____

RETENTION OF MATERIAL

Retention requires practicing the use of previously learned material. Apply the knowledge you have regarding pharmacology and contrast media to answer the following questions.

1. Who should sign a consent form and why?

2. Identify the four types of parenteral routes:

   _____

   _____

   _____

   _____

3. Discuss the ways in which oxygen can be administered to a pediatric patient and to an adult patient.

4. What steps should be taken by the RT if *extravasation* occurs during an IV drug administration?

5. Explain how radiolucent and radio-opaque materials will appear on a radiographic image with regard to density.

6. Discuss the usage for *negative* contrast agents and radiographic procedures in which they may be used.

7. Explain how *osmolarity* affects the process of osmosis.

8. Identify three common types of NE tubes.

9. Identify three common types of NG tubes.

10. Identify three contraindications for performing a radiographic procedure in which barium is required.

11. Discuss how the atomic number of human tissue and of contrast agents influences a radiographic image.

12. Differentiate between the following central venous catheters/lines:

    A PICC line

    B Groshong catheter

    C Swan-Ganz catheter

    D Infusion port *(Port-a-Cath)*

II

Equipment Operation and Quality Control

CHAPTER 6

Physics Terminology

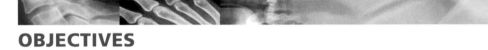

OBJECTIVES

Upon completion of this chapter, the reader will be able to:

- Identify the three subatomic particles of an atom and their associated electrical charge
- Describe various types of energy common to the imaging profession
- Describe the four nuclear arrangements in terms of similarities and differences
- Identify five types of matter interactions along with their respective energy level
- Discuss ionizing and nonionizing types of radiation
- Differentiate between bremsstrahlung and characteristic interactions
- List standardized units of measurement regarding ionizing radiation
- Explain the three requirements necessary to produce x-ray photons
- Discuss the properties or characteristics of x-ray photons

CONCEPT THINKING

Physics terminology is based on the understanding that terms are not isolated bits of information but are rather like puzzle pieces that, once connected, demonstrate a complete picture of the way that something works. To understand how x-ray production occurs, one must first have a thorough understanding of the atom and its components. Because the atom contains three subatomic particles with electrical charges, i.e., protons (+), neutrons (no charge), and electrons (−), we can see how having an equal number of protons and electrons would result in a stable or neutral atom, i.e., possessing no electrical charge. However, once an atom's stable environment is altered through ionization (either the gain or loss of an electron), several reactions can occur that can cause a modification of matter. It is through the process of ionization that x-ray production is possible. Remember, for x-ray production to occur, three requirements must be met: a source, a force, and a target. Through the process of thermionic emission, i.e., *boiling off of electrons at the cathode filament due to high current supplied by the step-down transformer*, a space charge *(cloud of electrons)* is created at the filament. The emitted electrons originating from the tungsten atoms of the cathode filament become the source for x-ray production; once acted upon by the kilovoltage (kVp), an electromotive force will initiate the acceleration of electrons from cathode to anode *(a distance of approximately 1–2 cm)* at nearly half the speed of light. The tremendous force at which these electrons impact the anode target causes the electron's kinetic energy to be converted to approximately 99% heat and 1% x-ray photons. Keep in mind, the x-ray photons are a direct result of both bremsstrahlung and characteristic interactions. It is this 1% of converted x-ray photons to which we attribute image production.

RELATED TERMS

absorption – Absorption is the total consumption of an x-ray photon *(energy)* by the matter with which it interacts.

acceleration – Acceleration is the change in velocity of an object in motion within a specified timeframe.

amplitude – Amplitude refers to one-half the range of height from valley to crest of a sinusoidal (or sine) wave *(see Figure 6–1)*.

angstrom (Å) – An angstrom is the unit to measure wavelength of radiant energy. (1 Å = 10^{-10} meters)

anode – *Refer to Chapter 8: X-ray Tube.*

atom – An atom is the smallest portion of matter, or the smallest portion of an element containing three fundamental particles: protons, neutrons, and electrons *(see Figure 6–2)*.

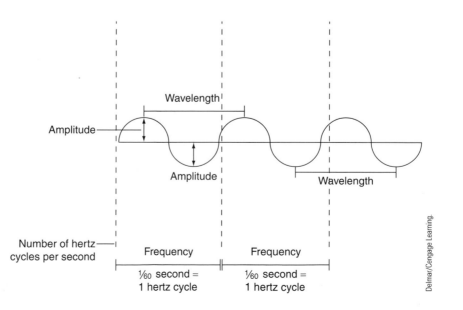

FIGURE 6–1. Sinusoidal wave form.

Delmar/Cengage Learning.

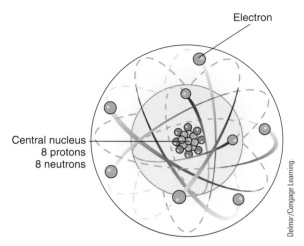

FIGURE 6–2. Bohr's atomic model.

atomic mass number, "A" number – The atomic mass number (A#) indicates the number of protons and neutrons *(nucleons)* found within an atom *(see Figure 6–3).*

atomic mass unit (amu) – An atomic mass unit (amu) is a definitive unit to measure the mass of subatomic particles *(protons, neutrons, electrons)* found within an atom. 1 amu = $1.66053886 \times 10^{-27}$ kilograms, or 1/12 of a carbon 12 atom, which is known to have six protons and six neutrons in its nucleus.

atomic number, "Z" number – The atomic number (Z#) indicates the number of protons found within the nucleus of an atom *(see Figure 6–3).*

attenuation – Attenuation is the partial absorption of x-ray photons as they travel through matter, resulting in a decrease of intensity of the exiting x-ray beam.

Bohr's atomic model – Physicist Neils Bohr, born October 7, 1885, in Copenhagen, Denmark, designed a model of an atom in 1913 resembling a solar system with a nucleus in the center and electrons in orbital shells revolving around the nucleus. This model, commonly referred to as "Bohr's atomic model," is perhaps the most frequently used scientific model depicting components that comprise an atom *(see Figure 6–2).*

cathode – *Refer to Chapter 8: X-ray Tube.*

current – Current is produced when electrons are in motion. Units to measure current are the ampere (A) or milliampere (mA).

■ **alternating current (AC)** – Current that changes direction from positive to negative during a complete hertz (Hz) cycle is referred to as alternating current or AC current *(see Figure 6–4A).*

■ **direct current (DC)** – Current moving in only one direction is referred to as direct current or DC current; the current has been rectified to ensure only a positive hertz (Hz) cycle *(see Figure 6–4B).*

diagnostic x-ray range – This term can be used to indicate the diagnostic range for exposure techniques, which would include ranges for kVp, mA, and time. However,

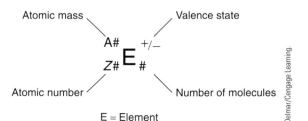

FIGURE 6–3. Element with superscript and subscript symbols identifying the A#, or number of protons and neutrons, the Z#, or number of protons, the valence state, and the number of molecules.

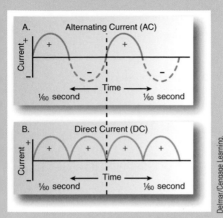

FIGURE 6–4. *A.* Alternating current (AC). *B.* Direct current (DC).

because this chapter pertains to physic concepts, only the approximate range of energy values associated with diagnostic x-ray procedures will be mentioned. Exposure technique used in diagnostic radiography will be discussed in *Chapter 10 - Image Production.*

■ **range of kVp values** – 25 kVp – 150 kVp

electrification – Electrification occurs when an object (matter) becomes electrically charged as the result of the atom gaining or losing electrons (matter with no electric charge is the result of an equal number of protons and electrons in the atom; this type of atom is considered to be stable or balanced). Electrification can occur by way of:

■ *contact* between two objects;

■ *friction*, the rubbing of two objects together to cause a concentration of electrons; or

■ *induction*, the transference of an electrical charge from a charged object with an electrical field to an uncharged object with no electrical field.

electrodynamics – Electrodynamics is the study of electrical charges (electrons) in motion, better known as current or electricity.

electromagnetic spectrum – The electromagnetic spectrum is a chart or graph depicting the three main types of electromagnetic radiation (radiofrequency, visible light, and x-radiation) and their subcomponents according to their range of energy, frequency, and wavelength *(see Figure 6–5).*

electron – An electron is a negatively charged particle positioned in an orbital shell that revolves around the nucleus of an atom *(see Figure 6–2).*

electrostatics – Electrostatics is the study of electrical charges that are stationary (not in motion). Matter, which is composed of atoms, consists of protons (subatomic particles that have a positive [+] charge) and electrons (subatomic particles that have a negative [–] charge) in a stationary form. However, when an atom gains an electron, or loses an electron, the matter becomes electrically charged, or electrified.

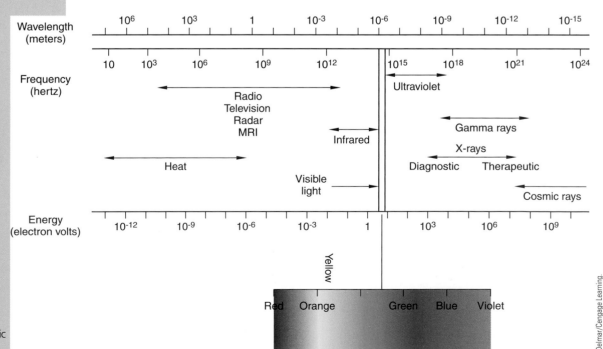

FIGURE 6–5. Electromagnetic spectrum.

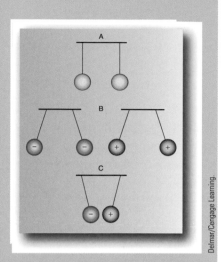

FIGURE 6–6. Laws of electrostatics. *A.* Neutral charge. *B.* Like charges repel each other (+ + and − −). *C.* One positive charge (+) and one negative (−) charge attracted to each other.

■ **laws of electrostatics** – The laws of electrostatics are the basic principles depicting the behavior of stationary charges. The four laws of electrostatics are as follows:

1. Like charges repel each other, and unlike charges attract each other *(see Figure 6–6).*

    (+) (+) repel each other

    (+) (−) attract each other

2. The electrostatic force existing between two electrical charges is directly proportional to the product of the quantity of charge present, and inversely proportional to the square of the distance between the two electrical charges. This phenomenon, known as *Coulomb's law,* is named after 18th-century French physicist Charles-Augustin de Coulomb. Coulomb discovered that creating distance between two electrical charges greatly affected the electrostatic force between the two electrical charges. Coulomb's law is mathematically depicted as:

    $$F = k \frac{Q_A \times Q_B}{d^2}$$

    where F = electrostatic force; k = constant of proportionality; Q_A and Q_B = two separate electrostatic charges; and d^2 = distance between electrostatic charges squared.

3. Only negative (−) electrical charges (electrons) flow through a conductor. Negative (−) electrical charges are located on the conductor's external surface and are concentrated in areas of curvature.

4. Electrical charges are uniformly distributed along the surface of conductors and uniformly distributed throughout nonconductors.

element – An element is a substance made up of identical atoms with the same number of protons (Z#). Currently, there are 117 known elements, which are arranged on the periodic table of elements according to their increasing Z# (atomic number) and the way in which they demonstrate similar chemical behavior *(see Figure 6–7).*

energy – Energy can be described as the ability to do work. The unit to measure energy is the joule (J). The electron volt (eV) is the unit used to represent various energies depicted within the electromagnetic spectrum. The eV is also the unit used to indicate the binding energy of electrons located in different orbital shells within an atom.

■ **law of conservation of energy** – Energy cannot be created or destroyed but can be transformed from one form to another. Various types of energy common to the imaging profession are:

● binding energy – Binding energy refers to the strength of energy associated with the electrons of orbital shells and their proximity to the nucleus. Electrons positioned close to the nucleus as in the K shell possess a higher binding energy and are more tightly bound to the nucleus than are electrons located in orbital shells further away from the nucleus, such as in the M or N shell *(see Figure 6–8).*

● chemical energy – Energy resulting from chemical reactions between bonds of atoms and molecules is known as chemical energy.

Delmar/Cengage Learning.

IUPAC Periodic Table of the Elements

Key:

atomic number
Symbol
name
standard atomic weight

Z	Symbol	Name	Standard atomic weight
1	H	hydrogen	1.007 94(7)
2	He	helium	4.002 602(2)
3	Li	lithium	6.941(2)
4	Be	beryllium	9.012 182(3)
5	B	boron	10.811(7)
6	C	carbon	12.0107(8)
7	N	nitrogen	14.0067(2)
8	O	oxygen	15.9994(3)
9	F	fluorine	18.998 4032(5)
10	Ne	neon	20.1797(6)
11	Na	sodium	22.989 769 28(2)
12	Mg	magnesium	24.3050(6)
13	Al	aluminium	26.981 538 6(8)
14	Si	silicon	28.0855(3)
15	P	phosphorus	30.973 762(2)
16	S	sulfur	32.065(5)
17	Cl	chlorine	35.453(2)
18	Ar	argon	39.948(1)
19	K	potassium	39.0983(1)
20	Ca	calcium	40.078(4)
21	Sc	scandium	44.955 912(6)
22	Ti	titanium	47.867(1)
23	V	vanadium	50.9415(1)
24	Cr	chromium	
25	Mn	manganese	54.938 045(5)
26	Fe	iron	55.845(2)
27	Co	cobalt	58.933 195(5)
28	Ni	nickel	58.6934(2)
29	Cu	copper	63.546
30	Zn	zinc	(3)65.409(4)
31	Ga	gallium	69.723(1)
32	Ge	germanium	72.64(1)
33	As	arsenic	74.921 60(2)
34	Se	selenium	78.96(3)
35	Br	bromine	79.904(1)
36	Kr	krypton	83.798(2)
37	Rb	rubidium	85.4678(3)
38	Sr	strontium	87.62(1)
39	Y	yttrium	88.905 85(2)
40	Zr	zirconium	91.224(2)
41	Nb	niobium	92.906 38(2)
42	Mo	molybdenum	95.94(2)
43	Tc	technetium	[98]
44	Ru	ruthenium	101.07(2)
45	Rh	rhodium	102.905 50(2)
46	Pd	palladium	106.42(1)
47	Ag	silver	107.8682(2)
48	Cd	cadmium	112.411(8)
49	In	indium	114.818(3)
50	Sn	tin	118.710(7)
51	Sb	antimony	121.760(1)
52	Te	tellurium	127.60(3)
53	I	iodine	126.904 47(3)
54	Xe	xenon	131.293(6)
55	Cs	caesium	132.905 451 9(2)
56	Ba	barium	137.327(7)
57–71		lanthanoids	
72	Hf	hafnium	178.49(2)
73	Ta	tantalum	180.947 88(2)
74	W	tungsten	183.84(1)
75	Re	rhenium	186.207(1)
76	Os	osmium	190.23(3)
77	Ir	iridium	192.217(3)
78	Pt	platinum	195.084(9)
79	Au	gold	196.966 569(4)
80	Hg	mercury	200.59(2)
81	Tl	thallium	204.3833(2)
82	Pb	lead	207.2(1)
83	Bi	bismuth	208.980 40(1)
84	Po	polonium	[209]
85	At	astatine	[210]
86	Rn	radon	[222]
87	Fr	francium	[223]
88	Ra	radium	[226]
89–103		actinoids	
104	Rf	rutherfordium	[261]
105	Db	dubnium	[262]
106	Sg	seaborgium	[266]
107	Bh	bohrium	[264]
108	Hs	hassium	[277]
109	Mt	meitnerium	[268]
110	Ds	darmstadtium	[271]
111	Rg	roentgenium	[272]

Lanthanoids

Z	Symbol	Name	Standard atomic weight
57	La	lanthanum	138.905 47(7)
58	Ce	cerium	140.116(1)
59	Pr	praseodymium	140.907 65(2)
60	Nd	neodymium	144.242(3)
61	Pm	promethium	[145]
62	Sm	samarium	150.36(2)
63	Eu	europium	151.964(1)
64	Gd	gadolinium	157.25(3)
65	Tb	terbium	158.925 35(2)
66	Dy	dysprosium	162.500(1)
67	Ho	holmium	164.930 32(2)
68	Er	erbium	167.259(3)
69	Tm	thulium	168.934 21(2)
70	Yb	ytterbium	173.04(3)
71	Lu	lutetium	174.967(1)

Actinoids

Z	Symbol	Name	Standard atomic weight
89	Ac	actinium	[227]
90	Th	thorium	232.038 06(2)
91	Pa	protactinium	231.035 88(2)
92	U	uranium	238.028 91(3)
93	Np	neptunium	[237]
94	Pu	plutonium	[244]
95	Am	americium	[243]
96	Cm	curium	[247]
97	Bk	berkelium	[247]
98	Cf	californium	[251]
99	Es	einsteinium	[252]
100	Fm	fermium	[257]
101	Md	mendelevium	[258]
102	No	nobelium	[259]
103	Lr	lawrencium	[262]

Notes

- 'Aluminum' and 'cesium' are commonly used alternative spellings for 'aluminium' and 'caesium'.
- IUPAC 2005 standard atomic weights (mean relative atomic masses) are listed with uncertainties in the last figure in parentheses [M. E. Wieser, *Pure Appl. Chem.* **78**, 2051 (2006)]. These values correspond to current best knowledge of the elements in natural terrestrial sources. For elements that have no stable or long-lived nuclides, the mass number of the nuclide with the longest confirmed half-life is listed between square brackets.
- Elements with atomic numbers 112 and above have been reported but not fully authenticated.

FIGURE 6–7. Periodic table of the elements.

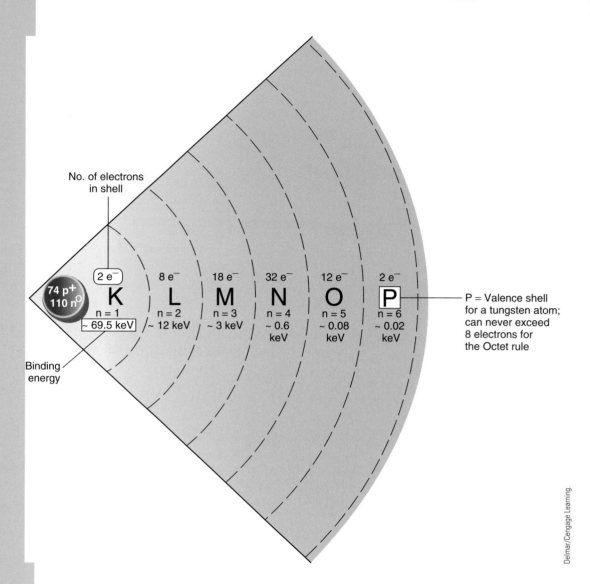

No. of electrons in shell

74 p+
110 n⁰

2 e⁻

K
n = 1
~ 69.5 keV

8 e⁻
L
n = 2
~ 12 keV

18 e⁻
M
n = 3
~ 3 keV

32 e⁻
N
n = 4
~ 0.6 keV

12 e⁻
O
n = 5
~ 0.08 keV

2 e⁻
P
n = 6
~ 0.02 keV

P = Valence shell
for a tungsten atom;
can never exceed
8 electrons for
the Octet rule

Binding energy

Delmar/Cengage Learning.

FIGURE 6–8. Atom with orbital shells (K, L, M, N, O, P) indicate binding energies, Octet rule, and valence shell with no more than eight electrons.

- electrical energy – Energy resulting from electrons in motion *(current)* is known as electrical energy.

- electromagnetic energy – Electromagnetic energy refers to the energy of photons within the *electromagnetic spectrum*. These energies possess both electrical and magnetic fields and are ranked according to their energy level (lowest to highest): *radio waves, microwaves, infrared light, visible light, ultraviolet light, x-rays, and gamma rays (see Figure 6–5).*

- mechanical energy – Energy resulting from physical exertion by a human or by a machine is known as mechanical energy; there are two types of mechanical energy:

  - kinetic energy – Kinetic energy is energy in motion.
    $KE = \frac{1}{2} (mass \times velocity)^2$

  - potential energy – Potential energy is energy that has the potential to be in motion, but is not actually in motion.

- nuclear energy – Nuclear energy is energy resulting from the nucleus of an atom being split apart; better known as *nuclear fission.*

- thermal energy – Thermal energy is energy resulting from atoms and molecules moving rapidly and generating heat.

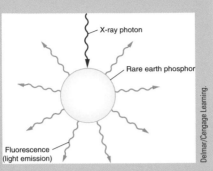

FIGURE 6–9. Fluorescence.

fluorescence – Fluorescence refers to light emitted by a phosphor when struck by x-ray photons *(see Figure 6–9)*.

frequency – Frequency, represented by the lower case letter *(f)*, refers to the number of sine-wave peaks (crests) or the number of sine-wave valleys (troughs) observed within a specified timeframe. The unit to measure frequency is the hertz (Hz) *(see Figure 6–1)*.

fundamental particles – A fundamental particle is a subcomponent of the atom. The three fundamental particles or subatomic particles found within an atom are protons, neutrons, and electrons *(see Figure 6–2)*.

half-life – Half-life refers to the length of time it would take for a radioactive material *(radioisotope)* to decay to half of its original quantity.

hertz – The frequency of a sine-wave is measured in the unit hertz (Hz). The Hz depicts the up and down movement (one complete peak and one complete valley), better known as one complete cycle. 1 Hz is equivalent to 1 cycle occurring within a 1 second timeframe.

incident electron – An incident electron or incoming electron is one that has been ejected from an atom and travels on a projected path with the capacity for interaction with matter *(see Figure 6–10)*.

ion – An ion is an unstable atom or molecule possessing an electrical charge, either (+) or (−). A stable atom has no electrical charge; it is considered to be neutral because it contains the same number of protons as it does electrons. However, when an atom loses an electron and becomes unstable, it takes on a positive (+) charge because of the fact that the atom contains more protons (+) than it does electrons (−). This charged particle is called a *"cation"* or positive ion. The same principle holds true if an atom gains an electron; causing the atom to contain more electrons than protons results in the atom having a negative (−) charge, which is referred to as an *"anion"* or negative ion *(see Figure 6–11)*.

ionization – Ionization is the addition or subtraction of electrons from an atom attributable to impingement of either electrons or x-ray photons *(see Figure 6–11)*.

ionizing radiation – Ionizing radiation is radiation that is capable of ionizing matter. This type of radiation has the potential to cause biological harm. Some forms of ionizing radiation have a greater linear energy transfer (LET) than others and therefore can be more damaging to biological tissue. There are two main types of ionizing radiation: *electromagnetic radiation* and *particulate radiation*.

■ **electromagnetic radiation** – Electromagnetic radiation possesses both electrical and magnetic fields, travels at the speed of light, and is capable

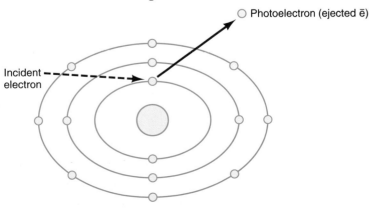

FIGURE 6–10. Incident electron interaction with matter.

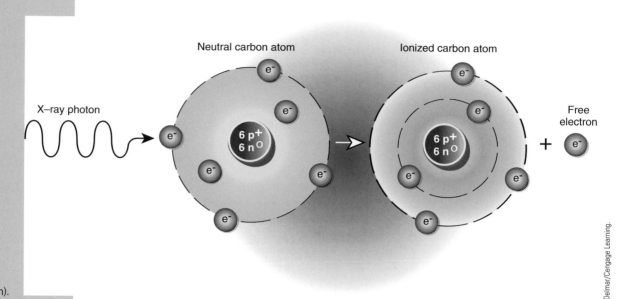

Delmar/Cengage Learning.

FIGURE 6–11. Ionization (knocking out an electron).

of ionizing matter. However, this type of radiation is considered to be less ionizing than *particulate radiation (see Figures 6–5 and 6–12).*

- **gamma rays** – Gamma rays originate from the nucleus of an atom and are considered to have a low LET and a low relative biological effect (RBE; *see Figure 6–13*).

- **x-rays** – X-rays originate outside the nucleus of an atom, either by the ejection of an electron from its orbital shell and the subsequent filling of the vacancy by electrons from outer orbit shells or by the slowing down (braking) of an electron and the altered path of deviation it takes as it encounters the positive force from the atom's nucleus. X-rays are also considered to have a low LET and a low RBE. X-rays are a human-made type of radiation and do not occur naturally in the universe; therefore, they should be examined separately and in greater detail under the categories of *human-made radiation* and *x-ray properties (see Figure 6–13).*

■ **particulate radiation** – Particulate radiation is associated with radioactive decay or spontaneous disintegration. As a radioactive atom attempts to become stable, the nucleus will emit photons and particles such as alpha and beta particles. This type of particulate radiation is considered to be highly ionizing and is therefore considered to have a high LET and a high RBE.

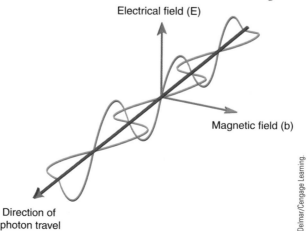

FIGURE 6–12. Photon traveling (sine-wave) electrical and magnetic fields.

Delmar/Cengage Learning.

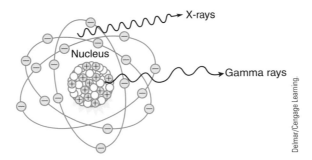

Delmar/Cengage Learning.

FIGURE 6–13. Gamma rays and x-rays.

- **alpha radiation** – Alpha radiation originates from heavy radioactive nuclei and is considered to be extremely ionizing, with low penetrating ability in matter.

- **beta radiation** – Beta radiation originates from radioactive nuclei and is less ionizing than alpha radiation with a higher penetrating ability in matter. However, beta radiation is still less penetrating in matter than x-rays or gamma rays.

StudyWARE™ CONNECTION

View the Ionizing Radiation animation on the StudyWARE™ CD-ROM to help build your understanding of this important concept.

isobar – An isobar is an atom that has the same A# (atomic mass number or number of nucleons) but a different Z# (atomic number or number of protons) and a different number of neutrons *(see Table 6–1).*

isomer – An isomer is an atom that has the same A# (atomic mass number), the same Z# (number of protons), and the same number of neutrons. These atoms appear identical with the exception of varying levels of energy *(see Table 6–1).*

isotone – An isotone is an atom that has the same number of neutrons, but a different A# (number of nucleons) and a different Z# (number of protons; *see Table 6–1).*

isotope – An isotope is an atom that has the same Z# (number of protons) but a different number of neutrons, causing a different A# (atomic mass number). Isotopes are the most common nuclear arrangement discussed in the field of radiology *(see Table 6–1).*

TABLE 6–1   Nuclear Arrangements

NUCLEAR ARRANGEMENT	ATOMIC NUMBER (Z#)	ATOMIC MASS NUMBER (A#)	NEUTRON NUMBER
Isobar	Different	Same	Different
Isomer	Same	Same	Same
Isotope	Same	Different	Different
Isotone	Different	Different	Same

From Bushong, S. C. (2008). *Radiologic science for technologists: Physics, biology, and protection* (9th ed.). St. Louis, MO: Elsevier. Copyright © Elsevier. Reprinted with permission.

isotropic – Isotropic refers to a uniform spreading in all directions from a single point of origin.

lambda (λ) – Lambda is the Greek letter representing a sinusoidal wavelength.

luminescence – Luminescence is the emission of light.

mass – Mass is the quantity of matter within an object.

matter – Matter is anything that has mass and occupies space.

matter interaction – The interaction of x-ray photons and matter is referred to as matter interaction; there are five different types of interactions between x-ray photons and matter:

- **coherent scattering, classical scattering, Rayleigh scattering, Thompson scattering, unmodified scattering** – This type of matter interaction is most commonly referred to as coherent scattering or classical scattering, although all five names are interchangeable. Coherent scattering is the result of a very low-energy incident photon (energy levels at or less than 10 keV), entering an atom and causing an electron to resonate or vibrate. This vibration is known as *excitation*. The energy passed on to the electron from the incident photon is not sufficient to remove it from its orbital shell. It is, however, enough energy for the electron to emit the energy in the form of a secondary photon possessing the same energy as the incident photon. The projected path of the secondary photon as it exits the atom is very different than the path of the incident photon; therefore, this photon is said to be a scattered photon. This type of matter interaction is typically not associated with diagnostic radiographic image formation due to insufficient energy values *(see Figure 6–14)*.

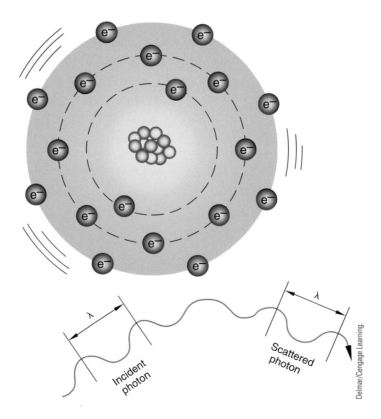

FIGURE 6–14. Coherent scattering interaction.

■ **Compton scattering** – This type of matter interaction is the result of a moderate-energy incident photon (energy levels in the moderate to high diagnostic x-ray range) knocking out an outer orbital shell electron, causing the atom to become ionized. The ejected electron, now known as a *recoil electron* or *Compton electron*, travels out of the atom with the ability to cause ionizing interactions with other atoms. The remaining kinetic energy from the incident photon resides with the deflected scattered photon, now known as a *Compton scattered photon.* However, it should be noted that the greater the angle of deflection *(angle of deflection can range from 0° to 180°)* between the Compton scattered photon and the recoil electron, the less kinetic energy is imparted to the Compton scattered photon and the more kinetic energy resides with the recoil electron. This type of matter interaction is associated with diagnostic x-rays due to the typical energy values necessary for radiographic image formation *(see Figure 6–15).*

■ **pair production** – This type of matter interaction is the result of a very high-energy incident photon (energy levels above 1.02 MeV) imparting all its energy to the nucleus of an atom. This transference of energy produces two particles, a *negatron* with a (–) electrical charge, and a *positron* with a (+) electrical charge. The negatron will exit the atom and continue on its projected path with the ability to cause ionizing interactions with other atoms. The positron will combine with an electron and undergo what is known as an *annihilation reaction* in which the two particles are annihilated, leaving in their place a pair of photons; each with an energy value of 0.51 MeV. These photons will move in opposite directions from one another. This type of matter interaction is not associated with diagnostic x-rays due to the high energy values used *(see Figure 6–16).*

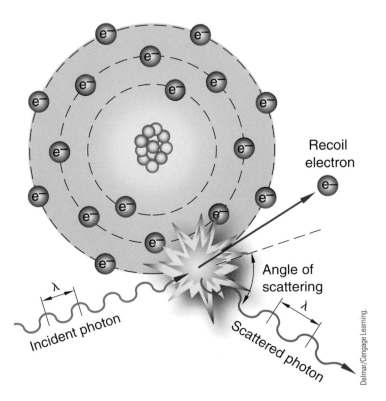

FIGURE 6–15. Compton scattering interaction.

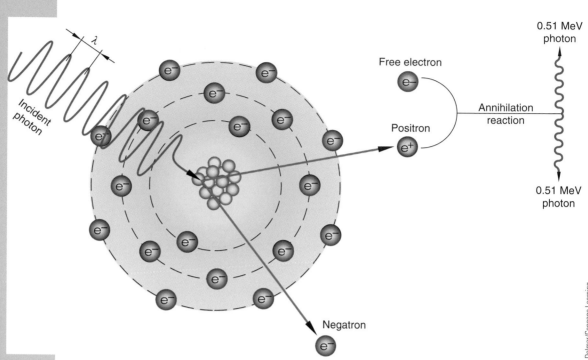

FIGURE 6–16. Pair production interaction.

Delmar/Cengage Learning.

■ **photodisintegration** – This type of matter interaction is the result of an extremely high-energy incident photon (energy levels greater than 10 MeV) imparting all its energy to the nucleus of an atom. This transference of energy excites the nucleus, causing it to eject a nucleon or nuclear fragment. This type of matter interaction is not associated with diagnostic x-rays because of the extremely high energy values used *(see Figure 6–17)*.

■ **photoelectric absorption** – This type of matter interaction is the result of a low-energy incident photon (energy levels in the lower diagnostic x-ray range) knocking out an inner orbital shell electron *(photoelectron)*. This interaction causes the atom to become ionized. The incident photon energy must be greater than the electron's binding energy for the electron to be

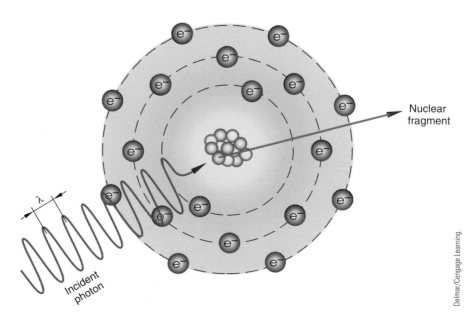

FIGURE 6–17. The photodisintegration interaction.

Delmar/Cengage Learning.

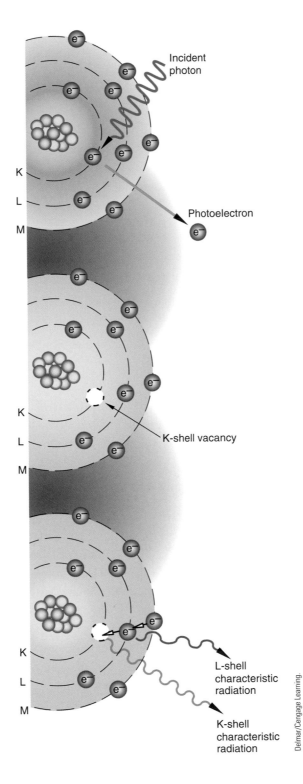

FIGURE 6–18. Photoelectric absorption interaction.

Delmar/Cengage Learning.

ejected from its orbital shell. This interaction will cause the incident photon to be completely absorbed, leaving a vacancy in the orbital shell where the ejected electron used to be. The atom will attempt to stabilize itself by having an outer shell electron fill the inner orbital shell vacancy. The process of outer shell electrons dropping into inner shell vacancies can occur several times as the atom attempts to stabilize itself. Each time a vacancy is filled, energy is released in the form of a low-energy photon *(see Figure 6–18).*

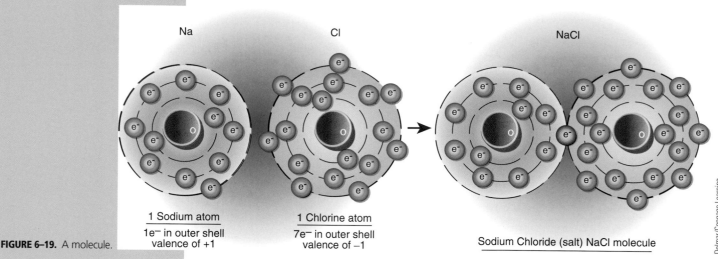

Na   Cl   NaCl

1 Sodium atom   1 Chlorine atom
1e⁻ in outer shell   7e⁻ in outer shell   Sodium Chloride (salt) NaCl molecule
valence of +1   valence of −1

FIGURE 6–19. A molecule.

Delmar/Cengage Learning.

molecule – A molecule is produced when two or more atoms of either the same element or of different elements combine *(see Figure 6–19)*.

neutron – A neutron is a fundamental particle or subatomic particle of an atom. The neutron is located within the nucleus of an atom and is considered electrically neutral; it has neither a positive (+) nor a negative (−) charge *(see Figure 6-2)*.

nonionizing radiation – Nonionizing radiation possesses insufficient energy to ionize an atom; examples include visible light, ultraviolet light, infrared light, microwave, radiofrequency, and extremely low-frequency radiation.

nucleons – Nucleon is the term used to refer to both protons and neutrons. Nucleons are located within the nucleus of an atom *(see Figure 6-2)*.

orbital shell – An orbital shell is best described as an elliptical or circular path rotating around the nucleus of an atom that contains a specified number of electrons *(see Figure 6-8)*.

■ **"K" shell** – The "K" shell is the orbital shell that is closest to the nucleus. Each consecutive orbital shell, moving further from the nucleus, is labeled "L" shell, "M" shell, "N" shell, and so on. Because of the close proximity of the "K" shell to the nucleus, any electrons found here will possess the highest binding energy and the lease potential energy *(see Figure 6-8)*.

■ **octet rule** – The octet rule states that no more than eight electrons can ever occupy the outermost orbital shell *(valence shell)* of an atom *(see Figure 6-8)*.

■ **valence shell** – The valence shell is the outermost orbital shell of an atom *(see Figure 6-8)*.

orbital shell formula – The orbital shell formula is a mathematical equation used to determine the maximum number of electrons that can occupy any orbital shell. $2n^2$ is the formula used to calculate the maximum number of electrons in any orbital shell. *(n)* represents the number of the orbital shell as determined by its proximity to the nucleus; starting with the K shell as the number one *(see Table 6-2)*.

photon – A photon is a small bundle of energy that has no mass and no electrical charge but possesses both an electrical and magnetic field moving in a sinusoidal manner *(sine-wave)* at the speed of light. There are different types of photons with varying energy values, which are noted on the electromagnetic spectrum *(see Figure 6-19)*.

TABLE 6–2 Orbital Shells with Corresponding Electrons

ORBITAL SHELL AND CORRESPONDING NUMBER	FORMULA AND MAXIMUM NUMBER OF ELECTRONS
K (1)	$2 \times n(1)^2 = \mathbf{2}$
L (2)	$2 \times n(2)^2 = \mathbf{8}$
M (3)	$2 \times n(3)^2 = \mathbf{18}$
N (4)	$2 \times n(4)^2 = \mathbf{32}$
O (5)	$2 \times n(5)^2 = \mathbf{50}$

From Bushong, S. C. (2008). *Radiologic science for technologists: Physics, biology, and protection* (9th ed.). St. Louis, MO: Elsevier. Copyright © Elsevier. Reprinted with permission.

Planck's constant – "Planck's constant" refers to the constant proportionality between photon energy and photon frequency; it is assigned a numerical value of 4.15×10^{-15} eV·s. The following mathematical equation depicts the direct relationship between photon energy and photon frequency, and the indirect relationship between photon energy and photon wavelength with the velocity remaining constant (*at the speed of light*).

■ **Planck's constant formula:** **E** (energy) = **h** (Planck's constant) × **f** (photon frequency)

- Energy represented in (eV) electron volts
- Planck's constant represented by 4.15×10^{-15} eV·s
- f represented in the unit hertz (Hz)

polyenergetic – Polyenergetic is a term describing many different energy values.

proton – A proton is a subatomic particle with a positive charge; it is located within the nucleus of an atom (*see Figure 6-2*).

quanta/quantum – A quantum is a photon or small bundle of energy traveling at the speed of light, which is 186,000 miles per second or 3×10^8 m/s (*meters per second*) or 3×10^{10} cm/s (*centimeters per second*).

quarks – Quarks are subnuclear components found in both protons and neutrons.

radiation (human-made), x-radiation, x-rays – Radiation that does not occur naturally within the universe is referred to as human-made radiation, artificial radiation, x-radiation, or x-rays. X-radiation is produced in an x-ray tube caused by *bremsstrahlung* or *characteristic interactions* and is typically referred to as *x-rays*. X-ray photons possess no mass or electric charge; they do, however, possess electrical and magnetic fields that run perpendicular to each other (i.e., at right angles to each other). These discrete bundles of energy travel at the speed of light in straight lines that diverge outward

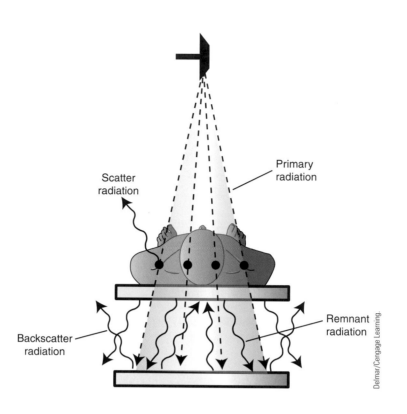

Scatter radiation

Primary radiation

Backscatter radiation

Remnant radiation

Delmar/Cengage Learning.

FIGURE 6–20. Primary radiation, remnant radiation, scatter radiation, and backscatter radiation.

isotropically from their point of origin *(target focal spot).* Both the electrical field and the magnetic field of an x-ray photon have sinusoidal movement, even though their respective wavelengths, frequencies, and amplitudes can vary greatly from one another. There are several terms that refer to human-made radiation (x-rays), which are often categorized by the behavior of the photons as they interact with matter; these are noted in the list to follow *(see Figure 6–20).*

◼ **backscatter radiation** – X-ray photons that have been directed back toward the point of origin are referred to as backscatter radiation. Backscatter can contribute to the patient's overall radiation dose as well as the technologist's occupational dose, if the technologist is present in the x-ray room during the procedure (i.e., fluoroscopy; *see Figure 6–20).*

◼ **extrafocal, off-focal, off-focus** – Radiation produced in areas of the target other than the focal spot are known as extrafocal, off-focal, or off-focus radiation *(see Figure 6–21).*

◼ **image forming radiation, exit radiation, remnant radiation** – Image forming radiation exits the patient and interacts with the image receptor. This type of radiation consists of both scatter x-rays and x-rays that transverse through the patient *(see Figure 6–20).*

◼ **primary radiation** – Radiation that is useful in forming a diagnostic image. This type of radiation is produced at the anode target, exits the x-ray tube window, and travels in a straight diverging path toward the patient *(see Figure 6–20).*

  • **bremsstrahlung radiation** – Approximately 80%–90% of the radiation produced at the anode target is attributable to bremsstrahlung

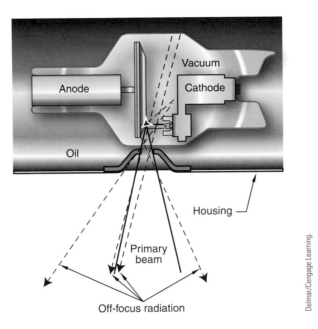

Delmar/Cengage Learning.

FIGURE 6–21. Off-focus radiation.

interactions. The high percentage of bremsstrahlung radiation is directly related to various energy values produced by the slowing down and deflection of the incident electrons. The kinetic energy (measured in keV) of bremsstrahlung radiation can range from zero to the kVp applied to the x-ray tube. Production of *"brems"* radiation occurs as the result of the strong attraction of the negative charge incident electron as it comes in contact with the positive force field of the tungsten atom nuclei (the positive force field is caused by the high number of protons *(Z # is 74)* within the nucleus of a tungsten atom). As the incident electron feels the "pulling" force from the nucleus, it slows and deviates from its straight-line path. It is at that moment the kinetic energy of the incident electron is converted to x-ray energy. This energy conversion results in the formation of an x-ray photon. The greater the deviation of the incident electron, the greater the kinetic energy of the x-ray photon produced. The various energy values produced through bremsstrahlung interactions (the braking or slowing of incident electrons) are the cause for a heterogeneous x-ray beam *(see Figure 6–22)*.

• **characteristic radiation** – Approximately 10%–20% of radiation produced at the anode target is caused by characteristic interactions. Characteristic radiation is produced at the anode target through the process of an incident electron *(produced by thermionic emission at the cathode filament)* knocking out an inner K shell electron from a tungsten atom of the target, at which point the vacancy is filled by an outer shell electron. The ejection and filling of a K shell electron is the only type of characteristic radiation important in diagnostic imaging; other characteristic radiation that may occur via the L or M shell is too low in energy to be of value in diagnostic imaging *(see Figure 6–23)*.

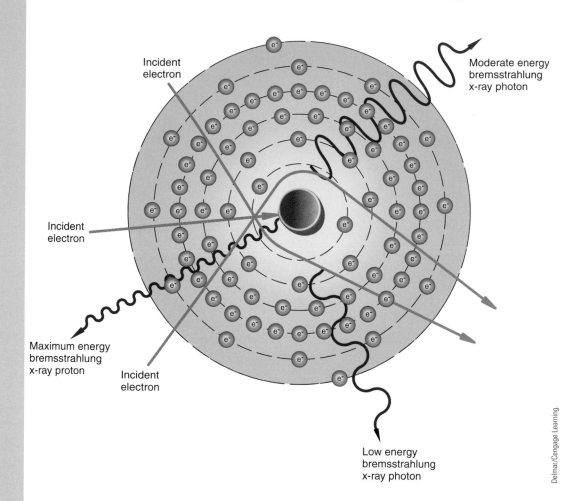

FIGURE 6–22. Bremsstrahlung interactions.

- **secondary radiation** – Radiation that is nonuseful in forming a diagnostic image is referred to as secondary radiation. The two types of secondary radiation are:

  - **leakage radiation** – *Leakage radiation* is radiation that exits through the protective metal tube housing. Leakage radiation cannot exceed 100 mR/hr at 1 meter from the source *(see Figure 6–24)*.

  - **scatter radiation** – Scatter radiation consists of x-ray photons that have deviated from their straight-line path of origin *(see Figure 6–20)*. Known facts of scatter radiation include:

    - The deviation of a photon from its original straight-line path causes a loss of energy (the exception is coherent scatter radiation).

    - Most scatter radiation occurs in the patient.

    - Scatter hinders visibility of recorded detail on the image by depositing unwanted densities on the image, often referred to as "fog."

    - Scatter can be best be reduced by lowering kVp, using a grid, and increasing collimation.

    - Scatter radiation contributes to the overall quantity of photons reaching the image receptor. Therefore, when attempting to reduce

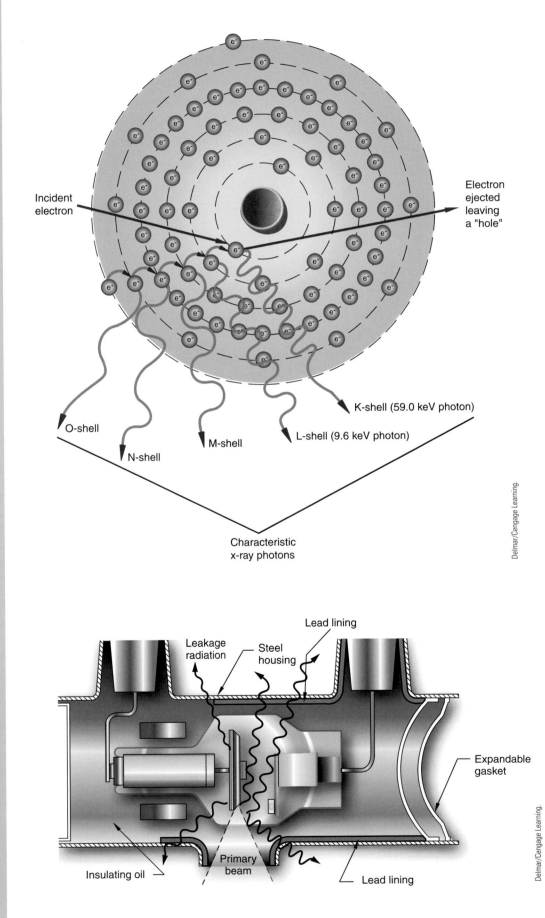

FIGURE 6–23. Characteristic interactions.

Incident electron

Electron ejected leaving a "hole"

K-shell (59.0 keV photon)

L-shell (9.6 keV photon)

M-shell

N-shell

O-shell

Characteristic x-ray photons

Delmar/Cengage Learning.

Lead lining

Leakage radiation

Steel housing

Expandable gasket

Insulating oil

Primary beam

Lead lining

FIGURE 6–24. Leakage radiation.

Delmar/Cengage Learning.

scatter, the technologist must consider an adjustment in exposure technique to compensate for the reduction in the overall quantity of photons initially produced.

radiation (natural) – There are three common types of radiation that exist naturally:

- **cosmic** – Cosmic radiation is produced naturally by the sun and stars.
- **radionuclide** – A radionuclide is a type of radiation naturally produced within the human body.
- **terrestrial** – Terrestrial radiation is naturally produced within the earth.

radioactivity – An unstable atom will attempt to become stable by emitting energy from its nucleus in the form of alpha particles, beta particles, or gamma rays; these emissions are known as radioactivity.

- **becquerel (Bq)** – The Bq is the International System (SI) unit to measure radioactive material. 1 Bq = 1 dps (disintegration per second of radioactive material)
- **curie (Ci)** – The Ci is the traditional unit to measure radioactive material. 1 curie = 3.7×10^{10} becquerel

sinusoidal wave or sine-wave – A sinusoidal wave is a wave of electrical and magnetic fields moving up and down to depict a photon's amplitude, frequency, and wavelength as it travels at the speed of light *(see Figure 6–1).*

speed of light – Traveling at the speed of light equates to 186,000 miles per second in a vacuum or, as listed in the SI system, 3×108 m/s *(meters per second)* or 3×10^{10} cm/s *(centimeters per second).*

units of ionizing radiation – The International Commission on Radiologic Units (ICRU) provides standardized units of measurement regarding ionizing radiation; they are known as traditional units, as opposed to *SI units*, which are the units of measurement for ionizing radiation derived from the French Système international d'unités. Traditional units for measuring radiation are the *rad* (radiation absorbed dose), the *rem* (radiation equivalent in humans), and the *Roentgen* (radiation in air). Note that a millirad, millirem, or milliRoentgen is 1/1000 of the unit rad, rem, or Roentgen, and a milligray (mGy) or millisievert (mSv) is 1/1000 of the unit gray or sievert. SI units for measuring radiation are the *gray* (radiation absorbed dose), the *sievert* (radiation equivalent in humans), and the *Coulomb/kilogram* (radiation in the air) *(see Table 6–3).*

velocity – Velocity refers to the rate of speed at which an object travels, which is the distant traveled within a certain timeframe; v = d/t *(velocity is equal to distance divided by time).* For radiology purposes, velocity refers to the speed at which a photon travels, which is the speed of light represented by the lowercase letter *(c).*

- velocity (c) = frequency (f) $\times$ wavelength (λ)

    - c = 186,000 miles per second or 3×10^{8} m/s (meters per second) or 3×10^{10} cm/s (centimeters per second)

    - frequency of wavelengths (f) – measured in hertz

    - wavelength (λ) – (measured in angstrom (Å) or meter (m))

TABLE 6-3 Conversions of Traditional Radiation Units to SI Units

TRADITIONAL UNITS – RADIATION	SI UNITS – RADIATION
• Radiation absorbed dose (patient)	
1000 mrad = 1 rad =	0.01 gray (Gy)
100 rad =	1 gray (Gy)
• Radiation equivalent dose (occupational exposure)	
1000 mrem = 1 rem =	0.01 sievert (Sv)
100 rem =	1 sievert (Sv)
• Radiation exposure (in air)	
1000 mR = 1 Roentgen (R)	2.58×10^{-4} Coulomb/kilogram (C/kg)
TRADITIONAL UNIT – RADIOACTIVITY	**SI UNIT FOR RADIOACTIVITY**
1 curie (Ci) =	$3.7\ 10^{10}$ Becquerel (Bq)

Data from Carlton, R. R., & Adler, A. M. (2006). *Principles of radiographic imaging: An art and a science* (4th ed.). Clifton Park, NY: Delmar Cengage Learning.

---

wavelength – Represented by the Greek letter lambda (λ), wavelength is the distance between two consecutive peaks (crests) of a sine-wave or the distance between two consecutive valleys (troughs) of a sine-wave. The unit to measure wavelength is either the meter *(m)* or the angstrom (Å) *(see Figure 6–1).*

wave-particle duality – Wave-particle duality describes the dual characteristics of an x-ray photon. X-ray photons travel through space in a wave-like manner and have the ability to ionize matter. Therefore, they resemble both a wave by their motion through space and a particle by their impact on atoms.

weight – Weight is the force an object possesses because of the earth's gravitational pull. Wt = m × gravity *(weight of an object is equal to the object's mass multiplied by the gravitational force of the earth).* Gravitational force in SI units is noted as 9.8 m/s^2.

work – Work as it relates to physics can be defined as an applied force over a specified distance. Mathematically, *work* (W) is equal to an applied *force* (F) multiplied by the *distance* (d) in which the force is applied (W = F × d). The unit to measure work is the joule (J).

x-ray circuit, x-ray unit – The basic x-ray circuit or x-ray unit is composed of three main sections: an operating console, a high-voltage generator, and an x-ray tube. X-ray units generally operate with a supply voltage *(incoming line of voltage)* of 210–220 volts. *(Refer to Chapter 7: Circuitry.)*

x-ray production – Three requirements are necessary to produce x-ray photons:

1. A source of electrons (thermionic emission)
2. A force to drive electrons from cathode to anode (kilovoltage)
3. An object for accelerated electrons to hit (anode target)

x-ray properties – X-ray photons:

- are a type of **electromagnetic radiation**.
- are **invisible**.
- are **highly penetrating**.
- are **polyenergetic** (consisting of various energies).
- are capable of **ionizing** matter.
- travel at the **speed of light** (186,000 miles per second or 3×10^8 m/s *(meters per second)* or 3×10^{10} cm/s *(centimeters per second)* in a vacuum.
- travel in **straight diverging lines**.
- **cannot be focused** by a lens.
- **cause fluorescence** (emit light) of certain types of phosphor crystals:
  - calcium tungstate (older intensifying screens)
  - rare earth phosphors, e.g., gadolinium, lanthanum, and yttrium (modern intensifying screens)
  - cesium iodide (image intensifier tube's input phosphor)
  - zinc cadmium sulfide (image intensifier tube's output phosphor)
- affect **photographic film**.
- cause **biological changes**.
- have **no mass**.
- have **no electrical charge**.
- produce **secondary radiation**.

StudyWARE™
CONNECTION

After completing this chapter, complete the Spelling Bee activity or another interactive game on your StudyWARE™ CD-ROM that will help you learn the content of this chapter.

CONCEPT THINKING QUESTIONS

When you answer the following questions, ask yourself to think beyond the question and see what other physics aspects come to mind. These questions are designed to stimulate thought beyond a single answer. Challenge yourself to apply the knowledge you have gained through your course of study to all content categories within the book and self-assess frequently to see what content areas in which you are strong and what areas may need improvement.

1. What does wave-particle duality mean?

2. Where does the majority of scatter radiation originate?

3. Why are bremsstrahlung interactions more prominent at the anode target than characteristic interactions?

4. Where does electron to photon conversion occur?

5. Does the velocity of x-ray photons remain constant? If so, what is the velocity?

6. What is the relationship between a photon's frequency and its wavelength?

7. What is the relationship between a photon's frequency and its kinetic energy?

8. What are the three necessary requirements for x-ray production to occur?

9. If a stable atom loses an electron, the atom would be considered unstable and would have a _____ charge.

10. Isotopes are considered to be atoms that have the same number of _____ but a different number of _____.

PRACTICE EXERCISES

1. What does the superscript for the element $^{127}_{53}I$ indicate?

2. What does the subscript for the element $^{127}_{53}I$ indicate?

3. Using the $2n^2$ formula, calculate the maximum number of electrons that could occupy the M orbital shell of $^{138}_{56}Ba$.

4. The element $^{184}_{74}W$ is a stable atom; therefore, the atom should contain _____ electrons.

5. What is the difference between an atom's A# and Z#?

6. Write the subscript for an isotope of barium possessing six fewer neutrons than indicated in $^{138}_{56}Ba$.

7. A positive ion has more _____ than it does _____, which is the reason for its positive charge.

8. What two subatomic particles constitute nucleons?

   Answer: _____ and _____

9. Which orbital shell of Ba would contain electrons that possess the highest binding energy? *(Why?)*

10. Which orbital shell of W would contain electrons that possess the highest potential energy? *(Why?)*

MATCHING

Match each term to the appropriate description.

proton	A#	alpha particles
wavelength	electron	kinetic energy
motor	binding energy	cathode
scatter	heat	work
x-ray	neutron	hertz
quark	Z#	isotope

Description   **Term**

1. 99% of kinetic energy is converted to   _____

2. Subatomic particle with no
   electrical charge   _____

3. Force applied over distance   _____

4. Number of protons and neutrons   _____

5. Particular radiation; highly ionizing   _____

6. Unit to measure frequency   _____

7. Number of protons in an atom   _____

8. Radiation deviated from a straight path _____

9. Energy associated with orbital shells   _____

10. Negatively charged electrode   _____

11. Energy in motion   _____

12. Is inversely related to photon frequency _____

RETENTION OF MATERIAL

Retention requires practicing the use of previously learned material. Try writing or drawing symbols and/or pictures to assist you in remembering specific concepts.

1. What does a high-energy sinusoidal wave look like? Draw it out. *(Clue: Remember the electromagnetic spectrum and the relationships between frequency, wavelength, and photon energy.)*

2. What does a low-energy sinusoidal wave look like? Draw it out. *(Refer to the clue in question 1.)*

3. Label the following atom and list the associated electrical charges of each subatomic particle.

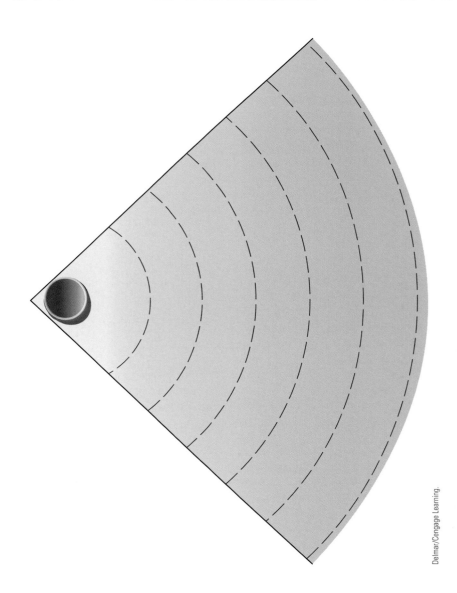

Delmar/Cengage Learning.

4. List five interactions with matter and identify the main two that directly contribute to forming the radiographic image.

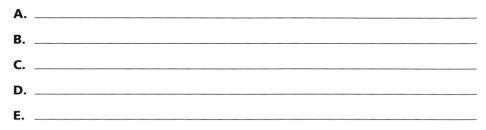

A. _____

B. _____

C. _____

D. _____

E. _____

5. See how many of the 14 properties of x-rays *(characteristic of x-ray photons)* you are able to remember.

    1. _____

    2. _____

    3. _____

    4. _____

    5. _____

    6. _____

    7. _____

    8. _____

    9. _____

  10. _____

  11. _____

  12. _____

  13. _____

  14. _____

CHAPTER 7

Circuitry

OBJECTIVES

Upon completion of this chapter, the reader will be able to:

- Identify common electric circuit symbols
- Differentiate between electrostatics and electrodynamics
- Discuss electromagnetism and its significance to the x-ray circuit
- Differentiate between a generator and a motor
- Explain the relationship between current, voltage, and resistance within the x-ray circuit
- Apply mathematical formulas for Ohm's law and transformer laws
- Identify various types of transformers
- Explain the function of the three primary components of a high-voltage generator
- Discuss voltage rectification and voltage ripple regarding high-voltage generators
- Identify basic x-ray circuit components and discuss their functions

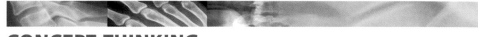

CONCEPT THINKING

When students begin to study x-ray circuitry, one of the first questions asked is "why do we need to know this—it's not as if we're going to be working on repairing x-ray machines." This is true; registered radiologic technologists do not repair x-ray units. However, they do select specific amounts of current and voltage to enable the production of x-ray photons. These photons will travel at the speed of light to interact with the patient and the image receptor, thus resulting in a radiographic image. The exposure technique selections made at the control console determine what takes place in the high-voltage generator and ultimately determines the *quantity* and *quality* of x-ray photons exiting the x-ray tube. One can think of the x-ray circuit as a chain of events necessary for producing optimal images for accurate interpretation by the radiologist. Image interpretation will play a significant role in the diagnosis and, oftentimes, prognosis of the patient. If we can visualize a sequential chain of events within the x-ray circuit, beginning at the console where the current (mA) and kilovoltage (kVp) selections are made, it will be easier to understand the actual processes occurring in the high-voltage section of the x-ray circuit. It is the high-voltage generator that permits voltage to be increased to kilovoltage, and milliamperage to be increased to amperage, for without high voltage and high amperage supplied to the x-ray tube, the production of x-ray photons would not be possible.

RELATED TERMS

automatic exposure control (AEC) devices – Automatic exposure control devices, often referred to as AEC devices, are x-ray imaging systems with special mechanisms designed to reduce repeat radiation exposure to patients while producing consistent quality radiographic images. The two types of AEC imaging systems common to diagnostic radiography are the *ionization chamber* and the *photomultiplier tube*; each operates differently, yet both produce quality standard images. AEC selectors are located on the x-ray control console and permit technologists to choose from an array of radiographic procedures in which the appropriate detection chamber (or photocell arrangement), mA station, and kVp value have been pre-set. The physicist or service engineer will take several phantom test exposures to determine the appropriate amount of radiation necessary to produce optimal radiographic images. The imaging system will then be calibrated to automatically terminate an x-ray exposure when a predetermined amount of radiation for a selected radiographic procedure (position/projection) has been detected. Therefore, AEC imaging systems terminate radiographic exposures by regulating the length of exposure times to coincide with predetermined quantities of radiation selected for producing optimal images of various anatomic structures. It is the responsibility of the radiologic technologist to precisely position the body part over the appropriate chamber (or photocell) for the AEC device to work properly; otherwise, underexposed or overexposed images can result. It should be noted that AEC imaging devices are designed for an average body habitus (sthenic patient). Therefore, the technologist may need to adjust the density settings (e.g., −3, −2, −1, +1, +2, +3) for patients whose body habitus is below average (hyposthenic or asthenic) or above average (hypersthenic).

■ **AEC imaging systems** – There are two main types of automatic exposure control imaging systems:

● **ionization chamber** – The ionization chamber is considered the most common AEC imaging system used today. The parallel-plate ion chamber operates by collecting ion pairs and, when a predetermined amount has been detected, the exposure timer will terminate the exposure. The ionization chamber is located between the patient and the image receptor *(see Figure 7–1).*

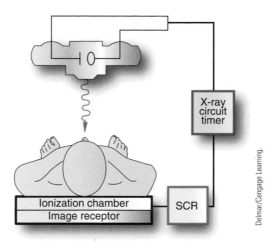

FIGURE 7–1. The ionization chamber is an automatic exposure control (AEC) device. SCR = silicon-controlled rectifier.

- **photomultiplier tube** – The photomultiplier tube is considered to be outdated and not common in modern-day imaging equipment. The photomultiplier tube operates by the use of a fluorescent screen, which gives off light when struck by radiation. When a predetermined amount of light (via radiation) has been detected, the exposure timer will terminate the exposure. The photomultiplier tube is located behind the image receptor (see Figure 7–2).

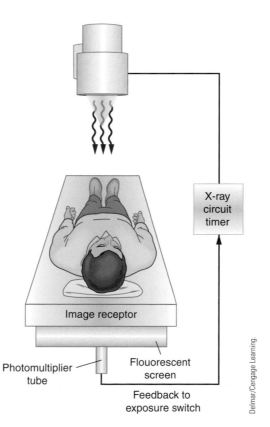

FIGURE 7–2. Photomultiplier tube – AEC.

automatic exposure control (AEC) selectors – There are various AEC selectors located on the console that play a significant role in the proper function of the AEC.

◼ **automatic exposure control terms** – There are terms specific to AEC imaging systems.

     ● **minimum reaction time** – Minimum reaction time refers to the shortest possible exposure time in which the radiation detectors can react to terminate the exposure. For most diagnostic AEC imaging systems, the minimum reaction time is 0.001 seconds.

     ● **phototime** – Phototime and/or phototiming are terms used interchangeably within the imaging profession. These two terms refer to the use of an AEC imaging system for radiographic images and do not distinguish between the two types of AEC systems *(ionization chamber* and *photomultiplier tube).*

◼ **backup time** – Backup time is a set amount of time on an AEC imaging system that is designed to serve as a safety device for the patient and for the x-ray tube. When an AEC imaging system is used, the backup time for each exposure should be set to 150%, or 1.5 times the amount of the anticipated milliampere-seconds required to produce an optimal image. Should an equipment malfunction occur when an exposure is taken, the machine will automatically terminate the exposure at the backup time set and not allow excess radiation exposure or tube overload to occur.

◼ **chambers or photocell arrangements** – Chambers (ionization chamber device) or photocells (photomultiplier tube) are the two types of AEC imaging detection devices used to measure quantities of radiation and terminate exposures.

◼ **density settings** – Calibration of AEC devices are based on radiographic procedures for patients of average body habitus (sthenic). However, when a technologist encounters a patient that is above or below the average body habitus, various density settings (e.g., $-3, -2, -1, +1, +2, +3$) can be used. The $(-)$ settings are to be used on patients whose body habitus is below average, whereas the $(+)$ settings are to be used on patients whose body habitus is above average. Each $(-1$ or $+1)$ setting represents a 30% change in exposure time, resulting in either 30% less radiation or 30% more radiation to the patient, respectively. Each $(-2$ or $+2)$ represents a 60% change in exposure time, resulting in either 60% less radiation or 60% more radiation, respectively, and each $(-3$ or $+3)$ setting represents a 90% change in exposure time, resulting in either 90% less radiation or 90% more radiation, respectively. These density settings were named for their effect on radiographic film density. A 30% change in radiation quantity (mAs) results in a noticeable difference on a radiographic film. The principle of a 30% adjustment in mAs (via time) affecting image quality remains the same when using computed (CR) and digital radiography (DR), even though the term "density" technically cannot be applied to an image visualized on a TV display monitor.

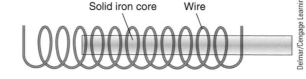

Solid iron core   Wire

Delmar/Cengage Learning.

FIGURE 7–3. Choke coil.

choke coil – A choke coil is a type of variable resistor that uses a fluctuating magnetic field (created by the forward and backward movement of an iron core within a solenoid) to create variations of resistance within an electrical circuit (see Figure 7–3).

circuit breaker – A circuit breaker is a safety device that interrupts the flow of current within a circuit when excessive heat is detected.

conductor – A conductor is a material that permits electrons to flow easily. Materials that serve as good conductors are typically metals such as aluminum, copper, graphite, iron, silver, and gold. However, water and concrete are also considered to be conductors.

coulomb – Named after French physicist Charles-Augustin de Coulomb, the coulomb is a unit to measure electric charge. 1 coulomb = 6.3×10^{18} electron charges (Refer to Chapter 6: Physics Terminology for electrostatics; laws of electrostatics).

current – Current is produced when negative (−) electrical charges (electrons) are in motion. Units to measure current are the ampere (A) or milliampere (mA). Conventional current or Franklin current is named after American inventor and scientist Benjamin Franklin, whose early experiments in electricity in the 1700s assumed positive electrical charges in motion produced current. It was some years later when it was determined that current was actually produced by negative electrical charges moving from a negative polarity to a positive polarity; this is termed actual electron flow. Both terms are used today; therefore, it is important to remember conventional current flows in the opposite direction of actual electron flow.

■ **actual electron flow** – Actual electron flow refers to negative electrical charges (electrons) moving from a negative (−) polarity to a positive (+) polarity.

■ **conventional current** – Conventional current refers to the assumed theory that current flows from a positive (+) polarity to a (−) polarity.

current types – There are two types of current necessary for the basic x-ray circuit to be operational; they are alternating current and direct current. Alternating current (AC) is required for mutual induction to occur at the circuit transformers, whereas direct current (DC) is required for the x-ray tube to be functional.

■ **alternating current/AC** – (Refer to Chapter 6: Physics Terminology.)

■ **direct current/DC** – (Refer to Chapter 6: Physics Terminology.)

electrical circuit wiring – Electrical circuit wiring is the pathway over which current flow is directed through the various components of the circuit. The main two types of electrical circuit wiring are parallel and series:

■ **parallel** – When an electrical circuit is wired in parallel, the voltage across the circuit will always be the same as the voltage across any component of the

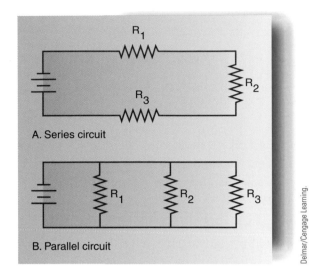

FIGURE 7–4. *A.* Circuit wired in series. *B.* Circuit wired in parallel.

circuit. Current flow in a parallel circuit does not travel in one continuous line along a conductor; rather, a circuit wired in parallel has bridges or connections that permit current to flow along various pathways within the circuit. There are three principles used to understand the parallel circuit *(see Figure 7–4)*:

- Total voltage across the circuit will be consistent with the voltage found at each circuit component, although current and resistance will vary. *(See Ohm's law.)*

- Total current across the circuit will be equal to the sum of individual current found at each circuit component.

- Total resistance across the circuit will always be less than the sum of the individual resistance found at each circuit component.

■ **series** – When an electrical circuit is wired in *series*, the current across the circuit will always be the same as the current across any component of the circuit. Current flow in a series circuit travels in one continuous line along a conductor. There are three principles used to understand the series circuit *(see Figure 7–4)*:

- Total current across the circuit will be consistent with the current found at each circuit component, although voltage and resistance will vary. *(See Ohm's law.)*

- Total voltage across the circuit will be equal to the sum of individual voltage found at each circuit component.

- Total resistance across the circuit will be equal to the sum of individual resistance found at each circuit component.

electrical grounding – Electrical grounding refers to a ground (earth) connection or pathway within a circuit that allows excessive electrical charges to be absorbed, thus preventing the user from experiencing an electrical shock *(see Figure 7-5).*

electric circuit – An electric circuit is a continuous pathway of current flow that begins and ends at the same point. Having an excess of electrons either at the start or end of the pathway will promote electron flow. *(Refer to Chapter 6: Physics Terminology.)*

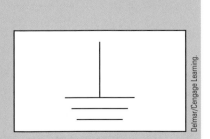

FIGURE 7–5. Electrical grounding symbol.

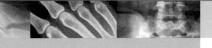

TABLE 7–1 Electric Circuit: Components, Symbols, and Functions

CIRCUIT COMPONENT	CIRCUIT SYMBOL	CIRCUIT COMPONENT FUNCTION
Battery		Source of electrical energy
Capacitor		Temporarily stores an electric charge
Diode/rectifier		Permits current to flow in only one direction
Meter		Measures electric current or voltage
(Ammeter)		Measures electric current and is wired in series
(Voltmeter)		Measures voltage and is wired in parallel
Resistor		Hinders the flow of electrons within the circuit
Rheostat		Varies amount of resistance within the circuit; known as a variable resistor
Switch (open)		Open switch halts the flow of electrons in the circuit
Switch (closed)		Closed switch permits the flow of electrons within the circuit
Filament transformer		Decreases voltage *(and increases amperage)* to secondary side of transformer
High-tension transformer (HTT)		Increases voltage *(and decreases amperage)* to secondary side of transformer

From Bushong, S. C. (2008). *Radiologic science for technologists: Physics, biology, and protection* (9th ed.). St. Louis: Mosby. Copyright © Elsevier. Reprinted with permission.

electric circuit symbols – Electric circuit symbols represent functions of specific devices within a circuit *(see Table 7–1).*

electrification – *(Refer to Chapter 6: Physics Terminology.)*

electrodynamics – *(Refer to Chapter 6: Physics Terminology.)*

electromagnet – An electromagnet consists of a current-conducting solenoid wrapped around an iron core (ferromagnetic material). When current passes through a solenoid, a magnetic field is induced *(see Figure 7–6).*

electromagnetic induction – Electromagnet induction refers to the ability of a changing magnetic field to induce or cause current to flow. In 1831, English physicist Michael Faraday discovered three ways in which a magnetic field could induce electrical current:

- ◼ move a conductor through a magnetic field
- ◼ move a magnetic field past a conductor
- ◼ vary the strength of a magnetic field while keeping the conductor stationary

> • **laws of electromagnets (Faraday's laws)** – There are four laws that govern the strength of the electrical current induced via change or movement of the magnetic field or movement of the conductor:
>
>> • strength of the magnetic field
>>
>> • speed of the magnetic field passing by the conductor
>>
>> • angle between the magnetic field and the conductor
>>
>> • number of turns or coils of the conductor
>
> • **mutual induction** – Mutual induction involves two coils, a *primary coil* wrapped around an iron core (referred to as an *electromagnet*) and a *secondary coil* placed in close proximity to the primary coil. When AC passes through the primary coil (electromagnet), a magnetic field will be produced. If a variation in AC occurs as it passes through the primary coil (electromagnet), a variation in the strength of the induced magnetic field will also occur. It is the continuous variation of the magnetic field that will cause AC to be induced in the secondary coil.
>
> • **self-induction** – Self-induction involves one coil wrapped around an iron core (referred to as an *electromagnet*). When AC passes though the primary coil, a magnetic field will be produced. It is the continuous variation of the magnetic field (caused by AC) that will induce an opposing voltage.

electromagnetism – Electromagnetism refers to the magnetic field that is produced when current is passed through a conductor *(see Figure 7-6).*

Magnetic field lines

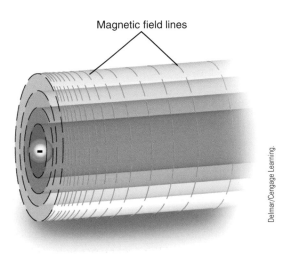

Delmar/Cengage Learning.

FIGURE 7–6. Electromagnet/ electromagnetism.

■ **Fleming's hand rules** – Fleming's hand rules are mnemonic hand techniques developed by British engineer Sir John Ambrose Fleming in the early 1900s. These techniques are extremely useful in reinforcing electromagnetic relationships regarding the direction of conventional current flow, electron flow, and magnetic lines of flux when current is permitted to pass through a conductor. It is important to remember that the direction of conventional current flow is opposite to the direction of actual electron flow.

StudyWARE™
CONNECTION

Review the Image Labeling exercises related to Fleming's hand rules on your StudyWARE™ CD-ROM.

• **left-hand rule** – The left-hand rule is often referred to as the left-hand motor rule. This hand technique mnemonic is very helpful in understanding electromagnetic relationships that arise when using a *motor*. The left hand is positioned with the thumb pointing in the same direction the conductor or armature is moving, the index finger points in the direction of the induced magnetic lines of flux and the third finger points in the direction of conventional current flow. To ensure proper positioning of the fingers, all three fingers should be held at a right angle to each other. *(The right-hand rule is used when the direction of actual electron flow is determined.)*

• **right-hand rule** – The right-hand rule is often referred to as the right-hand generator rule or right-hand dynamo rule. This hand technique mnemonic is very helpful in understanding electromagnetic relationships that arise when using a *generator*. The right hand is positioned with the thumb pointing in the same direction that the conductor or armature is moving, the index finger points in the direction of the induced magnetic lines of flux, and the third finger points in the direction of conventional current flow. To ensure proper positioning of the fingers, all three fingers should be held at a right angle to each other. *(The left-hand rule is used when the direction of actual electron flow is determined.)*

• **left-hand thumb rule** – The left-hand thumb rule is a hand technique mnemonic that calls for the *left thumb* to point in the direction of *actual electron flow* with the four fingers of the hand curled inward toward the palm, representing the direction of the magnetic lines of flux. The induced magnetic lines of flux will be perpendicular to the direction of actual electron flow.

• The left-hand thumb rule also applies to solenoids and electromagnets. With the fingers curled in the direction of actual electron flow, the thumb will point in the direction of the North Pole.

• **right-hand thumb rule** – The right-hand thumb rule is a hand technique mnemonic that calls for the *right thumb* to point in the direction of *conventional current flow* with the four fingers of the hand curled inward toward the palm, representing the direction of the magnetic lines of flux. The induced magnetic lines of flux will be perpendicular to the direction of conventional current.

• The right-hand thumb rule also applies to solenoids and electromagnets. With the fingers curled in the direction of conventional current flow, the thumb will point in the direction of the North Pole.

■ **Oersted experiment** – In 1820, a Danish scientist named Hans Christian Oersted discovered that there is a relationship between electrical current and magnetism. He found that a compass needle would change direction from pointing north to pointing toward the wire conductor whenever current was permitted to flow through the conductor. This phenomenon proved that electrical charges (electrons) in motion will induce a magnetic field perpendicular to the flow of current. To demonstrate the relationship between electrical current and magnetic lines of flux, the *right hand-thumb rule* is useful, whereas, to demonstrate the relationship between electron flow (which is opposite to the direction of current) and magnetic lines of flux, the *left hand-thumb rule* is used *(see Figure 7–7).*

electrostatic field – An electrostatic field exists wherever there is an electrical charge, positive ($+$) or negative ($-$). However, the force around a positive ($+$) electrical charge radiates outward from the charge, whereas the force around a negative ($-$) electrical charge is drawn inward to the charge. *(Refer to Figure 6–4.)*

EMF – EMF or electromotive force is the potential difference required to accelerate electrons across the x-ray tube from cathode to anode. EMF is measured in volts or kilovolts.

generator – A generator (also referred to as a dynamo) is a device that converts mechanical energy into electrical energy.

helix – A helix is a spiral coil of wire.

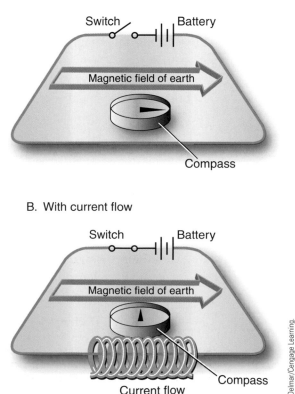

A. Without current flow

Switch   Battery

Magnetic field of earth

Compass

B. With current flow

Switch   Battery

Magnetic field of earth

Current flow   Compass

Delmar/Cengage Learning.

FIGURE 7–7. Oersted's experiment – magnet field and compass.

hertz – The frequency of a sine wave is measured in the unit hertz (Hz). The Hz depicts the up and down movement of current flow (one complete peak and one complete valley), better known as one complete cycle. One hertz is equivalent to one cycle occurring within 1 second. AC in the United States operates on a 60-Hz cycle, meaning that 60 cycles occur every second, producing two impulses per 1/60 of a second. The peak is the positive (+) or useful part of the cycle, whereas the valley is the negative (−) part or nonuseful part of the cycle. Therefore, unrectified AC produces one useful impulse (+) and one nonuseful impulse (−) every 1/60 of a second, yielding 60 useful impulses per second. If AC is rectified to DC (full-wave rectification) the nonuseful impulse becomes useful, and two useful impulses (+) (+) will be produced every 1/60 of a second, yielding 120 useful impulses per second.

horsepower (hp) – The horsepower (hp) is the British unit to measure electric power. 700 hp = 1 watt (W)

insulator – An insulator is a material that hinders the flow of electrons. Materials considered to be good insulators are glass, rubber, fiberglass, oil, and porcelain.

inverter circuit – An inverter circuit is special circuit device used in a high-frequency generator for the purpose of converting DC into a series of square pulses to create a nearly constant voltage waveform with minimal voltage ripple.

magnet – A magnet is a material capable of attracting iron and other ferromagnetic materials by way of the magnetic field that surrounds it. Magnets can be classified into three main categories according to their origin (see Table 7–2).

TABLE 7–2   Magnet Classifications

ORIGIN	EXAMPLES
Artificially produced permanent magnet	
■ typically made of iron	■ ALNICO (alloy of aluminum, nickel, and cobalt)
■ shaped like a bar or horseshoe	■ iron
■ permanent magnetic property can be destroyed via heat or hitting with a hammer	■ steel
Electromagnets	
■ helix of wire around an iron core	■ electric motor
■ current passed through the helix wire (conductor) produces a magnet field	■ induction motor in x-ray tube
	■ transformers
■ strength of magnetic field is proportional to the electric current	■ high-voltage generator
Natural magnet	
■ naturally found in the universe	■ lodestones (minerals in the earth)
	■ iron ore
	■ magnetite
	■ Earth (the planet)

Data from: Carlton, R. R., & Adler, A. M. (2000). *Principles of radiographic imaging: An art and a science.* (4th ed.). Clifton Park, NY: Delmar Cengage Learning; Bushong, S. C. (2008). *Radiologic science for technologists: Physics, biology, and protection* (9th ed.). St. Louis: Mosby. Copyright © Elsevier. Reprinted with permission; and http://www.themagnetguide.com.

TABLE 7–3   Reactions to Magnets

CLASSIFICATION	REACTION TO MAGNETIC FIELD
Diamagnetic material	Not attracted to a magnet field (e.g., copper, gold, and silver)
Ferromagnetic material	Strongly attracted to a magnet field (e.g., cobalt, iron, and nickel)
Nonmagnetic material	Unaffected by a magnetic field (e.g., glass and wood)
Paramagnetic material	Neither diamagnetic or ferromagnetic but classified as in between the two (e.g., gadolinium, magnesium, and molybdenum)

Data from: Carlton, R. R., & Adler, A. M. (2000). *Principles of radiographic imaging: An art and a science.* (4th ed.). Clifton Park, NY: Delmar Cengage Learning; and Bushong, S. C. (2008). *Radiologic science for technologists: Physics, biology, and protection* (9th ed.). St. Louis: Mosby. Copyright © Elsevier. Reprinted with permission.

magnetism – Magnetism refers to the magnetic field that surrounds a magnet and attracts ferromagnetic materials. Materials can be classified by how they react to a magnetic field *(see Table 7–3)*.

meter – A meter is an instrument used to measure the voltage or current flowing within an electrical circuit *(see Table 7–1)*.

- **ammeter** – An ammeter is a meter wired in series to measure the amperage (current) within an electrical circuit.

- **dynamometer** – A dynamometer is a meter that measures AC. When wired in *series*, it will measure the amperage within an electrical circuit; when wired in *parallel*, it will measure the voltage within an electrical circuit.

- **galvanometer** – A galvanometer is a meter that measures DC. When wired in *series*, it will measure the amperage within an electrical circuit; when wired in *parallel*, it will measure the voltage within an electrical circuit.

- **voltmeter** – A voltmeter is a meter wired in parallel to measure the voltage (electromotive force) within an electrical circuit.

motor – A motor is a device that converts electrical energy into mechanical energy.

- **induction motor** – The induction motor is considered part of the x-ray tube and consists of the rotor and several (electromagnetic) stators. Through mutual induction, the induction motor converts electrical energy to mechanical energy, causing the rotating anode to revolve (refer to *rpm*).

ohm (Ω) – The ohm, represented by the symbol Ω, is the unit to measure resistance within an electrical circuit.

Ohm's law – Ohm's law states that within a given circuit there is voltage (V), current (I), and resistance (R), and that the voltage within the circuit (total voltage or voltage at various points within the circuit) will always be equal to the amount of current flowing through the circuit, times the amount of resistance present.

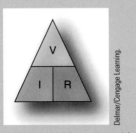

FIGURE 7–8. Ohm's pyramid.

Delmar/Cengage Learning.

Mathematically, Ohm's law can be depicted in any one of the following three ways (*see Figure 7–8*):

$$V = I \times R$$

$$I = V/R$$

$$R = V/I$$

> **Note**   *Current is measured in units of milliamperage (mA) or amperage (A); however, it is represented in Ohm's law as (I) for intensity.*

power – Power as it relates to physics is considered to be the rate of performing work. Units to measure power are the *watt* (W) or the *horsepower* (hp). Mathematically, power is depicted as *power* (P) equals *work* (W) divided by *time* (t):

$$P = W/t$$

power loss – Power loss is generally associated with transformers because of their ability to vary current (amperage) and voltage within a circuit. Power loss can be reduced significantly when a high-tension transformer (HTT) is used to increase voltage and decrease amperage. There is a direct relationship between amperage and power loss. An increase in amperage *(decrease in voltage)* is an increase in power loss; a decrease in amperage *(increase in voltage)* is a decrease in power loss. Using a circuit that uses high voltage and low amperage would prove to have the least amount of power loss.

■ **power loss formula** – Power loss is considered to be the amount of current in amperage squared, times the amount of resistance in ohms present within the electrical circuit. Mathematically, power loss is depicted as $I^{(2)} \times R$, where $I^{(2)}$ represents current in amperage squared and R represents resistance in ohms:

$$\text{Power Loss} = I^{(2)} R$$

■ **total power formula** – Total power (measured in watts) within an electrical circuit is the product of current (measured in amperage) multiplied by the amount of voltage present within the circuit. Mathematically, total power is depicted as $W = I \times V$, where (W) represents total power in watts, (I) represents current in amperage, and (V) represents voltage:

$$\text{Total power (W)} = I \times V$$

rectification – Rectification is the process of converting AC to DC. Within the x-ray circuit, this process takes place between the secondary side of the HTT and the x-ray tube, where a specified number of rectifying semiconductors (solid state diodes) permit current to flow in only one direction, from the cathode filament ($-$ charge) to anode target ($+$ charge). The number of diodes and the type of HTT determines the type of rectification that will occur, with the exception of the high-frequency x-ray generator. The high-frequency x-ray generator, considered to be the most efficient x-ray unit, uses *inverter circuits* to create small square impulses of DC to provide a nearly constant voltage waveform with less than 1% voltage ripple.

- **half-wave rectification** – A half-wave rectification unit may use one, two, or three diodes to ensure current flow in only one direction, from cathode (−) to anode (+). This is accomplished by eliminating the negative half of the Hz cycle, leaving only the positive half of the Hz cycle to create a useful waveform for x-ray production. This type of rectification method is very inefficient because it only permits a voltage waveform with 60 useful (+) impulses per second. With half-wave rectification, a100% voltage ripple occurs, creating a loss in voltage from maximum voltage peak to zero *(see Figure 7–9A).*

- **full-wave rectification** – A full-wave rectification unit uses four diodes to ensure current flow in only one direction, from cathode (–) to anode (+). Converting or rectifying the negative half of the Hz cycle into a positive half results in full-wave rectification. Therefore, full-wave rectification creates two useful (+) impulses per Hz cycle, or 120 impulses per second. Although this unit has a 100% voltage ripple, as does the half-wave rectified unit, the duration of time between maximum voltage peak and zero is half the time. This results in a unit that is twice as efficient in x-ray production as the half-wave rectification unit *(see Figure 7–9B).*

- **three-phase, six-pulse rectification** – A three-phase, six-pulse rectification unit uses six diodes to ensure current flow in only one direction, from cathode (−) to anode (+). Similar to full-wave rectification, the negative half of the Hz cycle is converted or rectified to a positive half, thus creating two useful (+) impulses per Hz cycle, or 120 impulses per second. Because of the type of HTT used (star, wye, or delta step-up transformer configuration) an overlap of three voltage waveforms synchronized 120° apart from one another is able to produce six useful (+) impulses per Hz cycle, or 360 impulses per second. This unit will have an estimated voltage ripple of 13%, making it approximately 35% more efficient at x-ray production than a full-wave rectified unit *(see Figure 7–9C).*

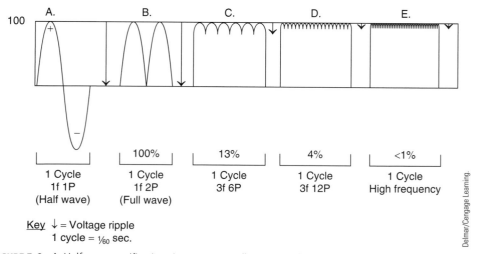

Key ↓ = Voltage ripple
1 cycle = 1/60 sec.

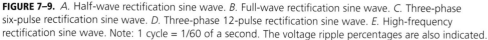

FIGURE 7–9. *A.* Half-wave rectification sine wave. *B.* Full-wave rectification sine wave. *C.* Three-phase six-pulse rectification sine wave. *D.* Three-phase 12-pulse rectification sine wave. *E.* High-frequency rectification sine wave. Note: 1 cycle = 1/60 of a second. The voltage ripple percentages are also indicated.

■ **three-phase, 12-pulse rectification** – A three-phase, 12-pulse rectification unit uses 12 diodes to ensure current flow in only one direction, from cathode (−) to anode (+). Similar to full-wave rectification, the negative half of the Hz cycle is converted or rectified to a positive half, thus creating two useful (+) impulses per Hz cycle, or 120 impulses per second. However, because of the type of HTT used (star, wye, or delta step-up transformer configuration), an overlap of three voltage waveforms synchronized 120° apart from one another is able to produce 12 useful (+) impulses per Hz cycle, or 720 impulses per second. This unit will have an estimated voltage ripple of 4%, making it approximately 41% more efficient at x-ray production than a full-wave rectified unit *(see Figure 7–9D)*.

■ **high-frequency rectification** – High frequency x-ray generators operate very differently than high-voltage type generators found in three-phase x-ray units. The incoming voltage line with 60-Hz cycle AC will be fully rectified to DC and greatly increased to a higher frequency (approximately 6–25 kHz) before the HTT. Through the use of inverter circuits, the high-frequency voltage waveform consisting of small square pulses of DC will be converted back to AC before entering the HTT transformer and will undergo rectification again after exiting the HTT for the x-ray tube to be operable. Having a greater Hz frequency voltage waveform supply to the HTT allows the use of a smaller, lighter step-up transformer that provides for a nearly constant potential waveform with less than 1% voltage ripple. The high-frequency x-ray generator is considered to be the most efficient unit for x-ray production. A high-frequency generator will permit technologists to use less radiation than required with three-phase units for producing optimal radiographic images. Less radiation exposure means less radiation dose to the patient *(see Figure 7–9E)*.

rectification formula – The rectification formula is a mathematical equation used to calculate new mAs necessary for maintaining consistent density between two images produced by two different types of rectified x-ray units (e.g., single-phase full wave rectification versus three-phase, six-pulse rectification). The formula is based upon assigning a multiplier factor or *phase conversion factor (PCF)* to three main types of rectification processes associated with the basic x-ray circuit *(see Table 7-4)*.

$$\frac{\text{mAs}_1}{\text{mAs}_2} = \frac{\text{PCF}_1}{\text{PCF}_2}$$

mAs_1 = original mAs

mAs_2 = new mAs

PCF_1 = original rectified unit

PCF_2 = new rectified unit

■ **phase conversion factor (PCF)** – PCF represents the increase or decrease in mAs required to maintain density as one switches to an x-ray unit with either a more efficient type of rectification or a less efficient type of rectification. For example, with a single-phase full-wave rectified unit, 100% of the mAs set will provide for an image with optimal density. However, when shifting to a three-phase, six-pulse rectified unit and attempting to maintain the same density of the image made with the mAs setting (kVp remains constant) used on the single-phase full-wave rectified unit, the technique would need to be adjusted to 2/3 of the original mAs to have consistent density between the two images. Therefore, we can state that three-phase, six-pulse rectification is 1/3 more efficient at x-ray production than single-phase full-wave rectification, thus requiring 2/3 of the original mAs to maintain consistent density between the two images. The same concept is true regarding three-phase, 12-pulse rectification. This type of rectification is twice as efficient at x-ray production than single-phase full-wave rectification. Therefore, the mAs used to produce an image with a single-phase full-wave rectified unit would need to be reduced by 1/2 (0.5) when switching to a three-phase 12-pulse rectified unit in order to have consistent density between the two images. However, an increase in mAs would be required when switching from a more efficient rectified unit to a less efficient x-ray unit in maintaining a consistent density between the two images *(see Table 7–4). (Refer to rectification formula in Chapter 11.)*

TABLE 7–4 **Rectification and Phase Conversion Factors**	
RECTIFIED UNIT	**PHASE CONVERSION FACTOR (PCF)**
Full-wave rectification	1
Three-phase, six-pulse rectification	0.67
Three-phase, 12-pulse rectification	0.5
Source: Delmar/Cengage Learning	

rectifier – A rectifier is a silicon semiconductor solid-state diode that permits current to flow in only one direction through the electrical circuit. Rectifiers can be referred to as diodes or valve tubes. However, the term "valve tube" refers to diodes constructed within a vacuum tube, which are now considered obsolete for modern day x-ray equipment *(see Table 7-1).*

resistance – Resistance is an opposing force that hinders the flow of electric current. The unit to measure resistance is the ohm (Ω). There are five main variables that greatly impact the amount of resistance present within an electrical circuit:

■ **conducting material** – Materials that serve as good *conductors*, allowing current to flow easily, are typically metals such as aluminum, copper, graphite, iron, silver, and gold. Materials considered to be good *insulators* that hinder the flow of current are glass, rubber, fiberglass, oil, and porcelain.

■ **diameter of conductor** – The larger the diameter (cross section) of the conductor, the easier it is for current to flow. There is an inverse relationship between the diameter of the conductor and the amount of resistance present within the conductor.

- large diameter = little resistance
- small diameter = greater resistance

■ **length of conductor** – As the length of a conductor increases, more resistance occurs. There is a direct relationship between the length of a conductor and the amount of resistance present within the conductor.

- long conductor = greater resistance
- short conductor = little resistance

■ **straight-line conductor** – There is less resistance with a conductor that lies in a straight line. When a conductor has bends or curves, the amount of resistance increases. There is an inverse relationship between the straightness of a conductor and the amount of resistance present within the conductor.

- less straight (with curves) = greater resistance
- straight = little resistance

■ **temperature of conductor** – As the temperature of the conductor increases (heat), the amount of resistance increases. There is a direct relationship between conductor temperature and amount of resistance present within the conductor.

- decrease temperature = less resistance
- increase temperature = greater resistance

resistor – A resistor is a circuit component that creates opposition (resistance) to the flow of electric current *(see Table 7-1)*.

■ **variable resistor** – A variable resistor is a circuit component that creates variations of resistance within an electrical circuit.

rheostat – A rheostat is a type of variable resistor that provides variations of resistance within an electrical circuit *(see Table 7-1)*.

rpm – The standard abbreviation for "revolutions per minute" is *rpm*. This term is associated with rotating anodes. The typical rotational spin for a rotating anode of a single-phase unit is 3,400 rpm, whereas the typical rotational spin for a rotating anode of a three-phase unit is between 10,000 and 12,000 rpm.

solenoid – A solenoid is a helix (spiral coil of wire) serving as a conductor for current flow. The spiral coiling of conducting wire will greatly increase the strength of the magnetic field once current is permitted to flow through it *(see Figure 7–10)*.

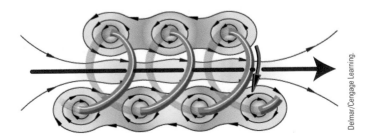

FIGURE 7–10. A solenoid.

Delmar/Cengage Learning.

transformer – A transformer, or x-ray generator, is an electrical circuit component that operates through the principles of electromagnetic induction. There are several types of transformers, and all require AC to be functional. Transformers are designed to vary the current within the electrical circuit, resulting in either an increase or decrease in voltage.

■ **types of transformers** – There are several types of transformers that operate either by self-induction or mutual induction. Only those that pertain to the basic x-ray circuit will be covered in this text.

  • **autotransformer** – The autotransformer is located within the control console panel and consists of one coil wrapped around an iron core (referred to as an *electromagnet*). When AC passes though the coil, a magnetic field is produced. It is the continuous variation of the magnetic field (caused by AC) that will induce an opposing voltage, which will be inversely related to the source voltage. This process allows for a limited range of voltage (100–400 V) to be supplied to the high-voltage section of the x-ray circuit, where the HTT (step-up transformer) and the filament transformer (step-down transformer) are located. The autotransformer has a primary side (input side) and a secondary side (output side). The primary side receives an incoming line of approximately 220 V, whereas the secondary side can provide output voltage up to 400 V depending on the points of connection used on the secondary side of the autotransformer. The primary connections on the autotransformer are there to ensure that the incoming line of voltage is maintained at 220 V *(see Figure 7–11)*.

  • **closed-core transformer** – The closed-core transformer can function as either an *HTT* (step-up transformer) or a *filament transformer* (step-down transformer) depending on the number of coil windings on both the primary and secondary sides of the transformer. This type of transformer is located in the high-voltage section of the x-ray circuit and consists of an iron core in the shape of a square or rectangle with an open cut out in the same shape. If the closed-core transformer has more coil windings or turns on the secondary side than it does on the primary side *(a step-up transformer)*, an increase in voltage (voltage converted to kilovoltage) and a decrease in amperage will result. If the closed-core transformer has more coil windings or turns on the primary side than it does on the secondary side *(a step-down transformer)*, a decrease in voltage and an increase in amperage will result *(see Figure 7–12A)*.

  • **filament transformer** – A filament transformer can also be referred to as a *step-down transformer*. This type of closed-core or shell-type transformer has more coils or windings on the primary side than it does on the secondary side. The purpose of a filament transformer is to step down or decrease voltage in order to greatly increase the current supply to the cathode filament. Therefore, the filament transformer functions to increase milliamperage to amperage. Keep in mind the cathode filament needs approximately 3–6 amperes to create thermionic emission for x-ray production in the diagnostic range to occur.

  • **high-tension transformer** – The HTT can also be referred to as a *step-up transformer*. This type of closed-core or shell-type transformer

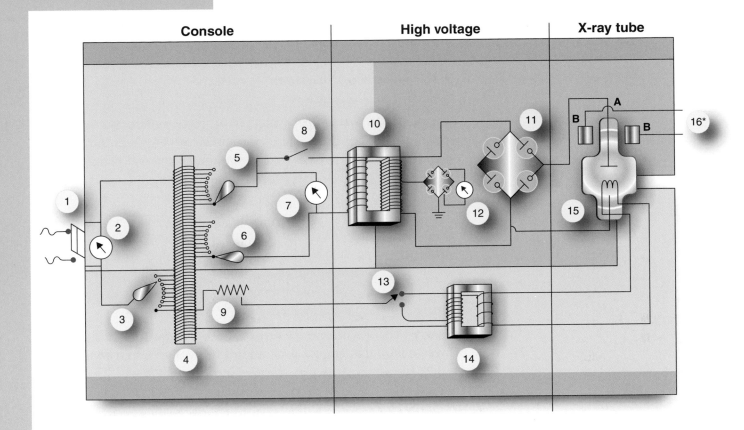

Console   **High voltage**   **X-ray tube**

FIGURE 7–11. X-ray circuit labeled to show its three main sections: control console, high-voltage generator, and x-ray tube.

I. Console

1. Main power switch
2. Line monitor
3. Line voltage compensator
4. Autotransformer
5. Major kVp selector
6. Minor kVp selector
7. Prereading kVp meter
8. Exposure timer circuit
9. mA selector

II. High-voltage section

10. High-tension transformer
11. Four diode rectification circuit
12. mA meter
13. Focal spot selector
14. Filament transformer

III. X-ray tube

15. X-ray tube
16. Induction motor
 A. Rotor
 B. Stators

*The induction motor is part of the x-ray tube.

Delmar/Cengage Learning.

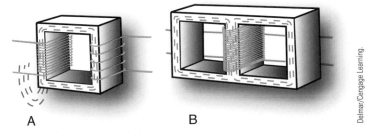

FIGURE 7–12. *A.* Closed core transformer. *B.* Shell type transformer.

Delmar/Cengage Learning.

has more coils or windings on the secondary side of the transformer than it does on the primary side of the transformer. The purpose of the HTT is to step up or greatly increase the voltage supply to the x-ray tube. Therefore, the HTT functions to increase voltage to kilovoltage while simultaneously decreasing current. Keep in mind that electrons produced via thermionic emission need a potential difference of approximately 25–150 kVp for acceleration across the tube to result in x-ray production for diagnostic purposes.

- **shell-type transformer** – The shell-type transformer can function as either an *HTT* (step-up transformer) or a *filament transformer* (step-down transformer) depending on the number of coil windings on both the primary and secondary sides of the transformer. This type of transformer is considered to be the most efficient (demonstrating the least amount of power loss) and is most common type of transformer found in today's basic x-ray unit. It is located in the high-voltage section of the x-ray circuit and consists of an iron core in the shape of a horizontal rectangle with a center piece down the middle, creating two vertical rectangular cutouts in the middle. Both the primary and secondary coil windings are wrapped around the center piece of the transformer, which greatly increases the strength of the induced magnetic field *(see Figure 7–12B)*.

transformer laws – Transformer laws are based on the fact that an inverse relationship exists between voltage and current *(Ohm's law)*. As voltage increases, a decrease in current results, and as voltage decreases, an increase in current results. The purpose of a transformer is to provide a variation in current and voltage flowing within the circuit. *A high-tension (or step-up) transformer* will have more coil windings on the secondary side of the transformer than on the primary side; therefore, current will decrease and voltage will increase (to kilovoltage) on the secondary side of the step-up transformer. *A filament transformer (or step-down transformer)* will have fewer coil windings on the secondary side of the transformer than on the primary side; therefore, current will increase and voltage will decrease on the secondary side of the step-down transformer. A *direct relationship* exists between *voltage* and number of *windings* on the secondary side of either a step-up or step-down transformer. An *inverse relationship* exists between *current* and the number of *windings* on the secondary side of either a step-up or step-down transformer. The direct relationship is known as the *transformer voltage law*, whereas the indirect or inverse relationship is known as the *transformer current law*. Mathematically, these laws are depicted as follows:

- **transformer current law** – This law is a mathematical equation depicting the indirect or inverse relationship between the number of turns on the secondary side of a step-up or step-down transformer and the amount of current produced:

$$N_p/N_s = I_s/I_p, \quad \text{where}$$

  N_p = number of turns or coil windings on the primary side

  N_s = number of turns or coil windings on the secondary side

  I_s = current on secondary side

  I_p = current on primary side

- **transformer voltage law** – The transformer voltage law is a mathematical equation depicting the direct relationship between the number of turns on the secondary side of a step-up or step-down transformer and the amount of voltage produced:

$$N_p/N_s = V_p/V_s, \quad \textbf{where} \quad N_p = \text{number of turns or coil windings on the primary side}$$

N_s = number of turns or coil windings on the secondary side

V_p = voltage on primary side

V_s = voltage on secondary side

transformer power loss – The three most common types of power loss associated with transformers include: copper loss, eddy current loss, and hysteresis loss.

■ **copper loss** – Copper loss refers to the loss of power that is inherent to the transformer material copper. Although copper is considered a great conductor, there is still a certain amount of resistance present, as with all conductors. This loss of power is referred to as copper loss. (For ways to reduce resistance, refer to the term *resistance*.)

■ **eddy current loss** – Eddy current loss refers to power loss as a result of the induced current opposing the magnetic lines of flux.

■ **hysteresis loss** – Hysteresis loss refers to power loss as a result of AC changing the magnetic field. The constant fluctuation of the magnetic field produces heat, which increases resistance and causes power loss.

transformer turns ratio/turns ratio (TR) – The TR of a high-tension or filament transformer indicates the ratio of coil windings on the secondary side to the number of coil windings on the primary side of the transformer. The increase or decrease in voltage (and current) is proportional to the difference in the number of coil windings between the primary and secondary sides of the transformer. A TR of 500:1 for a *HTT* would indicate that for every 1 turn (or coil winding) on the primary side of the transformer, 500 turns would be present on the secondary side of the transformer. This would result in an increase in voltage (and a proportional decrease in current) on the secondary side of the transformer by 500 times the voltage on the primary side. A TR of 1:10 for a *filament transformer* would indicate that for every 10 turns (or coil windings) on the primary side of the transformer, one turn would be present on the secondary side of the transformer. This would result in a decrease in voltage (and a proportional increase in current) on the secondary side of the transformer by 10 times the voltage on the primary side.

volt, voltage – The unit volt can be defined as a potential difference, or an electromotive force (EMF), that causes one ampere to flow in a circuit with a resistance of one ohm.

■ **kilovolt, kilovoltage (kV)** – 1000 volts are equal to 1 kilovolt (1 kV). Kilovoltage is produced within an x-ray circuit by the HTT (high-tension transformer, also referred to as a step-up transformer). Kilovoltage is a necessary requirement for x-ray production to occur.

voltage ripple – Voltage ripple refers to a percentage of voltage lost during the rectification process. A high voltage ripple indicates a high degree of voltage loss, which makes for an inefficient x-ray unit *(see Figure 7–9)*.

- **half-wave rectification** – Half-wave rectification produces a 100% voltage ripple as AC produces a voltage waveform that goes from peak to zero and remains nonuseful during the negative half of the Hz cycle.

- **full-wave rectification** – Full-wave rectification also produces a 100% voltage ripple as AC produces a voltage waveform that goes from peak to zero. However, full-wave rectification is able to take the nonuseful negative half of the Hz cycle and convert it to become a useful positive half. Two positive halves or impulses per Hz cycle *(full-wave rectification)* make x-ray production twice as efficient as x-rays produced utilizing only one positive half of the Hz cycle *(half-wave rectification)*. Full-wave rectification, therefore, requires half the amount of mAs as needed with a half-wave rectified x-ray unit.

- **three-phase, six-pulse rectification** – The three-phase, six-pulse rectified x-ray generator produces an approximate 13% voltage ripple, which means an estimated 87% of voltage is constantly supplied to the x-ray tube. This unit is more efficient at x-ray production than the full-wave rectified unit and will require two-thirds of the mAs utilized with a full-wave rectified unit.

- **three-phase, 12-pulse rectification** – The three-phase, 12-pulse rectified x-ray generator produces an approximate 4% voltage ripple, which means an estimated 96% of voltage is constantly supplied to the x-ray tube. This unit is more efficient at x-ray production than the full-wave rectified unit and will require half the amount of mAs used with a full-wave rectified unit.

- **high-frequency rectification** – The high-frequency generator produces less than 1% voltage ripple, which means an estimated 99% of voltage is constantly supplied to the x-ray tube. This unit is considered to be the most efficient at x-ray production and will require slightly less than half the amount of mAs used with a full-wave rectified unit.

watt (W) – The watt (W) is a unit to measure electric power. Mathematically, it can be depicted as: 1 W (watt) is equal to 1 A (ampere) of current flowing through an electric potential of 1 V (volt): $1 W = 1 A \times 1 V$

x-ray circuit – The basic x-ray circuit is composed of three main sections: *the control console*, the *high-voltage section*, and the *x-ray tube*. The x-ray circuit can also be examined through a classification of subcircuits on the basis of the location of high and low voltage and amperage regulation. For example, the *primary subcircuit* or *low-voltage subcircuit* contains electrical components that operate by means of low voltage. Therefore, we could classify the control console as the primary or low-voltage circuit because kilovoltage is not produced in this section of the circuit. The *secondary subcircuit* or *high-voltage subcircuit* is composed of electrical components found in the high-voltage section of the x-ray unit, where kilovoltage and waveform rectification occur. The *filament subcircuit* is where amperage is increased to provide sufficient heat for thermionic emission to take place at the x-ray tube filament. However, for ease of understanding the basic x-ray circuit, circuit components and their functions will be grouped accordingly to three main sections: the control console, the high-voltage section, and the x-ray tube *(see Figure 7–11)*.

- **control console components** – The control panel is considered the low-voltage section of the x-ray unit where exposure technique selections are made by the registered technologist. The control console consists of the following components *(see Figure 7–11):*

- **autotransformer** – The autotransformer is a variable transformer that operates through the principles of self-induction and serves to supply a range of voltage (approximately 100–400 V) to the HTT. The autotransformer is also designed to assist the line voltage compensator should the incoming line of voltage deviate from the 220-V requirement necessary to operate the unit.

- **circuit breakers** – Circuit breakers are safety devices designed to interrupt the flow of current when an overload of current/heat is detected within the circuit. Circuit breakers can be reset once the overload has been corrected.

- **exposure timer circuit** – The exposure timer circuit or exposure switch is a circuit device that initiates and terminates the x-ray exposure as determined by the selections made at the control console. Three main types of exposure timer circuits common to the basic x-ray unit include electronic timers, mAs timers, and synchronous timers *(see automatic exposure control [AEC] devices).*

  - **electronic timers** – Electronic timers are considered the most efficient and most common type of x-ray exposure timer circuit in modern imaging equipment (i.e., three-phase or high-frequency generators). This type of exposure timer circuit can terminate an exposure in as little as 0.001 second *(minimum reaction time)* and therefore is capable of providing rapid successions of exposures resulting in static images that capture functional mechanisms of anatomical organs and/or structures.

  - **mAs timers** – mAs timers operate by monitoring tube current (mA) and exposure time (s) on the secondary side of the HTT and terminating the exposure when the product of the two values (mAs) reach a designated level of mAs in keeping with *ALARA* principles. *(Refer to Chapter 13: Radiation Protection.)* mAs timers are intended to provide the shortest possible exposure time with the highest safe tube current (mA) for any given mAs setting.

  - **synchronous timers** – Synchronous timers are synchronized to the frequency of the hertz (Hz) cycle of current (AC producing 60 impulses per second in the United States). Synchronous timers are slow in comparison to electronic timers and offer a limited range of exposure times. The minimum or shortest exposure time capable with a synchronous timer using a 60-Hz cycle of current frequency is 1/60 of a second. Increasing increments of exposure times are offered in multiples of 1/60 of a second and do allow for long exposures of several seconds to accommodate breathing techniques.

- **line monitor** – The line monitor is a meter indicating the amount of incoming voltage supply to the x-ray unit.

- **line voltage compensator** – The line voltage compensator alters the line of voltage as necessary to maintain a constant 220-V supply to the unit.

- **main power switch** – The main power switch allows the user to turn on and off the incoming line of (220 V) voltage supply to the x-ray unit; allowing the unit to be operable or inoperable.

- **major kVp selector** – The major kVp selector is a voltage control adjustment permitting kVp to be increased or decreased by increments of 10 kVp.

- **mA selector** – The mA selector is a variable resistor (rheostat), which provides the registered technologist with a variety of tube currents to consider when setting exposure techniques. These tube currents appear on the control console panel as mA stations (typically ranging between 25 and 1600 mA) and ultimately will determine the amount of current supplied to the filament transformer.

- **minor kVp selector** – The minor kVp selector is a voltage control adjustment permitting kVp to be increased or decreased by increments of 2 kVp.

- **prereading kVp meter** – The prereading kVp meter is a meter that measures the voltage supply to the HTT and provides the registered technologist with a read-out of the anticipated kVp.

- **high-voltage section components** – The high-voltage section of the x-ray unit is where the *HTT* (also referred to as a step-up transformer) and the *filament transformer* (also referred to as a step-down transformer) are located. This section of the x-ray unit is where voltage is converted to kilovoltage and milliamperage is converted to amperage. The *rectification circuit* is also located in the high-voltage section and serves to convert AC to DC. The high-voltage section consists of the following components *(see Figure 7–11)*:

  - **HTT (high-tension transformer)** – The HTT can also be referred to as a step-up transformer. The HTT or step-up transformer is a transformer that operates through the principles of mutual induction to convert voltage to kilovoltage.

  - **filament transformer** – The filament transformer can also be referred to as a step-down transformer. The filament or step-down transformer is a variable transformer that operates through the principles of mutual induction to convert mA to amperage.

  - **focal spot selector** – When a dual-focus tube is used, the focal spot selector determines which filament (small or large) will be heated for thermionic emission. Filament selection is typically correlated to the selection of mA stations available on the control console, with lower mA stations designed for the small filament and higher mA stations designed for the large filament.

  - **mA meter** – The mA meter or milliammeter is connected at the midpoint of the secondary side of the HTT where x-ray tube current can be easily measured. Because kilovoltage is present at the secondary side of the transformer, the tube current reading will be low (inverse relationship between voltage and current). However, with the mA meter having a connection to the control console panel, it is necessary for the meter to be *grounded* to provide protection against electrical shock.

- **rectifier (rectification circuit)** – The rectification circuit design for a basic x-ray unit to provide full-wave rectification (meaning current will flow in the same direction during both halves of a hertz cycle) requires 4, 6, or 12 rectifiers. The number of rectifiers indicates the type of rectification used within the x-ray generator *(single-phase vs three-phase)*. The purpose of the rectifiers is to convert existing (AC) current to (DC) current, ensuring current supply to the x-ray tube flows in only one direction. This process protects the x-ray tube from a backflow of current, which would cause damage to the x-ray tube.

x-ray tube – The x-ray tube is the section of the x-ray circuit at which high-speed electrons (produced at the cathode's filament) travel at the speed of light (when an electromotive force [kVp] is applied) within a vacuum enclosure to forcefully strike an anode target, causing the production of x-ray photons *(see Figure 7–11)*.

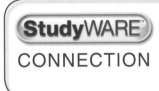

StudyWARE™
CONNECTION

After completing this chapter, review the flashcards or play an interactive game on your StudyWARE™ CD-ROM that will help you learn the content in this chapter.

CONCEPT THINKING QUESTIONS

1. What are the three main sections of the basic x-ray circuit?

2. Explain the three ways in which a magnetic field could induce electrical current.

3. Differentiate between self-induction and mutual induction.

4. Explain the function of a conductor and provide two examples of materials that make good conductors.

5. Explain the function of an insulator and provide two examples of materials that make good insulators.

6. Identify the three types of transformers found in a basic x-ray unit.

7. What is the relationship (direct or indirect) between the current and voltage?

8. What is the purpose of an autotransformer?

9. What is the purpose of the HTT and what is the purpose of a filament transformer?

10. Identify the x-ray circuit component that operates by the principles of self-induction and identify the component(s) that operate by the principles of mutual induction.

11. Explain what resistance is and identify variables impacting the amount of resistance in a given circuit.

12. Explain the relationship between voltage and number of coil windings on an HTT. Explain the relationship between voltage and number of coil windings on a filament transformer.

PRACTICE EXERCISES

1. Identify each component of the x-ray circuit console and explain its function.

2. Identify each component of the x-ray circuit high-voltage section and explain its function.

3. Identify each component of the x-ray circuit tube and explain its function.

4. Draw the pyramid representing Ohm's law and write the three mathematical formulas that depict this law.

5. Apply Ohm's law to solve the following problem: What is the voltage across a circuit that has 6 A of current and 2 ohms of resistance?

6. Apply Ohm's law to solve the following problem: How much resistance is present in a household appliance that operates on 110 volts and 3 A of current?

7. Write the transformer law formulas for both voltage and current. Explain the relationships that are apparent by the way the formulas are written.

8. Calculate the amount of voltage on the secondary side of an HTT with a turns ratio of 1:1000 and an incoming line of 220 V.

9. Calculate the amount of current on the secondary side of a filament transformer with a TR of 1:10 and an incoming line of current at 300 mA.

10. Explain the type of current necessary for transformers located in the high-voltage section of the x-ray circuit to be operational.

MATCHING

Match each term to the appropriate description.

rheostat	motor	(A) or (mA)
ohm	three-phase, six-pulse	copper
diode	step-down transformer	inverter circuit
EMF	100% voltage ripple	no voltage ripple
hysteresis loss	autotransformer	three-phase, 12-pulse
dielectric oil	step-up transformer	generator

Description   **Term**

1. Unit to measure current   _____

2. Self-induction   _____

3. Variable resistor   _____

4. Unit to measure resistance   _____

5. High-frequency generator   _____

6. 4% voltage ripple _____

7. Potential difference _____

8. Rectifier _____

9. Electrical energy to mechanical energy _____

10. Full-wave rectification _____

11. Filament transformer _____

12. Power loss _____

RETENTION OF MATERIAL

Retention requires practicing the use of previously learned material. Apply the knowledge you have of the x-ray tube to answer the following questions.

1. List the two main types of AEC devices, explain their location, and explain how they function.

2. Approximately how much force is needed to accelerate the liberated electrons from the cathode filament across the tube to the tungsten target?

3. Define a helix, solenoid, and choke coil.

4. Explain the difference between circuits wired in series and circuits wired in parallel.

5. Explain when to use Fleming's right-hand rule and what electromagnetic relationships are depicted.

6. Draw a voltage wave-form that would correctly depict the voltage ripple associated with various types of power supplies:

   ◾ single-phase, half-wave

   ◾ single-phase, full-wave

   ◾ three-phase, six-pulse

   ◾ three-phase, 12-pulse

   ◾ high-frequency

7. Write the mathematical formula for *power loss* and explain the best scenario for reducing power loss as it pertains to voltage and current.

8. What was the voltage supply to the HTT if the turns ratio was 1:500 and the following exposure was produced 75 kVp, 300 mA, and 1/20 sec?

9. A filament transformer with a TR of 1:15 produced 6 A to the cathode filament. What was the current supply from autotransformer?

10. A HTT with a turns ratio of 1:500 has an input supply of 240 V and 50 A. What is the output supply of voltage and current provided to the x-ray tube?

11. An optimal anteroposterior image of the lumbar spine was produced with the use of a single-phase full-wave rectified x-ray unit with an exposure technique of 75 kVp at 30 mAs. What would the new mAs have to be to produce a consistent density of the same image when a three-phase, 12-pulse unit is used?

12. A lateral projection of the shoulder was taken with 75 kVp at 8 mAs using a three-phase, six-pulse x-ray unit. If the technologist wanted to produce an identical image using a single-phase full-wave rectified unit, what adjustment in mAs would be necessary?

CHAPTER 8

X-ray Tube

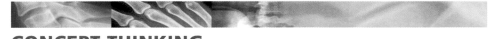

OBJECTIVES

Upon completion of this chapter, the reader will be able to:

- Identify x-ray tube components and their functions
- Explain the role of current and voltage in the operation of the x-ray tube
- Differentiate between inherent filtration and added filtration
- Discuss the factors that control and influence heat dissipation
- Discuss the importance of line focus principle
- Calculate heat units for various types of x-ray generators
- Describe mobile x-ray units and their usage
- Identify reasons for x-ray tube failure

CONCEPT THINKING

The x-ray tube, in simple terms, consists of two electrodes, one positive (anode), and one negative (cathode). The laws of electrostatics *(refer to Chapter 7)* come into play; unlike charges, such as $+/-$, attract, and like charges, such as $-/-$ or $+/+$, repel. Thus, the positive electrode (the anode) attracts the negatively charged electrons, which are produced by the negative electrode (the cathode). Because the function of the x-ray tube is to create x-ray photons, three key conditions must be present. First, there must be a **source** to create x-ray photons *(electrons liberated from the tungsten atoms of the cathode's filament, via high current)*. Second, there must be an electromotive **force** to accelerate the electrons across the tube, from cathode to anode *(kVp setting the technologist chooses at the console)*. Third, there must be a suitable **target** or object *(the anode focal track)* to stop the accelerated electrons, permitting the conversion of electrons to x-ray photons. When this process is initiated, there will be approximately 1% x-ray photon production and 99% heat production. Because of the extreme degree of heat produced at the target, the material of choice must be suitable to withstand a high thermal transfer of energy without melting. The element tungsten has a high atomic number (74 and a melting point of approximately 3410°C, and it therefore serves to dissipate heat well. Other considerations for increasing x-ray production efficiency include the degree of target angle, speed and diameter of the rotating anode, filament size, and temperature. Heat is extremely hazardous to the x-ray tube, and therefore conducting and insulating materials are chosen for their ability to withstand and dissipate heat rapidly.

RELATED TERMS

ampere (A) – An ampere is a unit to measure current *(electrons in motion)*. One ampere is equal to one coulomb flowing through a circuit in a period of one second.

anode – The anode is a positively charged electrode *(located within the x-ray vacuum tube)* that serves as a target for the accelerated electrons produced by the cathode's filament. The most common anode materials used in diagnostic x-ray units are copper, graphite, and molybdenum.

- ■ **rotating anode** – A rotating anode is much more efficient at dissipating heat than a stationary anode. The rotating anode of a single-phase full-wave rectification x-ray unit spins at approximately 3400 rpm *(revolutions per minute)*, whereas the rotational spin of an anode located in a three-phase full-wave rectification x-ray unit is much faster, spinning at approximately 10,000–12,000 rpm. The faster the anode rotates, the more heat is dissipated *(see Figure 8–1)*.

- ■ **stationary anode** – A stationary anode does not spin and therefore is limited in its ability to dissipate heat. This type of anode is more often found in portable x-ray machines and dental x-ray units, which do not require high-exposure techniques *(see Figure 8–1)*.

anode heel effect – The anode heel effect is a phenomenon in which a nonuniform density occurs across an image from anode side to cathode side. This phenomenon is attributable to the target angle of the x-ray tube anode and the greater occurrence of x-ray absorption at the heel of the anode. A 45% difference in x-ray intensity is

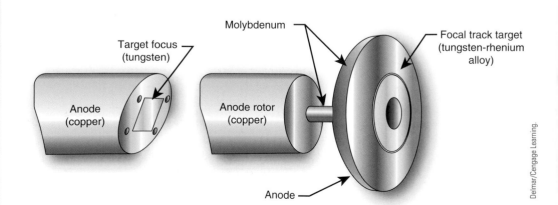

FIGURE 8–1. A stationary anode *(left)* and a rotating anode *(right)*.

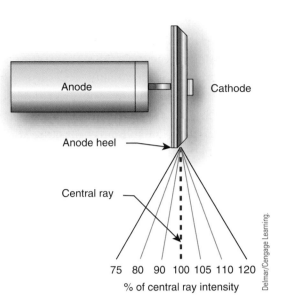

75 80 90 100 105 110 120
% of central ray intensity

FIGURE 8–2. Anode heel effect.

estimated along the longitudinal axis of the image, from anode side to cathode side, with greater radiographic density at the cathode side of the image. Although variation of radiation intensity occurs during every x-ray exposure, the anode heel effect can be used to an advantage by positioning thinner anatomic body parts toward the anode side of the x-ray tube and thicker anatomic body parts toward the cathode side of the x-ray tube. Increasing collimation *(decreasing field size)* will also help reduce the appearance of the anode heel effect *(see Figure 8–2).* Factors contributing to a more noticeable anode heel effect include:

- short SID
- large image receptor size (14 inch × 17 inch)
- small (steep) anode target angle
- small effective focal spot size

anode target – The anode target is a portion of the anode at which the focal track resides *(see focal track).*

cathode – The cathode is a negatively charged electrode *(located within the x-ray vacuum tube)* composed of a filament *(serves as a source of electrons)* and a focusing cup *(see Figure 8–3).*

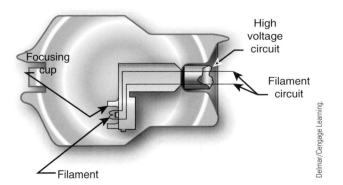

FIGURE 8–3. A cathode.

compensating filters – Compensating filters compensate for inconsistent tissue density of anatomic structures being radiographed. Compensating filters contain a varying degree of absorbing material (typically aluminum). Proper placement of the compensating filter (less absorbing material over the thicker body part and more absorbing material placed over the thinner body part) will result in an image with more uniform radiographic density. Compensating filters are generally constructed of aluminum or plastic *(materials with a low atomic number)* with various shapes and forms to accommodate a range of radiographic procedures. The two most common types of compensating filters in diagnostic radiography are a *trough filter* and a *wedge filter*:

- **trough filter** – The trough filter is typically used for imaging the chest. It is designed to have more absorbing material on the sides with a thinner layer of absorbing material in the center, thus allowing for a more uniform density between the lung fields and the vertebra of the thoracic spine.

- **wedge filter** – A wedge filter is triangular in shape. The smaller, thinner angle of the wedge is to be positioned over the thicker body part, whereas the thicker section of the wedge is to be placed over the thinner body part as a means to absorb more useful radiation and create a less noticeable difference between densities of thinner and thicker anatomical structures. Common radiographic procedures in which a wedge filter might be used include anteroposterior projection of the foot, anteroposterior projection of the thoracic spine, lateral projection of the cervical spine, and a left lateral decubitus abdomen.

current – Current occurs when electrons are in motion. Current within the x-ray tube consists of both alternating current (AC) and direct current (DC). The units to measure current are the ampere and the milliampere.

dead-man switch – The dead-man switch is a type of x-ray exposure switch that acts as a safety feature because it is designed to only permit radiation exposure while the switch is depressed.

detent position – A detent position is a fixed position of the x-ray tube in which the tube is centered horizontally to the either the x-ray table bucky or wall bucky. The technologist still has freedom to move the tube longitudinally and vary the source to image distance.

dielectric oil – Dielectric oil is an insulating oil that surrounds the x-ray vacuum tube and serves to protect the electrical conductor components by absorbing a great deal of the heat produced during x-ray production.

dual-focus tube – A dual-focus x-ray tube houses two filaments, creating two focal spots, a large one to be used with exposure techniques that produce a large amount of heat and a small one for exposure techniques producing lesser amounts of heat that require high definition or resolution of the image.

field size – The size of the restricted primary beam is known as the field size.

filament – The filament is a component of the cathode assembly portion of the x-ray tube. It is a tiny coil of wire, approximately 2 cm long and 2 cm in diameter, typically made of thoriated tungsten and possessing a negative electrical charge. It receives a current of approximately 3–6 amperes from the filament transformer. The high current passing through the filament generates a high degree of heat, resulting in a boiling-off of electrons, referred to as *thermionic emission*. The filament serves to provide a source of electrons (via *thermionic emission*) for x-ray production. Most diagnostic x-ray units are dual-focus, meaning they have two filaments, a large and a small to accommodate various types of radiographic procedures. Typically, small focal spots are used with mA stations of 300 mA or less, whereas large focal spots can sustain larger amounts of heat and therefore can be used with mA stations greater than 300mA. mA selections at the console typically determine which filament size will be used *(see Figure 8–3)*.

filament vaporization – The cathode filament is typically made of tungsten (W) and serves as a source of electrons (thermionic emission) for x-ray production. Because of the extreme heat imparted on the filament during thermionic emission, vaporization of the tungsten atoms will begin to occur; this is referred to as filament vaporization.

filtration – Filtration is the removal of low-energy photons by an absorbing material such as aluminum (Al). Removing low-energy photons from the useful beam results in a higher-quality beam and a decrease in patient dose. There are two types of filtration, *added* and *inherent*; together, they are referred to as *total filtration (see Figure 8–4)*.

■ **added filtration** – Added filtration consists of a thin layer or layer(s) of aluminum positioned between the x-ray tube housing and the collimator assembly as a means of maintaining the correct amount of total filtration determined for the maximum kVp value of the x-ray unit.

■ **inherent filtration** – Inherent filtration is a type of filtration that naturally occurs as the result of the structural composition of the materials comprising the x-ray tube, surrounding dielectric oil, and tube housing. Approximately 0.5 mm of inherent filtration is present within a general diagnostic x-ray tube, with

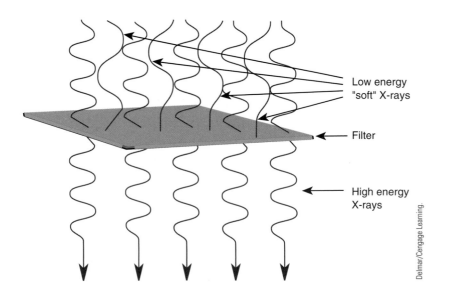

Low energy "soft" X-rays

Filter

High energy X-rays

Delmar/Cengage Learning.

FIGURE 8–4. Filtration hindering low-energy photons.

the glass envelope accounting for the majority of inherent filtration (0.5 mm of Al equivalent). As the tube ages, inherent filtration increases as a result of the vaporization of both the tungsten cathode filament and the tungsten anode target.

■ **total filtration** – Total filtration is the sum of added filtration and inherent filtration. The minimum amount of total filtration for a diagnostic x-ray unit is 2.5 mm of aluminum or aluminum equivalent. Total filtration is determined by the maximum kVp value of the x-ray unit. The Department of Health, Education, and Welfare has mandated a minimum amount of total filtration to correspond to specific ranges of kVp values:

- >70 kVp = 2.5 mm aluminum or aluminum equivalent
- 30–70 kVp = 1.5 mm aluminum or aluminum equivalent
- <30 kVp = 0.5 mm aluminum or aluminum equivalent

focal spot – The focal spot is the area of the anode target where high-speed electrons strike and where the conversion of electrons to x-ray photons occur. This conversion process is referred to as x-ray production. The focal spot size provided by the x-ray tube manufacturer and those listed on radiographic rating charts refer to the effective focal spot size, not the actual focal spot size.

■ **actual focal spot** – The actual focal spot is determined by the stream of electrons produced by *thermionic* emission at the cathode filament, which impacts the focal track of the anode. The size of the actual focal spot is determined by the length, diameter, and temperature of the cathode filament *(see Figure 8–5)*.

■ **effective focal spot** – The effective focal spot is determined by the stream of x-ray photons produced by the impingement of electrons on the anode focal spot. The effective focal spot is determined by the size of the actual focal spot and the degree of the anode target angle. The smaller the actual focal spot and the smaller the anode target angle, the smaller the effective focal spot size. The

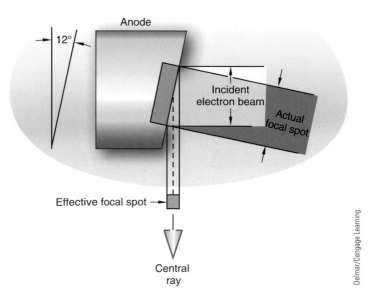

FIGURE 8–5. Actual focal spot and effective focal spot.

Delmar/Cengage Learning.

smaller the effective focal spot, the better the image's recorded detail. However, a small focal spot size will produce a more noticeable *anode heel effect*. Effective focal spot sizes for diagnostic x-ray tubes generally range from 0.1 mm to 3.0 mm. The effective focal spot will always remain smaller than the actual focal spot as long as the anode angle does not exceed 45°. A typical diagnostic x-ray tube has a rather small target angle, approximately 11° or 12°, well within the 7°–21° target angle range designated for diagnostic x-ray tubes *(see Figure 8–5)*.

focal track – The focal track is a circular beveled track on a rotating anode target, which provides the focal spot area for x-ray production *(see Figure 8–6)*.

focusing cup – The focusing cup is a metal component of the cathode. The focusing cup possesses a negative electrical charge, which serves to keep the electrons (produced at the filament via thermionic emission) from drifting apart. This focused stream of electrons is directed toward the anode target. The focusing cup can also serve as an exposure switch for a grid-controlled tube from which a rapid succession of x-ray exposures is made possible.

fractional-focus tube – A fractional-focus tube is a type of x-ray tube used for magnification purposes; it has the ability to produce extremely small focal spots (0.1–0.3 mm) to reduce the unsharpness or loss of recorded detail that occurs when magnifying a structure.

half-value layer (HVL) – A half-value layer is the amount of absorbing material placed in the path of the x-ray beam to reduce the x-ray beam's intensity to half of its original value.

heat – Heat occurs when molecules move rapidly. As the motion of molecules increase, so does the amount of heat generated. Heat is the transference of kinetic energy to thermal energy. The amount of heat produced within an x-ray tube is extremely high due to the electrons' speed and their rapid conversion to x-ray photons. Only 1% of the conversion taking place at the anode results in x-ray production; the other 99% results in heat.

heat dissipation – Heat dissipation refers to the cooling of the x-ray tube. Because approximately 99% of x-ray production generates heat, it becomes necessary to dissipate the heat quickly and efficiently. Reducing heat reduces the chance of equipment

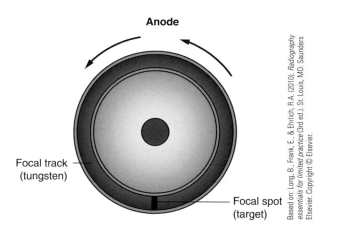

Anode

Focal track
(tungsten)

Focal spot
(target)

Based on: Long, B. Frank, E. & Ehrlich, R.A. (2010). *Radiography essentials for limited practice* (3rd ed.). St. Louis, MO: Saunders Elsevier. Copyright © Elsevier.

FIGURE 8–6. Focal track.

malfunctions and permits radiographic examinations to continue in succession, without interruption. Heat dissipation is contingent upon the following factors:

- **anode angle** – The lesser the degree of the anode angle, the greater the ability of the anode to dissipate heat.

- **anode mass** – The lesser the anode mass, the greater the ability of the rotating anode to spin and dissipate heat. The rotating anode will be composed of materials such as graphite or molybdenum that lie just below the tungsten focal track. The incorporation of these materials makes for a lighter rotating anode, resulting in faster rotational spin and quicker heat dissipation.

- **heat transfer** – There are three main ways to transfer heat:

    - **conduction** – Conduction is the transfer of heat through the touching of two objects.

    - **convection** – Convection is the transfer of heat through the movement of gas or liquid molecules.

    - **thermal radiation** – Thermal radiation is the transfer of heat attributable to the kinetic energy of charged particles being converted to electromagnetic radiation.

- **rotating anode diameter** – The greater the diameter of the rotating anode, the greater the ability of the anode to dissipate heat.

- **rotational speed** – The faster the rotating anode spins, the greater the ability of the anode to dissipate heat.

- **target material** – The greater the atomic number of the anode target material, the greater the ability of the anode to dissipate heat.

heat unit (HU) – A heat unit (HU) is a unit used to measure the amount of thermal heat generated within the x-ray tube during x-ray production. Most of x-ray production (99%) results in heat. To protect the x-ray tube from excess heat and possible tube overload, the technologist should be familiar with the process of calculating heat units for various types of x-ray generators. HUs can be calculated for a single x-ray exposure or for multiple x-ray exposures. Formulas for calculating heat units (HUs) are dependent upon the type of generator equipment used *(multiplier factors included)*, along with the technical factors selected. Listed are the formulas for calculating heat units based on the type of generator used:

- **fluoroscopic unit** – kVp × ma × time × multiplier factor of generator used × **60** *(multiplier factor for fluoroscopy)*
    Fluoroscopy tends to be tracked in minutes as opposed to seconds; therefore, the value of time represented in the formula indicates the number of fluoroscopic minutes and the multiplier factor of **60** in the formula represents the time in seconds (60 seconds equals 1 minute). Because each formula calls for the amount of kVp used as opposed to the amount of voltage used (1 kilovoltage = 1000 volts), the total amount of heat units produced will be in the thousands, which means that the unit to measure thousands of heat units will be **kHU**.

    - kilovolt heat unit (kHU) – 1000 heat units are equal to 1 kiloheat unit (1000 HU = 1 kHU).

- **high-frequency generator equipment** – kVp × mA x time × **1.45** *(multiplier factor for generator type)*

- **single-phase generator equipment** – kVp × mA × time × **1** *(multiplier factor for generator type)*

- **three-phase, six-pulse generator equipment** – kVp × mA × time × **1.35** *(multiplier factor for generator type)*

- **three-phase, 12-pulse generator equipment** – kVp × mA × time × **1.41** *(multiplier factor generator type)*

heterogeneous beam – The primary radiation beam is composed of many different energy values; therefore, it is said to be heterogeneous or polyenergetic. Energy values within the heterogeneous beam range from nearly zero to the applied kVp across the x-ray tube. The large variation of energy values is due to the wide range of bremsstrahlung interactions occurring at the anode target.

induction motor – The induction motor consists of a rotor and stators and operates by mutual induction as a means of spinning the rotating anode to enable heat dissipation *(see Figure 8–7)*.

isotropic – Isotropic refers to the dispersion of light or x-ray photons in all directions from a single point of origin.

kilovolt (kV) – 1000 volts are equal to 1 kilovolt (1000 volts = 1kV).

- **kV and kVp** – Kilovoltage and kilovoltage peak are terms used interchangeably within the imaging profession and refer to the penetrating ability of the x-ray beam. The greater the kVp, the more energetic and penetrating the x-ray beam. The use of a more penetrating x-ray beam permits x-ray photons to transmit through the patient rather than be absorbed by the patient. Increasing kVp while remaining within the optimal kVp range for the specific body part being imaged allows the technologist to use less mAs and therefore lower the patient's radiation dose.

kilovoltage peak (kVp) – Volt peak or voltage peak refers to the greatest energy produced from a specified amount of kilovoltage applied across the x-ray tube.

line focus principle – X-ray tube anodes are designed with an angled beveled edge in which the focal track resides. Line focus principle states that if the angle of the anode is less than 45°, the effective focal spot size will always be smaller than the actual focal spot size, thus creating better image resolution and a greater surface area for heat dissipation. The relationship between actual focal spot size and effective focal spot size is a direct relationship, i.e., increasing the actual focal spot size will result in an increase in the effective focal spot size; however, the effective

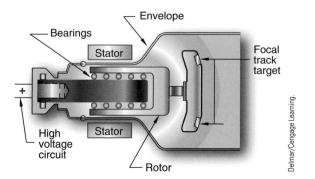

FIGURE 8–7. The induction motor consists of a rotor and stators.

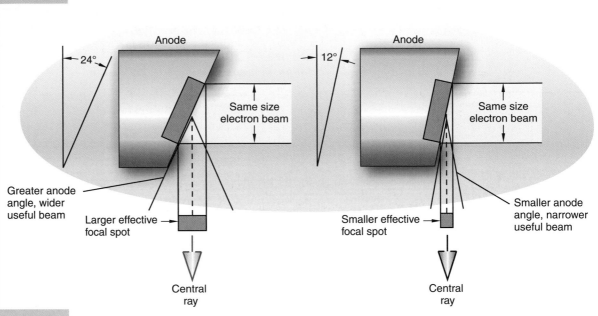

FIGURE 8–8. Line focus principle (a decrease in the anode angle results in a smaller effective focal spot size).

focal spot size will still remain smaller than the actual focal spot size as long as a 45° anode target angle is not exceeded *(see Figure 8–8).*

mA – A milliampere *(or milliamp)* is 1/1000 of 1 ampere of current. X-ray tube currents have correlating mA stations, which allow technologists to choose at the control console a specific quantity of current for a given exposure. Typical mA stations range between 25 mA to 1600 mA (milliamperes).

mAs – The sum of mA (milliamperes) multiplied by the exposure time yields mAs. mAs is a chosen amount of current flowing for a specified period of time. When calculating for mAs, the technologist must consider whether to create the shortest possible time to reduce involuntary motion or to increase time as a means of creating motion for blurring out structures that otherwise would hinder anatomic areas of interest, such as the sternum, ribs, and lateral thoracic spine. mAs is the controlling factor for determining the quantity of x-ray photon production.

mobile x-ray unit – A mobile x-ray unit is a portable unit utilized for imaging procedures on patients who are physically unable to be transported to the radiology department. There are two main types of mobile x-ray units (battery-operated and capacitor discharge) and a portable fluoroscopic unit, better known as a c-arm, that are commonly found in modern-day radiology departments.

■ **battery-operated unit** – A battery-operated unit is a type of mobile x-ray unit that operates by the use of a nickel-cadmium battery. These units are known for their high x-ray production efficiency, whereas voltage is maintained throughout the x-ray exposure. The batteries can be recharged as needed to maintain the units' maximum potential voltage.

■ **capacitor discharge unit** – A capacitor discharge unit, rarely used today, is a type of mobile x-ray unit that operates by the use of a capacitor. A capacitor is a device that temporarily stores an electrical charge. These units are typically plugged into a wall outlet overnight, causing the capacitor circuit to be charged to maximum potential for use the next day. With each x-ray exposure, the tube voltage falls approximately 1 kV/mAs.

- **c-arm unit** – A c-arm is a portable fluoroscopic unit primarily used in the operating room to aid physicians/surgeons in visualizing various projections of anatomic structures and internal hardware (pacemaker, stent, ORIF [i.e., open reduction internal fixator]) and other internal devices that may need to be evaluated for proper placement during the imaging procedure. *(Refer to Chapter 9: Fluoroscopy.)*

penetrability – Penetrability refers to the x-ray beam's ability to penetrate through matter. The greater the kVp, the greater the "quality" of the beam, and the more penetrating the x-ray beam. High penetrability equates to low patient dose because increasing KVp permits the technologist to decrease the mAs.

protective housing – The protective housing is a metal structure with a lead lining that surrounds the x-ray tube and serves four primary functions *(see Figure 8–9)*:

- protects the glass vacuum x-ray tube from harsh handling
- protects the patient and technologist from electrical shock
- protects the patient and technologist from excess radiation exposure by limiting the amount of leakage radiation to less than 100 mR/hr at 1 meter from the source
- assists in the dissipation of heat via air fans and/or circulating dielectric oil. The dielectric oil surrounds the x-ray tube and is contained within the protective steel housing.

saturation current, filament saturation – Saturation current occurs when an increase in kVp no longer has an effect on the percentage of electrons accelerated across the x-ray tube. Typically this occurs at 100 kVp or greater. At intensities less than 100 kVp, an increase in kVp affects the percentage of thermionic emitted electrons accelerated from cathode to anode.

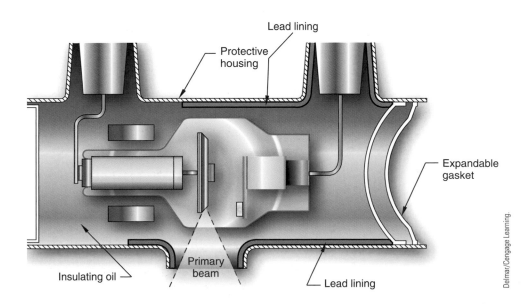

FIGURE 8-9. Protective housing in a diagnostic x-ray tube.

Lead lining

Protective housing

Expandable gasket

Insulating oil

Primary beam

Lead lining

Delmar/Cengage Learning.

space charge – A space charge is the accumulation of electrons around the cathode filament caused by thermionic emission. A space charge can also be referred to as a *thermionic cloud (see Figure 8–10).*

space charge effect – The negative (–) force created by a space charge makes it difficult for additional electrons (possessing a negative [–] charge) to be boiled off the filament; this phenomenon is known as a space charge effect. This is a good example of the *laws of electrostatics*: unlike charges attract one another, and like charges repel one another.

target – The target is the area of the anode that electrons strike as they are accelerated across the x-ray tube from cathode to anode. The element tungsten (W) with a high atomic number of 74 has been found to be the most common target material for basic diagnostic x-ray units. This is attributable to its ability to enhance thermal conductivity, dissipate heat, and efficiently convert high-speed electrons to x-ray photons *(see Figure 8–6).*

thermionic cloud – A thermionic cloud is composed of boiled off electrons from the tungsten atoms of the cathode filament. This cloud of electrons is kept from drifting away by the negative force of the focusing cup. The thermionic cloud will then be accelerated across to the anode target when kVp is applied.

thermionic emission – Thermionic emission is the term used to describe the boiling off of electrons from the tungsten atoms of the cathode filament. This boiling off phenomena occurs due to the high current (approximately 3–6 A) supplied to the filament.

tomography – Tomography is an imaging technique that permits the technologist to image a section or plane of anatomical structure while blurring out areas above or below the area of interest. This area of interest, better known as the object plane, often requires the use of calipers (a device used to measure body part thickness) to determine the correct *fulcrum* setting for placing the object plane in focus.

■ **linear tomography** – Linear tomography is the most basic type of tomography and perhaps the most common type of tomography used for radiographic imaging. It is referred to as linear because the x-ray tube and the image receptor move in opposite directions simultaneously along the longitudinal axis of the x-ray table during the x-ray exposure. It is the degree of tomographic angle that determines the thickness of the body section or body plane. The larger the tomographic angle (greater movement of the tube and image receptor), the thinner the slice of anatomical area or object plane.

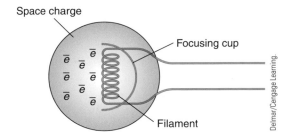

FIGURE 8–10. Space charge.

- fulcrum – The fulcrum is the imaginary pivot point at which the x-ray tube and the image receptor cross each other's path as they move longitudinally to the x-ray table from opposite directions.

■ **panoramic tomography** – Panoramic tomography, often referred to as a "panorex," requires the use of a specialized dedicated tomographic unit in which the patient either stands or is seated upright and the chin is placed on a resting guard while the x-ray tube and image receptor circle the patient's head during the x-ray exposure. This type of tomographic imaging is primarily used to visualize the mandible, TMJs (i.e., temporal mandibular joints), and the teeth.

■ **pluridirectional tomography** – Pluridirectional tomography is a more sophisticated type of tomography than linear tomography. With pluridirectional tomography, the x-ray tube moves in a hypocycloidal or spiral fashion to create better resolution of the object plane. However, due to a higher dose of radiation associated with this type of imaging technique, pluridirectional tomography is rarely seen in modern diagnostic imaging departments; computed tomography and magnetic resonance imaging have become the modalities of choice for visualizing detail of thin body sections or fine anatomical structures.

■ **zonography** – Zonography is a type of tomography that deals with a large or thick section of anatomical area. Because the tissue section or zone of tissue is so thick, the tomographic angle is very small, approximately 10° or less.

tungsten – Tungsten (W) is the choice of material used for the anode target area of a diagnostic x-ray tube for the following three reasons:

■ high atomic number (74) – increased efficiency of diagnostic x-ray production caused by the binding energy (69.5 keV) of the K shell electrons.

■ high melting point of 3410°C – withstands a high degree of heat before melting occurs. Typical diagnostic exposure techniques do not produce heat high enough to cause the tungsten to melt.

■ high thermal conductivity – it can dissipate heat quickly.

vacuum tube – X-ray tubes are made to have no air inside, which allows electrons to travel from the cathode to the anode without interruption from air or gas molecules. This vacuum permits a more efficient means of x-ray production.

volt, voltage – The unit volt can be defined as a potential difference, or an electromotive force (EMF), that causes one ampere to flow in a circuit with a resistance of one ohm.

warm-up procedure – Manufacturers typically recommend a warm-up procedure for x-ray tubes as a means to prolong the life of the tube. Damage can occur when a large amount of heat is applied to a cold anode. Although many modern x-ray tubes have built in devices that automatically warm up the tube, the standard rule of thumb is to take three x-ray exposures with one-second intervals between exposures, and a technique consisting of a moderate mA station, moderate kVp selection, and a time of 1 second.

x-ray tube – The x-ray tube consists of two electrodes encased within a vacuum tube. The positive anode attracts the electrons from the negative cathode. The vacuum tube serves to enhance x-ray production by keeping air molecules out of the path of the accelerated electrons. X-ray tubes possess either a stationary anode or rotating anode. More commonly used in diagnostic imaging departments is the rotating anode x-ray tube, for it is more efficient at dissipating heat than is the stationary anode x-ray tube *(see Figure 8–11).*

■ **Coolidge tube** – William D. Coolidge, an American physicist, developed a more advanced x-ray tube in 1913. The Coolidge tube was a *vacuum* x-ray tube, which served to greatly increase the efficiency of x-ray production. After the invention of the Coolidge tube, the Crookes tube was no longer utilized.

■ **Crookes' tube** – Sir William Crookes, a British physicist, is credited for developing the first x-ray tube in the early 1870s. It was while conducting cathode ray experiments with this type of x-ray tube when, on November 8, 1895, German physicist Wilhelm Conrad Roentgen accidentally discovered x-rays. This discovery earned Roentgen the first Noble Prize in physics in 1901.

■ **grid-biased tube** – *See grid-controlled tube.*

■ **grid-controlled tube** – A grid-controlled tube is a type of x-ray tube that permits a rapid succession of x-ray exposures; most commonly used with DSA (digital subtraction angiography), cineradiography, or with capacitor discharge generators. Grid-controlled tube can also be referred to as a grid-biased tube or a grid-pulsed tube.

■ **grid-pulsed tube** – *See grid-controlled tube.*

x-ray tube failure – X-ray tube failure occurs when the x-ray tube no longer operates under the conditions set forth by the manufacturer. Over extended time and with daily use, an x-ray tube may begin to lose its efficiency due to intense heat and vaporization build-up. Common types of tube failure include:

■ **anode cracking** – Cracking of the anode can occur when a high degree of heat is placed on a cold anode.

■ **anode melting** – Anode melting, or small surface melting, can occur when the induction motor ceases to rotate properly, causing the anode to receive a high degree of heat to a limited area on the focal track.

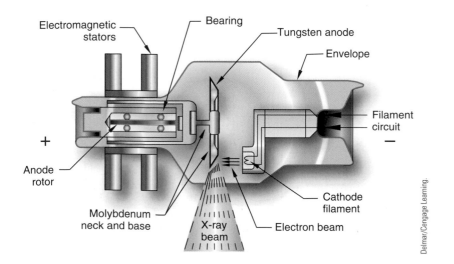

FIGURE 8–11. Vacuum x-ray tube with labeled components.

■ **arcing** – Arcing can occur when vaporized gas molecules interrupt the path of accelerated electrons traveling from anode to cathode; this change of direction is hazardous to the x-ray tube.

■ **malfunction of rotor assembly** – If the rotor bearings are not evenly rotating the anode, a "wobbling" of the anode can result in a malfunction of the x-ray tube.

■ **pitting** – Tiny numerous indentations on the surface of the anode focal track are referred to as "pitting." Pitting is known to occur with the use of high techniques over an extended period of time or with a single exposure that produces excessive heat, such as those involved with breathing techniques where time is measured in seconds as opposed to fractions of a second.

■ **vaporization** – Vaporization occurs when the cathode filament and anode target receive a tremendous amount of heat, causing some of the tungsten atoms to transform from a solid to a gas. This gas adheres to the inside of the vacuum x-ray tube and exhibits the same characteristics of filtration in that low energy photons are absorbed causing a decrease of x-ray photons exiting the window port. This type of tube is often referred to as a "gassy tube." Vaporization is considered the most common reason for tube failure.

x-ray tube life – X-ray tube life refers to the period of time in which the x-ray tube functions properly, producing optimal images without increasing exposure techniques as the tube ages.

x-ray tube rating charts – There are three types of rating charts available to assist technologists in protecting the x-ray tube from the damaging effects of heat production from either a single x-ray exposure and/or multiple x-ray exposures.

■ **anode cooling chart** – This type of tube rating chart is used by technologists to determine the cooling time necessary to protect the anode from excessive heat after a series of x-ray exposures has been performed. This requires the technologist to calculate the total number of heat units produced in the series *(see heat unit [HU] for formulas; see Figure 8–12).*

■ **housing cooling chart** – This type of rating chart closely resembles an anode cooling chart. However, instead of evaluating thousands of heat units (kHU) and the cooling time, the technologist evaluates millions of heat units (MHU) and the cooling time.

■ **radiographic rating chart** – This type of rating chart is used by technologists to determine whether the kVp, time, or mA selected for a single exposure is safe for the x-ray tube. Because x-ray units vary with heat-loading capability, manufacturers provide a tube-rating chart specific to each x-ray unit. When using a radiographic rating chart, the technologist must know kVp, mA, the exposure time, the speed of the rotating anode, the size of the anode angle, the focal spot size, and the type of rectification *(see Figure 8–13).*

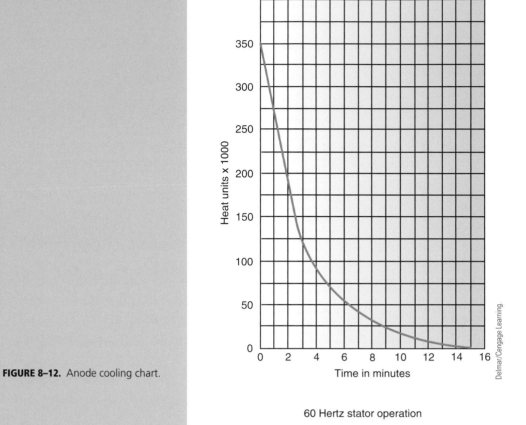

FIGURE 8–12. Anode cooling chart.

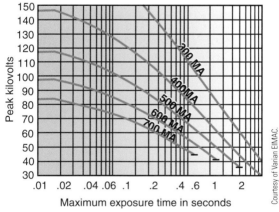

FIGURE 8–13. Radiographic rating chart.

StudyWARE™

CONNECTION

After completing this chapter, complete the Hangman activity or another interactive game on your StudyWARE™ CD-ROM that will help you learn the content in this chapter.

CONCEPT THINKING QUESTIONS

1. What purpose does a vacuum tube serve in the production of x-rays?

2. What electrical charge does the focusing cup have and why?

3. Why does a rotating anode have a beveled edge?

4. What degree of target angle is most common to a diagnostic x-ray tube?

5. What is the relationship (direct or indirect) between the actual focal spot and the effective focal spot?

6. What happens to the heat-loading capabilities of the x-ray tube when you increase the target angle?

7. What happens to the effective focal spot size when the degree of the target angle is decreased?

8. Explain the line focus principle and its importance.

9. Explain the anode heel effect and what variables make it more noticeable.

10. What is the controlling factor for determining the "quantity" of radiation produced?

PRACTICE EXERCISES

1. Label each component of the x-ray tube. Explain each component's function.

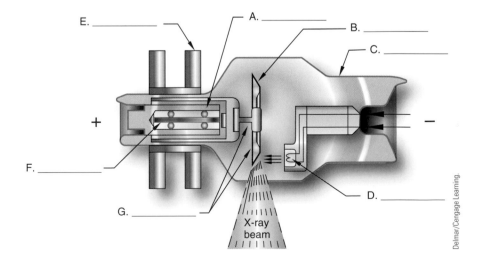

E. _____   A. _____   B. _____

C. _____

+

F. _____

G. _____

X-ray beam

D. _____

Delmar/Cengage Learning.

2. Label the large and small filaments, actual focal spot, and effective focal spot. Then indicate what takes place when you change from a large focal spot to a small focal spot regarding recorded detail, penumbra, anode heel effect, and the heat-loading capability of the anode.

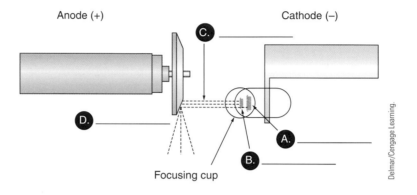

3. List the two components that make up the induction motor.

4. Use the radiographic tube-rating chart provided to determine whether the following conditions are safe for the x-ray tube.

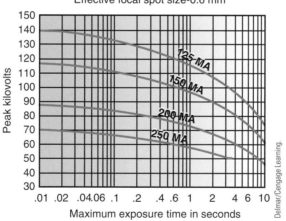

A. 200-mA station at 100 kVp with a 0.4-second exposure.

B. 200-mA station at 80 kVp with a 0.2-second exposure.

C. 125-mA station at 100 kVp with a 1-second exposure.

5. Calculate the number of heat units produced when using the following x-ray units.

A. Single-phase full-wave rectified unit with an exposure of 85 kVp, 300 mA, 0.4 second.

B. Three-phase, six-pulse rectified unit with an exposure of 110 kVp, 200 mA, 0.2 second.

C. High-frequency unit with an exposure of 95 kVp, 400 mA, 0.4 second.

6. Use the anode-cooling chart shown in Figure 8–12 to solve the following equations involving heat unit calculations:

   A. Determine the time necessary for the tube to completely cool down from a series of exposures that produced 250 kHU.

   B. How long would it take for the tube to cool down from 275 kHU to 50 kHU?

   C. How many exposures of 80 kVp, 400 mA, 0.4 second could be taken with a three-phase, six-pulse rectified unit without exceeding the maximum number of heat units for this cooling chart?

7. Differentiate between a space charge and a space charge effect.

8. Explain what the fulcrum point is regarding linear tomography.

9. What causes the primary x-ray beam to be heterogeneous?

10. What causes vaporization to occur within the x-ray tube?

MATCHING

Match each term to the appropriate description.

fulcrum	vaporization	cathode
focusing cup	anode	polyenergetic
Coolidge tube	milliampere	conduction
heat	focal spot	filament
stators	kilovoltage	Crookes tube
attract	tungsten	aluminum

Description	Term
1. Electromotive force	_____
2. Repels electrons	_____
3. Part of the induction motor	_____
4. Choice of target material	_____
5. Choice of filtration material	_____
6. 99% produced during x-ray production	_____
7. Vacuum x-ray tube	_____
8. Many different energies	_____
9. Attracts electrons	_____
10. Area where x-rays are produced	_____
11. Unit to measure current	_____
12. Transference of heat when objects touch	_____

RETENTION OF MATERIAL

Retention requires practicing the use of previously learned material. Apply the knowledge you have of the x-ray tube to answer the following questions.

1. List the three conditions necessary for x-ray production to occur.

_____

_____

_____

2. What is the name given to an x-ray tube that has two filaments?

3. What is the approximate range of amperage needed for thermionic emission to occur?

4. What tube components contribute to inherent filtration? What is the largest contributor to inherent filtration?

5. Explain the line focus principle. What would happen if the target angle was greater than 45°?

6. Describe the anode heel effect and how it could best be used to an advantage.

7. List the two main parts of the x-ray tube induction motor.

_____

_____

8. Write the HU (heat unit) formula that would correspond to each type of rectified x-ray unit.
- Single-phase (full-wave rectification)
- Three-phase, six-pulse unit
- Three-phase, 12-pulse unit
- High-frequency unit
- Fluoroscopic unit

9. What anode characteristics would best accommodate high-exposure techniques that produce a great amount of heat?

10. How does vaporization affect x-ray tube output?

11. Explain two ways in which a smaller effective focal spot could be achieved.

12. Explain how linear tomography works.

CHAPTER 9

Fluoroscopy

OBJECTIVES

Upon completion of this chapter, the reader will be able to:

- Explain the difference between static images and dynamic images
- Discuss fluoroscopy and its role in the imaging profession
- Identify the components of an image intensifier tube
- List the function of each component of the image intensifier tube
- Discuss the chain of events that occur in converting incident x-ray photons to a lighted visible image
- Identify and discuss various operation modes and ancillary devices associated with the typical fluoroscopic system

CONCEPT THINKING

Fluoroscopic procedures typically are scheduled in the morning hours by most imaging departments. Therefore, radiologic technologic students while on clinical externship will spend a great deal of their learning experience performing hands-on manipulation of fluoroscopic equipment. Acquiring a basic understanding of the operations of fluoroscopic imaging systems is essential for demonstrating a complete dynamic study of anatomical structures relevant to each fluoroscopic procedure. Fluoroscopy is used to see form and function of internal anatomical structures in real time. Because various tissue densities within the body can appear similar, making it difficult to distinguish one tissue type from another, the use of contrast media (positive and/or negative – *Refer to Chapter 2: Abbreviations and Word Parts)* is often necessary. Both fluoroscopy and digital fluoroscopy require the use of an image intensifier tube. The role of the image intensifier tube is to increase the brightness level of fluoroscopic images to allow the operator and others to view the dynamic study in real time on a video display monitor. The brightness level is maintained throughout the study by the automatic brightness control (ABC), which self-adjusts the mA and/ or kV according to the tissue density of the part being examined. Because fluoroscopy is a dynamic study of anatomical structures, it requires the operator to use more *time* when delivering radiation. To compensate for the lengthy radiation exposure times typically involved with fluoroscopic procedures, a very low mA range of 0.5 to 5.0 is used. Fluoroscopic units use a 5-minute audible timer as a safety feature to remind the operator of elapsed radiation exposure time. In keeping with patient safety, the NCRP (Nuclear Council on Radiation Protection) provides recommendations for limiting patient dose with a minimum distance requirement for both fixed (stationary) and portable (mobile) fluoroscopic units. Fixed fluoroscopic units require a minimum distance from x-ray source to patient skin of 15 inches, and a portable fluoro-unit requires a minimum distance from x-ray source to patient skin of 12 inches. In accordance with radiation protection guidelines, the average table top exposure rate for fluoroscopy is 1–3 R/min and should never exceed 2.1 R/min/mA at 80 kVp. The tabletop x-ray exposure rate (or x-ray intensity) for fluoroscopy should not exceed 10 R/min; when high-level fluoroscopy is used, tabletop exposure intensity should not exceed 20 R/min.

RELATED TERMS

analog-to-digital converter (ADC) – An ADC is a device used to convert the fluctuating analog signal into a discrete digital signal, thus allowing data to be recorded in binary code for computer manipulation of a radiographic image.

analog signal – An analog signal is an electrical signal that continually fluctuates in amplitude, frequency, and degree of noise.

audible (5-minute) timer – An audible timer is equipped on a fluoroscopic unit to sound off when 5 minutes of fluoroscopic time (actual time of radiation exposure to the patient) has elapsed. The timer serves as a safety device to remind the health care team of the amount of time the patient has been exposed to primary radiation (and themselves to secondary radiation if they are in the immediate area of the radiation source).

brightness control – Brightness control or image illumination is maintained as the kVp and mA self-adjust during the fluoroscopic procedure. There are several terms that refer to the control system that holds the brightness level at a constant as the fluoro carriage (or c-arm) is moved over a range of varying tissue densities (e.g., bone, muscle, solid organ, adipose tissue, hollow organ, air).

■ **ABC** – automatic brightness control

■ **ABS** – automatic brightness stabilization

■ **AGC** – automatic gain control

c-arm – The portable fluoroscopic unit is often referred to as a c-arm because of its shape, which resembles the letter "c." It should be noted that the configuration of this type of mobile unit allows the x-ray tube and the image intensifier tube *(located at opposite ends of the "c")* to remain in constant alignment while

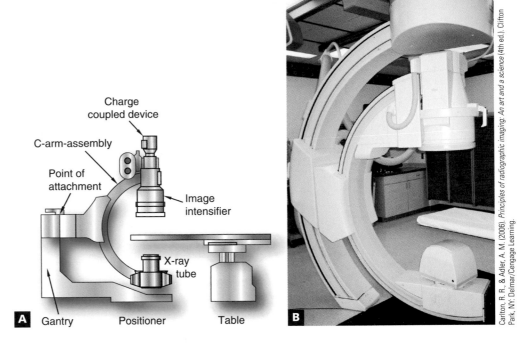

Carlton, R. R., & Adler, A. M. (2006). *Principles of radiographic imaging: An art and a science* (4th ed.). Clifton Park, NY: Delmar/Cengage Learning.

FIGURE 9–1. A fixed fluoroscopic unit with c-arm assembly.

permitting the equipment to move directly over the patient and to rotate from a vertical position to a horizontal position. The increased flexibility of up, down, and side-to-side movement provides a multitude of imaging perspectives for anatomical structures being viewed *(see Figure 9–1)*.

carriage – The carriage or tower is the support system for the x-ray tube and image intensifier tube on a fixed fluoroscopic unit. The carriage can be easily moved by the technologist or radiologist to allow the patient easy access to and from the x-ray table. It also permits a free range of movement (up, down, and side to side) to view anatomical structures as the patient is moved into various positions. Fluoroscopic adjustment controls (brightness level, collimation, magnification, and image recording selections) are also located on the carriage for ease of image manipulation *(see Figure 9–2)*.

cathode ray tube (CRT) – A cathode ray tube, or TV picture tube, permits real-time viewing of the fluoroscopic procedure on a TV display monitor. It works by receiving the electronic signal from the TV camera tube and converting it to a lighted image *(see Figure 9–3)*.

charge-coupled device – A charge-coupled device is a semiconducting device that converts light photons from the image intensifier tube into numerous electron charges (analog signal), which, with the aid of an ADC adaptor (analog-to-digital converter), can be interpreted and displayed as a visible image on a display monitor *(see Figure 9–4)*.

computed radiography – Computed radiography, often referred to as CR imaging, uses imaging plates containing photostimuable phosphors inside an imaging cassette receptor. These plates replace conventional film and can be exposed to light without harming the latent image. There is no need to open the cassette because the imaging process calls for the cassette to be placed in an image plate reader, where the imaging plate is removed and scanned by laser. Information

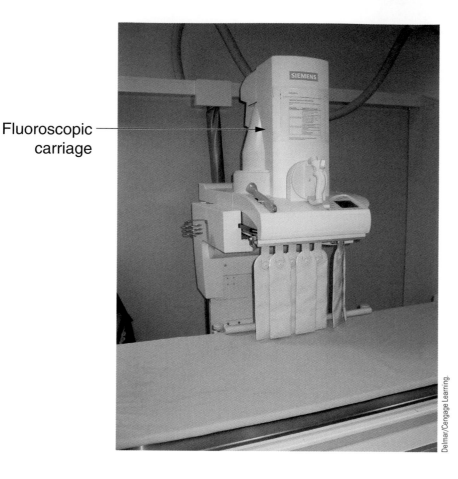

Fluoroscopic carriage

Delmar/Cengage Learning.

FIGURE 9–2. Fluoroscopic carriage.

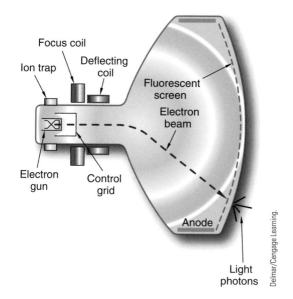

Focus coil

Ion trap

Deflecting coil

Fluorescent screen

Electron beam

Electron gun

Control grid

Anode

Light photons

Delmar/Cengage Learning.

FIGURE 9–3. Cathode ray tube (CRT).

depicting the latent image is then transferred in the form of several energy conversions to produce a visible image to be viewed on a display monitor where electronic manipulation for quality enhancement can occur. The image can then be directly sent to the radiologist for interpretation and/or archived for future reference. *(Refer to Chapter 10: Image Production.)*

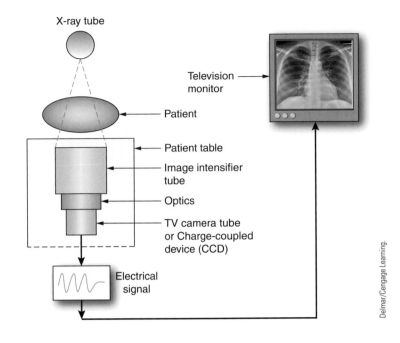

X-ray tube

Television monitor

Patient

Patient table

Image intensifier tube

Optics

TV camera tube or Charge-coupled device (CCD)

Electrical signal

Delmar/Cengage Learning.

FIGURE 9–4. Charge-coupled device (CCD) is part of the fluoroscopic system.

contrast resolution – The ability to visually distinguish between anatomical structures of similar tissue density.

dead-man foot pedal – The dead-man foot pedal requires the fluoro operator to have their foot placed on the pedal for fluoroscopic imaging to occur. This type of foot pedal acts as a safety feature because it is designed to only permit radiation exposure while the pedal is depressed, thus preventing the operator from using excess radiation for visualization of internal structures. The dead-man foot pedal promotes intermittent fluoroscopic images as the operator steps on and off the pedal to provide a brief view of anatomical structures. An interspersed image can remain on screen as a static image until the next dynamic image is initiated or it can be saved in electronic format or hard copy to become part of the patient's permanent medical records file.

digital fluoroscopy (DF) – Digital fluoroscopy uses a charge-coupled device connected to an image intensifier output phosphor in conjunction with an ADC adaptor (analog-to-digital converter) to convert the analog signal to a digitized signal that can then be displayed in pixel formation for viewing on a display monitor.

direct digital radiography – Direct digital radiography, often referred to as digital radiography or DR imaging, uses image detectors, eliminating the need for cassettes. This method of image acquisition permits remnant x-rays (those exiting the patient) to directly interact with digital detectors to produce visible images on a display monitor where electronic manipulation for quality enhancement can occur. Therefore, direct digital imaging is considered a more efficient (and more expensive) method of producing images because it eliminates the need for several energy conversion processes to occur as necessary when using film/screen combination and computed radiography. The image can then be directly sent to the radiologist for interpretation and/or archived for future reference. (*Refer to Chapter 10: Image Production.*)

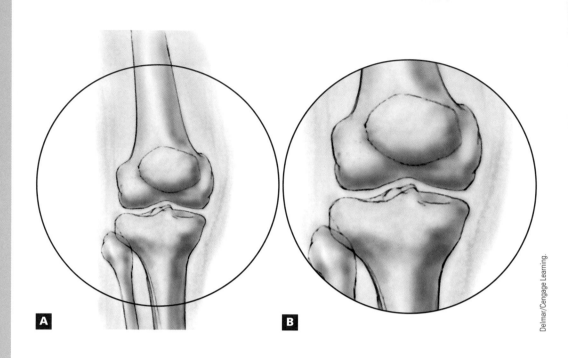

A

B

FIGURE 9–5. Magnification mode results in a smaller FOV. *A.* larger FOV. *B.* smaller FOV.

dynamic image – A dynamic *(moving)* image is a radiographic image that demonstrates the functional ability of internal structures in real time.

field of view (FOV) – Field of view, or FOV, refers to the actual area of anatomical structures seen on a display monitor. Magnification mode results in a decrease of the image intensifier's input phosphor diameter, resulting in a decrease in the FOV and an increase in the size of the structure imaged *(see Figure 9–5).*

film-screen combination – A film-screen combination refers to an imaging cassette that has either one intensifying screen *(to be used with single-emulsion film)* or two intensifying screens *(to be used with double-emulsion film)* and a sheet of radiographic film. This type of imaging system requires a film processor to develop the radiographic image *(see Figure 9–6).*

fluoroscope – The fluoroscope was invented in 1896 by Thomas A. Edison. It is a radiographic device consisting of an x-ray tube and a fluorescent screen designed to permit real-time viewing of internal structures within the human body.

fluoroscopic image – A fluoroscopic image refers to the dynamic image that appears on the video monitor or on the flat screen panel(s) when anatomical structures are being radiographed through the use of a fluoroscope.

fluoroscopic mA range – The range of mA for film fluoroscopic examinations is between 0.5 and 5.0 mA. This low range of mA is attributable to the increase in time (minutes) of actual radiation exposure to the patient and serves to keep radiation dose to a minimum. Direct fluoroscopic examination requires greater mA because of the pulsed beam.

fluoroscopic system – The fluoroscopic system is a fixed unit consisting of several components working together to provide dynamic images for viewing. Typically, the x-ray tube is located underneath the x-ray table and underneath the patient, with the image intensifier tube suspended above the patient. However, it should

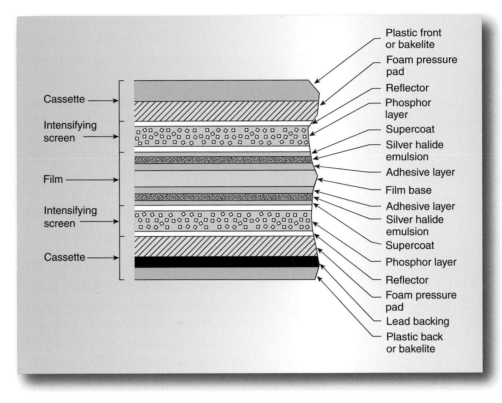

FIGURE 9–6. Cross-section of intensifying screen and film.

Delmar/Cengage Learning.

be noted there are *remote fluoroscopic systems* in which the opposite arrangement of x-ray tube and image intensifier exists. *(For ease of understanding component function of a fluoroscopic system, we will focus on the more common under-table unit, which positions the x-ray tube underneath the x-ray table and underneath the patient.)*

■ **auxiliary imaging devices** – Auxiliary imaging devices are operational devices located on the fluoro carriage that permit various methods for viewing fluoroscopic images. With the exception of the cassette-loaded spot-film, all other modes of viewing fluoroscopic images require a direct connection (via fiber optics or lens optics) between the TV camera tube (vidicon or Plumbicon) or charge-coupled device and the image intensifier output phosphor.

■ **bucky slot cover** – The bucky slot cover is a lead cover that conceals the opening of the bucky tray, which tends to run the length of the x-ray table. It serves as a radiation protective device to reduce radiation exposure to radiologic technologists and other health care members present during fluoroscopic procedures. All fluoroscopic imaging systems are required to possess a minimum of 0.25 mm of lead (Pb) for the bucky slot cover.

■ **bucky tray** – Invented by Gustov Bucky in 1921, a bucky tray can be found on both a flat and upright imaging system. The bucky tray is a movable tray that holds imaging cassettes of various sizes for overhead radiography. It can be moved to any position along the length of the x-ray table and is moved to the foot of the x-ray table during fluoroscopic procedures as to not interfere with the production and/or viewing of dynamic images. The bucky tray also enables the *grid* to move backward and forward during a radiographic exposure. This back-and-forth motion of the grid assists in reducing scatter radiation from reaching the image receptor while simultaneously blurring grid lines to make them less noticeable on a radiographic image.

- **cassette-loaded spot-film** – A cassette-loaded spot-film uses conventional radiography to make static images during a fluoroscopic procedure. A single exposure or multiple exposures (2, 4, and 6) can be achieved on one film when the fluoroscopic portion of the procedure is interrupted for conventional radiography to take place. This is easily achieved because the spot-film cassette is positioned on the lower portion of the fluoroscopic carriage, placing it between the patient and the image intensifier tube.

- **cine camera** – *see cinefluorography.*

- **cine film imaging** – *see cinefluorography.*

- **cinefluorography** – Cinefluorography is a static recording of images taken in rapid succession (up to 90 frames per second) on either 16-mm film or 35-mm film that, when viewed at high speeds, appear as a dynamic study. Cinefluorography was primarily used in cardiac catherization and has since been replaced with digital equipment.

- **image intensifier tube *(suspended above the patient)*** – The image intensifier tube serves to convert image-forming x-ray photons (those that have exited the patient) to light photons with an increased brightness level for viewing fluoroscopic images in daylight. The range of brightness gain is approximately 1000–30,000. This amplified level of brightness permits viewers to visualize the image in daylight *(photopic vision)*, whereas conventional fluoroscopy (now discontinued) used a fluorescent screen that required total darkness *(scotopic vision)* for visualization of the image. The image intensifier's main components and their functions are listed in sequential order of the conversion process of x-ray photons to increased light photons *(see Figure 9–7).*

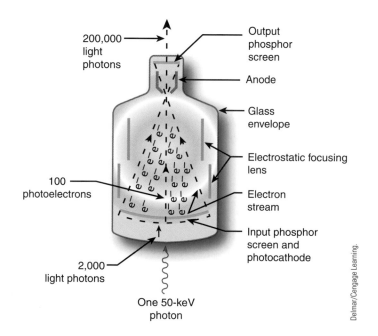

FIGURE 9–7. Image intensifier tube.

- **anode** – The anode is a small circular metal plate possessing a positive electrical charge of approximately 25,000 volts. It serves to accelerate electrons from the photocathode to the output phosphor. The anode has a small opening in the center to permit the accelerated electrons to pass through to the output phosphor *(see Figure 9–7)*.

- **electrons** – Electrons are negatively charged particles *(see Figure 9–7)*.

- **electrostatic focusing lenses** – Electrostatic focusing lenses guide the stream of electrons as they travel from photocathode to anode *(see Figure 9–7)*.

- **glass envelope** – The glass envelope is a vacuum tube typically made of Pyrex that serves to keep air molecules from interacting with accelerated electrons moving from the photocathode to the anode when a potential difference (approximately 25,000 volts) is applied *(see Figure 9–7)*.

- **input phosphor** – The input phosphor is composed of cesium iodide (CsI) and serves to convert the incoming x-ray photons (those that exit through the patient) to visible light photons. The input phosphor has a convex shape and a diameter of approximately 8–10 inches *(see Figure 9–7)*.

- **output phosphor** – The output phosphor is composed of zinc cadmium sulfide and serves to convert the accelerated electrons from the photocathode to a lighted image. The output phosphor has a flat surface and a diameter of approximately 1 inch. The dramatic increase in brightness at the output phosphor is directly due to *minification gain* and *flux gain (see Figure 9–7)*.

- **photocathode** – The photocathode is a thin metal composed of cesium and antimony compounds; it possesses a negative electrical charge. It is firmly attached to the back of the input phosphor and is responsible for converting the visible light photons emitted by the input phosphor to electrons. This process is better known as *photoemission (see Figure 9–7)*.

- **protective curtain** – The protective curtain is a lead-lined radiation protective device *(minimum of 0.25 mm Pb equivalent)* that attaches to the outside part of the fluoroscopic carriage to create a protective barrier between the patient and the fluoroscopic operator. It therefore serves to protect the fluoroscopic operator (technologist) from excessive radiation exposure during fluoroscopic procedures.

- **spot-film camera, photospot camera** – A spot-film camera or photospot camera uses 70-mm film or 105-mm film to rapidly *(12 images per second)* produce static images that resemble a dynamic image when viewed at high speed. The advantage of using a larger film format size is a greater degree of resolution; the disadvantage is greater radiation dose to the patient.

- **tilt table with footrest** – Fluoroscopic units incorporate tilt tables to permit the fluoroscopic operator to move the patient for better visualization of anatomical structures and, with the aid of gravity, move contrast media to specific locations within the body. For example, a 90/20 tilt table would permit the head of the table to be raised to a 90° angle or to an upright position.

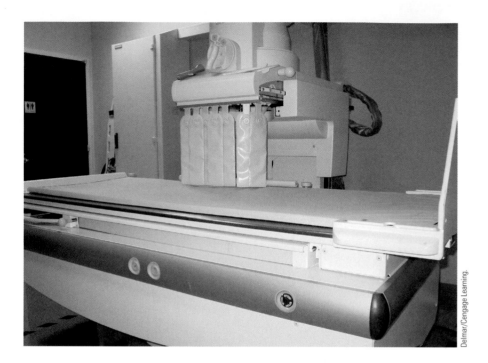

Delmar/Cengage Learning.

FIGURE 9–8. Tilt table with foot rest.

It would also permit the head to be lowered 20° (Trendelenburg position; *refer to Chapter15: Positioning Terms, Landmarks, and Lines*) from a supine position, placing the patient's feet at a higher level than their head. This type of table must have a foot rest located at the foot end of the table to allow patients to stand without falling off the table as the table is tilted toward a 90° angle *(see Figure 9–8).*

- **TV display monitor** – The TV display monitor is essentially a cathode ray tube (CRT) that serves to transform the electrical signal provided by the TV camera tube to a lighted visible image for viewing dynamic images in real time. It should be noted that modern imaging systems incorporate LCD and plasma technology by using flat panel display monitors to replace the conventional TV display monitor.

- **x-ray tube** – *Refer to Chapter 8: X-ray Tube.*

  - **fluoroscopic x-ray tube (positioned underneath table)** – The fluoroscopic x-ray tube is typically positioned underneath the table and the patient, with the image intensifier tube suspended above the patient. The fluoroscopic carriage easily moves, permitting the operator complete control over placement of the image intensifier tube and x-ray tube, as they are designed to remain in constant alignment with each other *(see Figure 9–9).*

  - **overhead x-ray tube (ceiling mounted)** – The overhead x-ray tube is typically mounted from the ceiling and permits the operator to take conventional radiographic images before and after the fluoroscopic procedure. If static images are requested during fluoroscopic procedures, a general radiographic imaging system (spot-film cassette, film/screen combination, computed radiography, and DR) would be initiated.

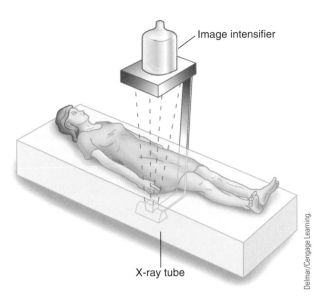

Image intensifier

X-ray tube

Delmar/Cengage Learning.

FIGURE 9–9. X-ray tube positioned under x-ray table.

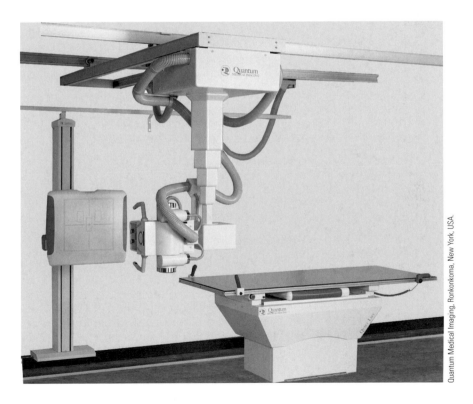

Quantum Medical Imaging, Ronkonkoma, New York, USA.

FIGURE 9–10. X-ray tube assembly positioned over x-ray table.

The overhead x-ray tube is moved out of the way during fluoroscopic procedures so that it does not interfere with the process of dynamic imaging *(see Figure 9–10).*

fluoroscopy – Fluoroscopy is a type of radiographic examination that uses an image intensifier tube to visualize dynamic studies of the body's internal structures.

flux gain – Flux gain refers to the increased amount of light photons from the image intensifier output phosphor in comparison to the number of x-ray photons striking

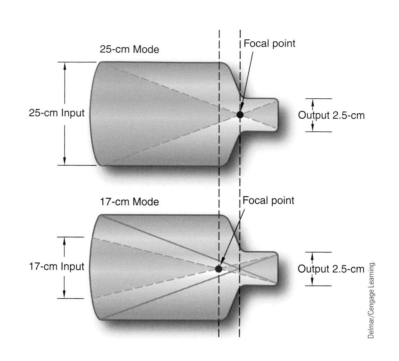

FIGURE 9–11. Focal point (enlarged).

the image intensifier input phosphor. This number can be calculated by using the following mathematical formula:

$$\text{Flux gain} = \frac{\text{\# of output light photons}}{\text{\# of input x-ray photons}}$$

focal point – The focal point is the area within the image intensifier tube that depicts the narrowest stream of electrons traveling from photocathode to anode. The narrowing of the electron beam is accomplished by the electrostatic lens positioned along the length of the image intensifier tube *(see Figure 9–11)*.

illumination – Illumination refers to the brightness level of the fluoroscopic image. Illuminations levels are typically measured in units of millilamberts (1000 mL = 1 L), and seldom exceed 1 L.

image recording – Image recording refers to an array of methods used to record both static and dynamic images *(see Table 9-1)*.

magnification – Anatomical structures visualized during a fluoroscopic procedure can be magnified by changing from a large input phosphor diameter to a smaller input phosphor diameter, thus creating a smaller FOV. The magnification factor can be determined by using the following mathematical formula:

$$\text{Magnification factor} = \frac{\text{large input phosphor diameter}}{\text{small input phosphor diameter}}$$

minification gain – Minification gain refers to the ratio of the diameter of the input phosphor squared to the diameter of the output phosphor squared. This number can be calculated by using the following mathematical formula:

$$\text{Minification gain} = \frac{(\text{diameter of input phosphor})^2}{(\text{diameter of output phosphor})^2}$$

multifield image intensification – Multifield image intensification refers to the use of more than one diameter input phosphor size, resulting in various

---

TABLE 9–1 Image Recording Methods

STATIC IMAGE RECORDING	DYNAMIC IMAGE RECORDING
■ Cassette-loaded spot-film	■ Cineradiography
■ Conventional film/screen	■ Spot-film or photo-spot camera*
■ Computed radiography (CR)	■ Video recording (super-VHS)
■ Direct digital radiography (DR)	■ Digital fluoroscopy
	• Last image hold feature**

When viewed at high speed, this format produces static images that resemble dynamic images.

**Displays a static image of the previously viewed dynamic study.*

Data from: Carlton R., & Adler, A. M. (2006). *Principles of radiographic imaging: An art and a science.* (4th ed.). Clifton Park, NY: Delmar Cengage Learning; Bushong, S. C. (2008). *Radiologic science for technologists: Physics, biology, and protection* (9th ed.). St. Louis, MO: Mosby. Copyright © Elsevier. Reprinted with permission.

---

magnification modes. When a smaller input phosphor is used, the focal point moves further away from the output phosphor, resulting in a magnified view. Common to diagnostic radiography are multifield image intensifier tubes with input phosphor diameter sizes ranging from 25 cm to 10 cm; 25/17 (dual-field) or 25/17/10 (trifield).

■ **dual-field image intensifier tube** – A dual-field image intensifier tube offers two selections of input phosphor diameters, resulting in two separate fields of view. When changing to a smaller input phosphor diameter, the FOV will become smaller and the anatomical structures of interest will be magnified *(see Figure 9–11).*

■ **trifield image intensifier tube** – A trifield image intensifier tube offers three selections of input phosphor diameters, resulting in three separate fields of view. When changing to a smaller input phosphor diameter, the FOV will become smaller and the anatomical structures of interest will be magnified. This type of image intensifier offers more flexibility for viewing fluoroscopic images.

noise – Noise is the interference of imaged information that appears on the recording medium or viewing system.

patient dose – Patient dose is considerably greater with fluoroscopic procedures as opposed to conventional radiographic procedures. The greater patient dose is attributed to a greater length of radiation exposure time required with dynamic studies. It should be noted that magnification during fluoroscopic procedures results in an increase in patient dose. To determine an increase in patient dose when employing the magnification mode, the following mathematical formula can be used:

$$\text{Patient dose (fluoro)} = \frac{\text{large input phosphor diameter}^2}{\text{small input phosphor diameter}^2}$$

photoemission – Photoemission refers to the production of electrons at the image intensifier's photocathode as a result of light photons from the input phosphor striking it. Photoemission is similar in concept to thermionic emission *(boiling off of electrons)*, which occurs at the cathode filament of an x-ray tube upon receiving high amperage *(see Figure 9–7)*.

photopic vision – Photopic vision or daylight vision permits visual acuity (i.e., how well we see detailed structures) to increase. The cones of the eye are responsible for photopic vision. Both static and dynamic radiographic studies are viewed in daylight conditions, permitting viewers to utilize their phototopic vision.

quantum mottle, quantum noise – Quantum mottle or quantum noise manifests as a grainy or blurry appearance on a radiographic image. This causes a loss of detail, primarily attributable to an insufficient quantity of x-ray photons striking the recording medium. This phenomenon can occur with the use of very low mA exposures, high-speed film-screen combinations, or with an imaging system that inherently produces a high level of signal interference. These variables cause a loss of anatomical information (data), resulting in a poor radiographic image. Reducing quantum mottle and/or quantum noise will result in an increase in spatial resolution.

raster pattern – A raster pattern is an electrical signal originating from the TV camera tube as it receives information from the output phosphor of the image intensifier tube. This electrical signal is sent to the CRT in the form of two electron beams. These electron beams synchronously move across the fluorescent screen of the CRT, creating a horizontal distribution of information (moving from top left corner to top right corner and descending downward across the CRT). This horizontal distribution of information, known as a raster pattern, appears as a lighted image on the TV monitor *(see Figure 9–12)*.

recording system, recording medium, viewing system – Recording system, recording medium, and viewing system all refer to the methods used in visualizing radiographic images. Such methods include film/ screen radiography, computed radiography, direct digital radiography, cineradiography *(16-mm and 35-mm film)*, spot-film (or *photospot*) camera *(70-mm film and 105-mm film)*, video camera with display monitor, and high-resolution video recording.

remote fluoroscopic system – A remote fluoroscopic system is a fluoroscopic room designed to be operational from the console panel, located behind

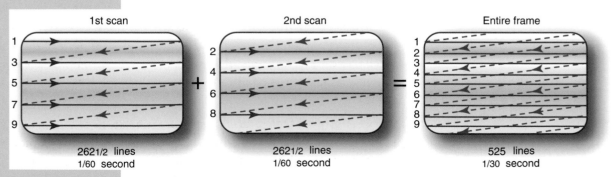

FIGURE 9–12. Raster pattern on monitor.

lead-glass shielding. The motorized controls permit the technologist and radiologist to conduct dynamic studies without being exposed to secondary radiation, for they are not present in the x-ray room during the radiographic procedure. Unlike a conventional fluoroscopic room where the x-ray tube is positioned beneath the x-ray table and the image intensifier is above the x-ray table, a remote fluoroscopic system places the x-ray tube above the x-ray table and the image intensifier underneath the x-ray table *(see fluoroscopic system)*.

scotopic vision – Scotopic vision or night vision is the ability to see in dimly lit conditions. A person's visual acuity declines with scotopic vision, making it difficult to differentiate small structures. The rods of the eye are responsible for scotopic vision. Early conventional fluoroscopy required viewers to be in total darkness and to use their scotopic vision; this limited their ability to detect fine anatomical structures. Today, both static and dynamic radiographic studies are viewed in daylight conditions, permitting viewers to use phototopic vision.

spatial resolution – Spatial resolution refers to the degree of sharpness *(detail)* recorded by the imaging medium (e.g., film-screen, computed radiography, digital radiography). Increased spatial resolution permits greater distinction between small structures that lie close to each other.

spot image, spot imaging – Spot imaging uses conventional radiography with film *(cassette with film/screen combination or 70-mm film and 105-mm film)* to provide static images of anatomical structures of interest viewed during a fluoroscopic procedure.

static image – A static image is an image caught in time; it is considered a still image of anatomical structures.

tabletop exposure rate – Tabletop exposure rate or x-ray intensity for fluoroscopic procedures should not exceed 10 R/min or 2 R/min/mA at 80 kVp. However, if high-level fluoroscopy is utilized, the tabletop exposure rate should not exceed 20 R/min.

total brightness gain – Total brightness gain refers to the increased amount of light or brightness of an image by the use of an image intensifier tube. It is the product of *minification gain* and *flux gain*. Total brightness gain can be calculated by using the following mathematical formula:

Brightness gain = minification gain − flux gain

TV camera tube – There are two types of TV camera tubes, the *vidicon* and the *plumbicon*. These TV camera tubes serve to convert light photons from the output phosphor of the image intensifier tube to an electrical signal that will then travel to the TV display monitor, where the electrical signal is converted to a lighted image for viewing purposes. For the imaging system to functionally operate, the diameter of the receiving end of the TV camera tube (approximately 1–2 inches) must match the diameter of the output phosphor and therefore is directly coupled to it *(see Figure 9–13)*.

vignetting – Vignetting is the term used to describe the loss of brightness around the periphery of the image being viewed. It is similar in concept to penumbra, which is a loss of spatial resolution around the periphery of an anatomical structure imaged on radiographic film.

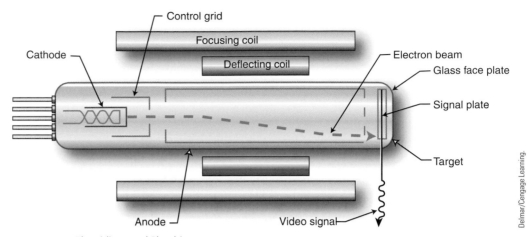

FIGURE 9–13. The vidicon and Plumbicon.

x-ray source to patient distance – Then NCRP (Nuclear Council on Radiation Protection) has established specific safety recommendations regarding distance between the x-ray source and the patient for both fixed and portable fluoroscopic units.

■ **fixed or stationary fluoroscopic units** – Fixed fluoroscopic units require a minimum distance of 15 inches between the x-ray source and the patient.

■ **portable or mobile fluoroscopic units** – Portable fluoroscopic units require a minimum distance of 12 inches between the x-ray source and the patient.

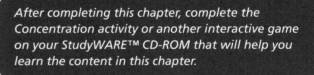

After completing this chapter, complete the Concentration activity or another interactive game on your StudyWARE™ CD-ROM that will help you learn the content in this chapter.

CONCEPT THINKING QUESTIONS

When answering the following questions and/or filling in the blanks, visualize the x-ray tube underneath the x-ray table and the image intensifier suspended over the patient. Remember that the brightness level automatically adjusts the mA and/or kVp (via the ABC system) to maintain a consistent level of brightness. Picture the vacuum tube image intensifier tube and other auxiliary imaging mode selectors located on the fluoro carriage. Think of each auxiliary mode of operation and its unique design in providing static and/or dynamic images. Keep in mind that patient dose is greater with fluoroscopy than with conventional radiography, and resolution or structural detail decreases with the use of fluoroscopy.

1. The ABC system maintains a consistent level of image brightness by increasing _____ and/or _____.

2. When magnifying a fluoroscopic image, the diameter of the input phosphor size is _____, causing the focal spot to shift away from the anode.

3. What happens to the FOV when an image area is magnified?

4. Why should the magnification mode not be used routinely?

5. What two devices can be directly coupled to the image intensifier output phosphor to enable the electrical signal to be received by a video display monitor?

6. What amount of voltage is required to accelerate electrons from photocathode to anode?

7. Which has a greater degree of noise or quantum mottle, conventional radiography (film-screen) or fluoroscopy?

8. Does the use of a cassette-loaded spot-film require the use of the image intensifier? Explain why or why not.

9. When an image is magnified, what happens to the spatial resolution?

10. When an image is magnified, what happens to the contrast resolution?

PRACTICE EXERCISES

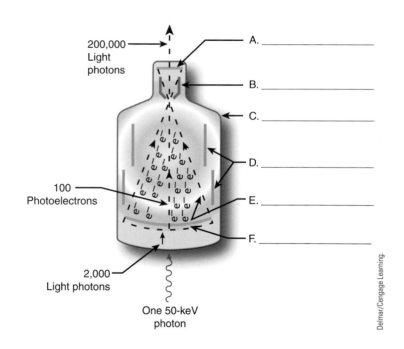

1. Label the components of the image intensifier tube.

2. List the function of each component of the image intensifier tube.

3. Identify the material or element associated with each of the following image intensifier components, and explain the conversions that occur at each component.

   A. input phosphor

   B. photocathode

   C. output phosphor

4. List at least seven components that comprise a fluoroscopic system.

5. Explain minification gain and write the mathematical formula depicting minification gain.

6. Explain flux gain and write the mathematical formula depicting flux gain.

7. Explain total brightness gain and write the mathematical formula depicting brightness gain.

8. Describe the term *photoemission* and explain how it closely resembles thermionic emission.

9. Explain the function of a spot-film or photospot camera and what type of fluoroscopic procedure(s) might it be used for.

10. When one uses the magnification mode, does the focal spot shift toward the anode or away from the anode? Explain what occurs.

11. What would be the total brightness gain for an image intensifier tube with a flux gain of 40, an input phosphor diameter of 25 cm, and an output phosphor diameter of 2.0 cm?

12. How much more magnified would an image be when switching from a 25-cm input phosphor diameter mode to a 10-cm input phosphor diameter mode?

MATCHING

Match each term to the appropriate description.

cones	electrostatic focusing lens	anode
mL	cesium and antimony compounds	dual-field tube
photocathode	zinc cadmium sulfide	rods
photoemission	vidicon	ABC
brightness gain	kVp	resolution
CsI	trifield tube	vignetting

Description	Term
1. Output phosphor	_____
2. Has a positive electrical charge	_____
3. Photopic vision	_____
4. Emits electrons when struck by light photons	_____
5. Controls stream of electrons	_____
6. 25/15	_____
7. Maintains brightness level	_____
8. Unit to measure illumination	_____
9. Loss of brightness at periphery	_____

10. Input phosphor   _____

11. Minification gain × flux gain   _____

12. TV camera tube   _____

RETENTION OF MATERIAL

Retention requires practicing the use of previously learned material. Apply the knowledge you have of the image intensifier tube to answer the following questions.

1. Kilovoltage applied to the image intensifier tube serves to _____ toward the anode.

2. The x-ray tube operates at what range of current during a fluoroscopic procedure?

3. Explain how the ABC maintains a consistent level of image brightness.

4. Illumination levels (image brightness) are measured in what units?

5. What is the typical range of illumination (image brightness) for dynamic studies?

6. What part of the eye is responsible for viewing fluoroscopic images on a TV display monitor?

7. Draw an image intensifier tube with all its components and briefly list their functions.

8. Explain why dynamic studies may be necessary and what they depict that static studies do not.

9. When decreasing the FOV on a TV display monitor, what happens to the resolution of the image being visualized? Why?

10. When increasing the FOV on a TV display monitor, what happens to the contrast resolution? Why?

11. Why is the lighted image at the output phosphor of the image intensifier tube more intense than the lighted image at the input phosphor?

12. What would be the difference in image resolution using a 70-mm film size as opposed to a 105-mm film size when using a photospot camera?

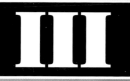

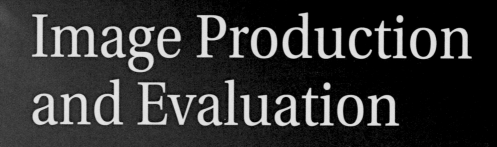

Image Production
and Evaluation

CHAPTER 10

Image Production

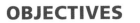

OBJECTIVES

Upon completion of this chapter, the reader will be able to:

- Explain the process involved in image acquisition via the use of various imaging systems
- Differentiate between a latent image and a manifest image
- Explain the cause of anode heel effect and influencing factors
- Differentiate between the actual focal spot and the effective focal spot
- Discuss the line-focus principle and its impact on focal spot size
- Identify controlling factors and influencing factors for contrast, density, detail, and distortion
- Compare and contrast computed radiography and direct digital radiography
- Differentiate between window width and window level

CONCEPT THINKING

Producing images of anatomical structures within the human body involves a technology that permits the conversion of x-ray photons to a visible image. Since the discovery of x-rays (November 8, 1895) to the present, technology has evolved tremendously. Within the past few decades, the imaging profession has transformed the way in which images are created and viewed. Although the most basic concept of image production remains constant (requiring a source, force, and target), the conversion process that converts remnant x-ray photons to a visible image is ever changing, The standard radiographic film, common for decades, is currently being replaced by more sophisticated technology known as computed radiography and/or digital radiography. The evolution of image production requires registered technologists to stay abreast of technological advancements regarding imaging equipment, technical skills, and patient care techniques. Imaging equipment has become very user friendly, with automatic settings that are designed to provide for more consistent image quality and fewer repeat patient exposures. However, this should not be misinterpreted to mean that the technologist requires less knowledge or technical skill in producing images via computed radiography (CR) and digital radiography (DR). These two methods of image acquisition permit for a greater *latitude* than does conventional radiography with the use of radiographic film. When an exposure technique error occurs, resulting in either an underexposed image (too light) or an overexposed image (too dark), the technologist must make corrections to the exposure technique and repeat the radiograph to produce a film of diagnostic quality. The use of CR or DR permits the supervising technologist (or in some instances the technologist) to manipulate an image that is slightly underexposed or overexposed through adjusting the *window level* and/or *window width* without repeating the image and causing additional radiation exposure to the patient. However, it should be noted that extreme cases of underexposure or overexposure will require the technologist to repeat the imaging process. The ability of CR and DR to provide technologists with greater latitude in image acquisition should not replace setting appropriate exposure factors that align to the ALARA principle. There are many controlling factors and influencing factors that the technologist must consider when setting exposure technique. Therefore, it is the responsibility of the technologist to apply critically thinking skills to devise an appropriate exposure technique, taking into account the unique variables that present with each and every patient.

RELATED TERMS

air-gap technique – The air-gap technique is the use of a 4- to 6-inch object-to-image distance (OID) to create enough space for scatter radiation to avoid interacting with the image receptor (IR). An air-gap technique may be used in place of a grid as it serves to reduce scatter and increase image contrast *(see Figure 10–1)*.

ALARA principle – The radiologic technologist should always adhere to the principle of using *as low as reasonably achievable* (ALARA) amounts of radiation to produce optimal images with the smallest dose to the patient.

attenuation – Attenuation is a reduction of x-ray beam intensity as it passes through an absorbing material (such as the patient).

beam-restricting devices – Beam-restricting devices restrict the field of radiation and are used to reduce patient dose. The use of a beam-restricting devise will enhance image contrast as the result of less scatter radiation interaction with the IR. Types of beam-restricting devices include collimation, aperture diaphragms (lead plate with cut-out shape), cones, and cylinders.

central ray – The central ray refers to the center of the x-ray beam. The center of the x-ray beam is the point that is used in the alignment of the x-ray tube, body part, and IR. In radiographic positioning, the radiologic technologist is required to know the central-ray placement (entry point and exit point) for every radiographic procedure and projection performed to provide optimal images demonstrating

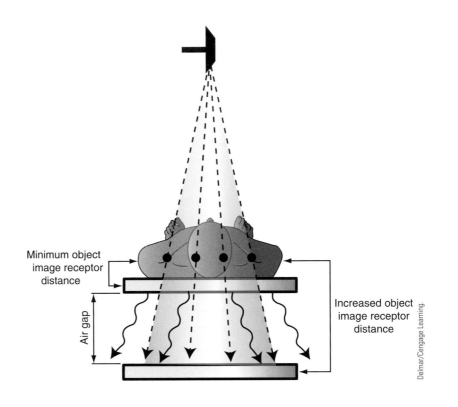

FIGURE 10–1. Air-gap technique.

Minimum object image receptor distance

Air gap

Increased object image receptor distance

Delmar/Cengage Learning.

appropriate anatomic structures. Anatomic structures perpendicular to the central ray (*umbra*) will demonstrate the greatest level of recorded detail. Images created primarily by the diverging part of the x-ray beam (*penumbra*) will show a decrease in recorded detail.

characteristic curve – A characteristic curve can also be referred to as an H&D curve (named after photographers Hurter and Driffield), a D log E curve (density and log relative exposure), or a sensitometric curve. This text will use the term "characteristic curve" as representational of each of the aforementioned alternative names. A characteristic curve may be created by taking several x-ray exposures via use of the same technique while revealing only a small portion of the radiographic film for each exposure, thus creating a doubling of density for every x-ray exposure taken. A better method of creating a gradient of x-ray exposures depicting a doubling of densities would be to use a penetrometer (step wedge) while taking one x-ray exposure. Perhaps the best way to produce a characteristic curve is not to use radiation but rather to use a sensitometer, which produces a gradient of densities (representing a doubling of radiographic densities) by exposing film to a variation of light exposure. The characteristic curve is a graph depicting specific density readings obtained from the film of gradient densities. These density readings depict three important aspects of a radiographic film: sensitivity to x-ray exposure (referred to as film speed), inherent contrast, and exposure latitude. The graph is designed to demonstrate density readings on the vertical axis in correlation to the log relative exposure noted on the horizontal axis. When density readings are obtained (via a densitometer), plotted, and connected, an "s"-shaped curve (characteristic curve) becomes apparent and can be used for characteristic comparisons of more than one film type. Areas of a characteristic

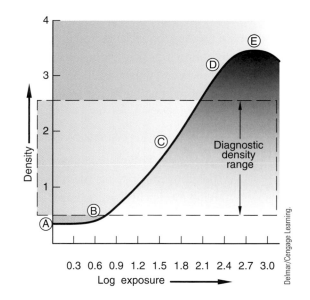

FIGURE 10–2. Characteristic curve.
A. Toe (includes base plus fog).
B. Threshold. *C.* Average gradient.
D. Shoulder. *E.* D-max.

curve are classified according to the amount of density present on a radiograph. The least amount of density is represented by the "toe" portion of the curve, whereas the greatest measurable density on a radiograph would found in the "D-max" portion of the curve. Variations of radiographic densities exist between the *toe* and *D-max*, with the useful range of densities located within the *average gradient* portion of the characteristic curve *(see Figure 10–2).*

- **toe** – The toe area indicates underexposure with densities less than 0.25 and includes the *base plus fog density* (inherent on all radiographic films).

  - **base plus fog** – The base plus fog density is considered an inherent density on a radiographic film that can be measured and recorded once it has undergone film processing. The base plus fog density is attributed to the way in which radiographic film is manufactured, the blue tint of the radiographic film, and the chemical processing the film undergoes in the transformation of latent image to manifest image. The typical range for base plus fog density is approximately 0.10–0.20.

- **threshold** – The threshold area on the curve is located between the toe and average gradient, where the useful density range begins.

- **average gradient/straight line portion** – The average gradient or straight line portion of the curve represents the useful densities of the film. The useful range of optical densities typically lies between 0.25 and 2.5.

- **shoulder** – The shoulder portion of the curve represents overexposure. Shoulder range of densities lie between 2.5 and 4.0.

- **D-max** – The D-max portion of the curve represents the highest degree of measureable density on a radiographic film. D-max is close to or at an optical density of 4.0.

collimation – Collimation is the restriction of the radiation field size by moving both sets of shutters *(longitudinal and horizontal)* on the collimator housing. Most fixed x-ray units have a PBL *(positive beam limiting)* device, which automatically collimates the field size to the IR size once the receptor is inserted into the Bucky tray. It should be noted, however, that even with the use of a PBL device, the technologist should adhere to the *ALARA principle* and further reduce radiation exposure to the patient by collimating on all four sides of an image. Collimation also improves visibility of recorded detail by hindering scatter radiation from reaching the IR. It should be noted that there is an indirect relationship between *collimation* and *collimation field size.*

- An increase in collimation equates to a decrease in the collimation field size.

- Increasing collimation means that the collimation field size gets smaller. Therefore, the opposite holds true: decreasing collimation means that the collimation field size gets larger. (Keep in mind that a change in collimation affects radiographic density and contrast.)

■ **collimation field size** – Collimation field size or just "field size" refers to the actual area of primary radiation distribution. Reducing the field size is the most effective way to decrease the amount of radiation a patient receives during a radiographic procedure. The collimator box is located just beneath the x-ray tube housing and contains two sets of shutters permitting multiple square and rectangular collimation field sizes. Circular beam restriction is possible through the use of cones and cylinders; other odd-shape beam restriction is possible with the use of unique cut-out aperture diaphragms. Cones, cylinders, and aperture diaphragms are designed to slide on and off a clip-like structure that lies just beneath the collimator box. These devices are held securely in place by the clip-like structure and are easily removed when desired (*see beam-restricting devices*).

compression – Compression of a body part will result in a decrease of part thickness. As body part thickness decreases, an increase in radiographic contrast will occur. Increasing radiographic contrast will improve the visibility of structural detail on the image. The saying often used to remember this concept is "less matter equals less scatter." Compression can be accomplished by the use of compression bands or by positioning the body in such a way as to use the weight of the body to compress the area of radiographic interest *(see Figure 10–3).*

computed radiography – Computed radiography, often referred to as CR imaging, uses imaging plates (IPs) containing photostimuable phosphors (PSP) inside an imaging cassette receptor. These plates replace conventional film and can be

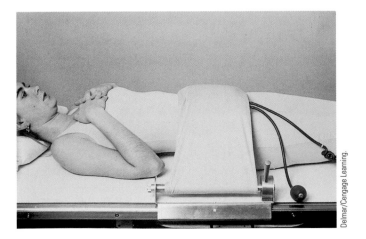

FIGURE 10–3. An example of a compression device. An intravenous urogram (IVU) compression device.

Delmar/Cengage Learning.

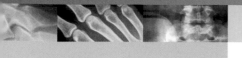

exposed to light without harming the latent image. However, there is no need to open the cassette because the imaging process calls for the cassette to be placed in an IP reader, where the IP is removed and scanned by laser. Information depicting the latent image is then transferred in the form of several energy conversions to produce a visible image to be viewed on a display monitor where electronic manipulation for quality enhancement can occur. The image can then be directly sent to the radiologist for interpretation or archived for future reference *(see Table 10–1)*.

TABLE 10–1 Comparison of Computed Radiography and Digital Radiography

COMPUTED RADIOGRAPHY (CR)	DIGITAL RADIOGRAPHY (DR)
Less expensive than a DR system	More expensive than a CR system
Requires cassettes with PSP IP(s) and a laser scanner reading device	No cassettes or PSP IPs required
IP is reusable	Requires flat panel detectors
Indirect acquisition: X-ray photons interact with the PSP plate; the laser reader scans the IP, and light emitted from the PSP is detected by the photomultiplier tube, which converts light photons to an electronic analog signal to be sent to the ADC (analog-to-digital converter) to be converted to a digital signal for postprocessing/enhancing on display monitor.	Direct acquisition: Includes both *direct amorphous selenium* and *indirect amorphous silicon* ■ *Direct amorphous selenium* (a-Se): Contains flat panel detectors with a layer of a-Se. Voltage is applied across detectors, followed by x-ray photon interaction with a-Se that causes ionization. Liberated electron charges are collected via a storage capacitor and converted to an electrical signal. The electrical signal is amplified and sent to the ADC; the digital signal is sent to a computer for processing the digital image. ■ *Indirect amorphous silicon* (a-Si:H) – Contains flat panel detectors composed of a-Si:H photodiodes with a cesium iodide (CsI) or rare earth scintillator. X-ray photons interact with the scintillator, and the scintillator converts x-ray photons to light photons. a-Si:H photodiodes convert light photons to an electrical signal. The electrical signal is amplified and sent to the ADC; the digital signal is sent to a computer for processing the digital image.
Wide dynamic range (greater latitude than film)	Wide dynamic range (greater latitude than film)
More noise than DR system	Less noise than a CR system
Cassettes with PSP plates can be used with existing portable radiography units	Cannot be used with existing portable radiography units; instead, it would require a DR portable unit
Can be used with existing film/screen radiographic systems	Cannot be used with existing film/screen radiographic systems
Delayed image display	Immediate image display
Reduce repeat exposures with postprocessing enhancement	Reduce repeat exposures with postprocessing enhancement

Data from Carlton, R. R., & Adler, A. M. (2006). *Principles of radiographic imaging: An art and a science* (4th ed.). Clifton Park, NY: Delmar Cengage Learning; Bushong, S. C. (2008). *Radiologic science for technologists: Physics, biology, and protection* (9th ed.). St. Louis, MO: Mosby.

contrast – Contrast describes the difference between adjacent densities on a radiograph. High-contrast images have very noticeable differences between adjacent densities, whereas low-contrast images have little noticeable differences between adjacent densities. The following table depicts the *controlling factors* and the *influencing factors* for radiographic contrast *(see Table 10–2)*.

Image *contrast* and *scale of contrast* are two separate entities with an indirect relationship. Therefore, the controlling and influencing factors that cause an increase in contrast will cause a decrease in the scale of contrast.

■ **long scale of contrast** – A long scale of contrast refers to many shades of densities on a radiographic image, with little noticeable differences between each shade *(see Figure 10–4A)*.

■ **scale of contrast** – Scale of contrast refers to the number of density shades apparent on a radiographic image. The longer the scale of contrast, the more

TABLE 10–2   Controlling and Influencing Factors for Contrast

FACTORS	FACTOR ADJUSTMENT	RESULT OF FACTOR ADJUSTMENT
Controlling factor for contrast		
kVp	Decrease kVp =	Increase in contrast
	Increase kVp =	Decrease in contrast
Influencing factors for contrast		
Collimation	Increase collimation =	Increase in contrast
	Decrease collimation =	Decrease in contrast
Collimation field size	Decrease collimation field size =	Increase in contrast
	Increase collimation field size =	Decrease in contrast
Object-to-image distance (OID)	Increase OID =	Increase in contrast
	Decrease OID =	Decrease in contrast
Film speed	Increase film speed =	Increase in contrast
	Decrease film speed =	Decrease in contrast
Intensifying screen speed*	Increase or decrease =	No effect on contrast
Filtration	Decrease filtration =	Increase in contrast
	Increase filtration =	Decrease in contrast
Grid ratio	Increase grid ratio =	Increase in contrast
	Decrease grid ratio =	Decrease in contrast

*However, when used in conjunction with film as a *film/screen combination*, an increase in film speed will cause an increase in contrast

Data from Carlton, R. R., and Adler, A. M. (2006). *Principles of radiographic imaging: An art and a science* (4th ed.). Clifton Park, NY: Delmar Cengage Learning; Long, B.W., Frank, E. D., and Ehrlich, R. A. (2006). *Radiography essentials for limited practice* (2nd ed.). St. Louis, MO: Mosby; and Wallace, J. (1995). *Radiographic exposure principles & practice*. Philadelphia, PA: F. A. Davis Co.

shades of density there are with less noticeable differences between each shade. The shorter the scale of contrast, the fewer shades of density there are on a radiographic image with more noticeable differences between each shade. Note the inverse relationship between the "scale of contrast" and image "contrast."

- increasing the scale of contrast = a decrease in image contrast
- decreasing the scale of contrast = an increase in image contrast

■ **short scale of contrast** – A short scale of contrast refers to few shades of densities on a radiographic image, with more noticeable differences between each shade *(see Figure 10–4B).*

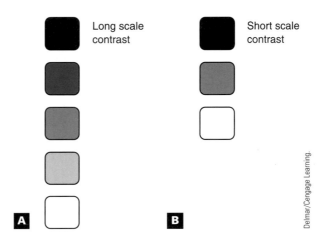

FIGURE 10–4. *A.* Long-scale contrast. *B.* Short-scale contrast.

controlling factors – Controlling factors are the primary technical factors used to adjust either a single radiographic property or several of the four radiographic properties: radiographic density, contrast, detail, and distortion. Controlling factors for each radiographic property vary and are identified separately under each of the four radiographic properties.

crossover, crosstalk – Crossover or crosstalk (also referred to as *parallax*) refers to the loss of detail that occurs on a film with double emulsion. Because the image is created from both emulsion sides and a diverging x-ray beam, the image on the side furthest from the x-ray tube will be slightly misaligned with the image on the emulsion side closest to the x-ray tube. Although this misalignment is minimal, it does cause a slight loss of recorded detail compared to an image produced with single-emulsion film. No crossover occurs with single-emulsion film.

densitometer – A densitometer is a device used to measure radiographic densities on a radiographic film *(see Figure 10–5).*

density – Density is a term used to describe the overall blackness of a radiographic film, or the percentage of light transmitted through a radiographic film when viewed by an illuminator device, most commonly referred to as a viewbox. This definition can be further clarified in the following mathematical equation in which optical density is determined by dividing the incident light intensity by the amount of light transmitted through the processed film.

$$OD = \log_{10} \frac{I_o \text{ (incident light intensity)}}{I_i \text{ (transmitted light intensity)}}$$

A *densitometer* is a device used to measure incident light intensity on radiographic film *(see densitometer)*. However, because optical density (OD) is calculated in a logarithmic manner, one can set up the following chart to easily determine the OD when given a percentage of illuminator light *(see Table 10–3)*. OD ranges as depicted on a characteristic curve begin at zero and go to a maximum of 4. Keep in mind that a processed film will inherently exhibit a small amount of density, known as *base plus fog*, and therefore a density reading of zero will not occur. The typical range for *base plus fog* density is approximately 0.10–0.20. The useful OD ranges of 0.25–2.5 lie within the *straight-line* portion of the characteristic curve, and OD ranges of 3 and 4 are found toward the upper part of the characteristic curve where the shoulder (and D-max) lie.

To know the exact densities on a radiographic film, a densitometer is required. The *controlling factors* for density are mA, exposure time, and mAs. mA multiplied by the exposure time provides a given mAs. The relationship between density and mAs (or any component of mAs) is direct, whereas the relationship between mA and time is indirect. There are numerous *influencing factors* affecting density, including kVp. The relationship between kVp and density is direct. The term "density," however, should not be used regarding digital images because these images involve a computer language (binary code) that allows for manipulation of bits of information (*window*

TABLE 10–3   Transmitted Light and Radiographic Density

% OF ILLUMINATOR LIGHT (TRANSMITTED THROUGH FILM)	OD READING	CHARACTERISTIC CURVE
100%	0	A zero OD reading can never occur because even a film with no x-ray exposure will exhibit a small amount of density once processed; this amount of density is referred to as *base plus fog* density.
10%	1	This OD range lies at the bottom of the *straight-line portion* of the characteristic curve, above the *toe* portion.
1%	2	This OD range lies within the *straight-line portion* of a characteristic curve between the toe and *shoulder* portions of the characteristic curve.
0.1%	3	This OD range lies close to the *shoulder* portion of the characteristic curve, where overexposure is demonstrated.
0.01%	4	This OD range demonstrates overexposure progressing toward *D-max*, where maximum radiographic density occurs.

Data from Carlton, R. R., & Adler, A. M. (2006). *Principles of radiographic imaging: An art and a science* (4th ed.). Clifton Park, NY: Delmar Cengage Learning; Bushong, S. C. (2008). *Radiologic science for technologists: Physics, biology, and protection* (9th ed.). St. Louis, MO: Mosby; and Long, B. W., Frank, E. D., & Ehrlich, R. A. (2006). *Radiography essentials for limited practice* (2nd ed.). St. Louis, MO: Mosby.

leveling and *window width*), resulting in an image that can be lightened or darkened on the display monitor. The *controlling factors* and the *influencing factors* for radiographic density are described in Table 10–4.

TABLE 10–4 Controlling and Influencing Factors for Radiographic Density

FACTORS	FACTOR ADJUSTMENT	RESULT OF FACTOR ADJUSTMENT
Controlling factors for density		
mAs	Increase mAs = Decrease mAs =	Increase in density Decrease in density
mA	Increase mA = Decrease mA =	Increase in density Decrease density
Exposure time	Increase exposure time = Decrease exposure time =	Increase in density Decrease in density
Influencing factors for density		
kVp	Increase kVp = Decrease kVp =	Increase in density Decrease in density
Collimation	Decrease collimation = Increase collimation =	Increase in density Decrease in density
Collimation field size	Increase collimation field size = Decrease collimation field size =	Increase in density Decrease in density
Object-to-image distance (OID)	Decrease OID = Increase OID =	Increase in density Decrease in density
Film/screen combination speed	Increase speed = Decrease speed =	Increase in density Decrease in density
Filtration	Decrease filtration = Increase filtration =	Increase in density Decrease in density
Source-to-image distance (SID)	Decrease SID = Increase SID =	Increase in density Decrease in density
Optimal developer temperature	Increase temperature = Decrease temperature =	Increase in density Decrease in density
Tube angulation*	Decrease tube angle = Increase tube angle =	Increase in density Decrease in density

Tube angulations cause a decrease in density unless compensation in SID is made.

Data from Carlton, R. R., & Adler, A. M. (2006). *Principles of radiographic imaging: An art and a science* (4th ed.). Clifton Park, NY: Delmar Cengage Learning; Long, B. W., Frank, E. D., & Ehrlich, R. A. (2006). *Radiography essentials for limited practice* (2nd ed.). St. Louis, MO: Mosby; and Wallace, J. (1995). *Radiographic exposure principles & practice.* Philadelphia, PA: F. A. Davis Co.

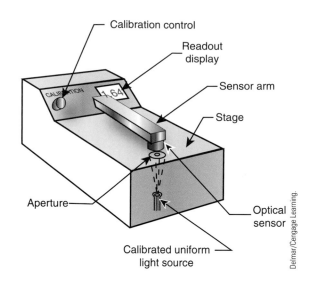

Delmar/Cengage Learning.

FIGURE 10–5. Densitometer.

TABLE 10–5   Options to Double or Halve Radiographic Density

4 OPTIONS TO DOUBLE DENSITY	4 OPTIONS TO HALVE DENSITY
1. Double the mAs.	1. Halve the mAs.
2. Double the mA.	2. Halve the mA.
3. Double the exposure time.	3. Halve the exposure time.
4. Increase kVp by 15%.	4. Decrease kVp by 15%.

Data from Carlton, R. R., & Adler, A. M. (2006). *Principles of radiographic imaging: An art and a science* (4th ed.). Clifton Park, NY: Delmar Cengage Learning; Long, B. W., Frank, E. D., & Ehrlich, R. A. (2006). *Radiography essentials for limited practice* (2nd ed.). St. Louis, MO: Mosby; and Wallace, J. (1995). *Radiographic exposure principles & practice.* Philadelphia, PA: F. A. Davis Co.

■ **doubling density or halving density** – A doubling or halving of density on a radiograph will occur when adjusting the controlling factors of mA or time or by using the influencing factor of kVp *(see Table 10–5).*

> **Note** *Density (overall blackness of a radiographic film) cannot exist on an image produced via CR/DR; rather, areas of darkness on a computed/digital image are due to* image receptor exposure, *with mAs as the controlling factor. Replace the term* density *with* image receptor exposure *when referring to the degree of darkness present on an image produced via a CR or DR imaging system.*

density maintenance formula – *See exposure maintenance formula.*

diagnostic x-ray range – Diagnostic x-ray range refers to the typical ranges of exposure factors selected for diagnostic procedures. These prime exposure factors include time, mA stations, and kVp values; ranges are as follow:

$$\text{exposure times} = 0.001\text{--}10 \text{ seconds}$$
$$\text{mA stations} = 25 \text{ mA--}1200 \text{ mA}$$
$$\text{kVp values} = 25 \text{ kVp--}150 \text{ kVp}$$

digital image acquisition – Digital image acquisition involves acquiring image data and converting the data into a computer language to allow electronic manipulation (post processing enhancement). Image information in the form of picture elements, or *pixels,* is displayed on a monitor for viewing purposes. The number of pixels depicted in rows and columns, along with the *field of view (FOV),* determines the *matrix* size. The larger the matrix size, the smaller the pixels are and the more detailed the image. Matrix sizes can vary greatly from a small matrix size of 256 × 256 to a large matrix size of 4096 × 4096. The 256 × 256 matrix size has large pixels in comparison to the matrix size of 4096 × 4096, which has very small pixels that provide greater image detail.

■ **field of view (FOV)** – Field of view, or FOV, refers to the actual area of anatomical structures seen on a display monitor. Magnification mode results in a decrease of the image intensifier's input phosphor diameter, resulting in a decrease in the FOV and an increase in the size of the structure imaged. FOV and pixel size have a direct relationship; an increase FOV equates to an increase in pixel size *(see Figure 10-6).*

■ **matrix** – A matrix consists of rows and columns of pixels. The larger the matrix size, the better the resolution of the image. Matrix size and resolution have a direct relationship; an increase matrix size equates to an increase in image resolution *(see Figure 10-7).*

■ **pixel** – A pixel represents image data in the form of a brightness level (similar to a density recorded on film). The smaller the pixel size, the better the resolution of the image. Pixel size is determined by dividing the FOV (in the unit of millimeters) by the matrix size. Pixel size and resolution have an indirect relationship; an increase pixel size equates to an decrease in image resolution *(see Figure 10-7).*

Larger FOV

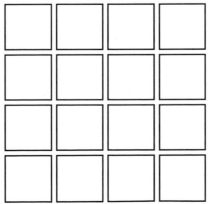

Smaller FOV

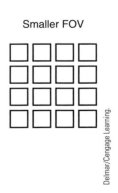

FIGURE 10–6. An increase in field of view (FOV) causes an increase in pixel size.

Delmar/Cengage Learning.

■ **voxel** – A voxel is a three-dimensional representation of tissue volume evident in a pixel *(see Figure 10–7C).*

direct digital radiography – Direct digital radiography, often referred to as digital radiography or DR imaging, employs image detectors, eliminating the need for cassettes. This method of image acquisition permits remnant x-rays (those exiting the patient) to directly interact with digital detectors to produce visible images on a display monitor where electronic manipulation for quality enhancement can occur. Therefore, DR is considered a more efficient (and more expensive) method for producing images because it eliminates the need for several energy conversion processes to occur as is necessary when using film/screen combination and computed radiography. The image can then be directly sent to the radiologist for interpretation and/or archived for future reference *(see Table 10–1).*

direct square law – *See exposure maintenance formula.*

distortion – Distortion refers to a misrepresentation of the true size or shape of an object being imaged. Distortion can be categorized into three main types: *size distortion* (referred to as magnification), *shape distortion*, and *spatial distortion*. The *controlling factors* and the *influencing factors* for distortion are described in Table 10–6.

■ **shape distortion** – Shape distortion, otherwise known as *elongation* or *foreshortening*, occurs as a result of the body part not lying parallel to the IR or

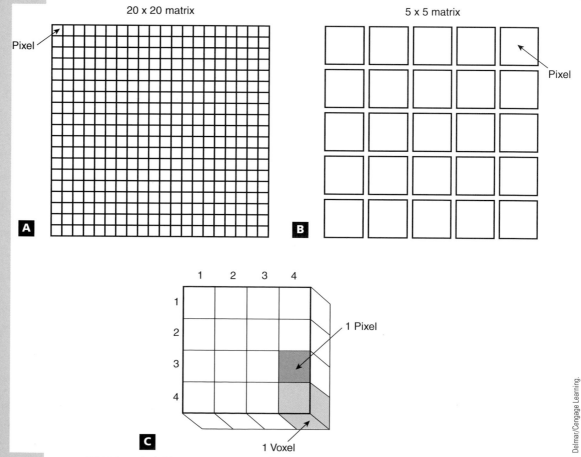

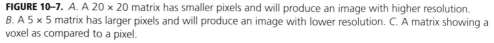

FIGURE 10–7. *A.* A 20 × 20 matrix has smaller pixels and will produce an image with higher resolution. *B.* A 5 × 5 matrix has larger pixels and will produce an image with lower resolution. *C.* A matrix showing a voxel as compared to a pixel.

TABLE 10–6   Controlling and Influencing Factors for Distortion

FACTORS	FACTOR ADJUSTMENT	RESULT OF FACTOR ADJUSTMENT
Controlling factors for size distortion		
Object-to-image distance (OID)	Decrease OID =	Increase in recorded detail
	Increase OID =	Decrease in recorded detail
Source-to-image distance (SID)	Decrease SID =	Decrease in recorded detail
	Increase SID =	Increase in recorded detail
Controlling factors for shape distortion		
Central ray/body part/IR alignment	Central ray perpendicular to body part and IR (with body part and IR parallel to each other) =	Decrease in shape distortion
Influencing factors for size distortion		
Part thickness	Decrease part thickness (compression) =	Decrease in size distortion
	Increase part thickness (compression) =	Increase in size distortion
Body part position	Body part positioned closest to IR =	Decrease in size distortion
	Body part positioned away from IR =	Increase in size distortion

Data from Carlton, R. R., & Adler, A. M. (2006). *Principles of radiographic imaging: An art and a science* (4th ed.). Clifton Park, NY: Delmar Cengage Learning; Long, B. W., Frank, E. D., & Ehrlich, R. A. (2006). *Radiography essentials for limited practice* (2nd ed.). St. Louis, MO: Mosby; and Wallace, J. (1995). *Radiographic exposure principles & practice.* Philadelphia, PA: F. A. Davis Co.

by improper alignment of the x-ray tube, body part, and IR. Ideally, the central beam should be perpendicular to the body part and the IR, with the body part and IR placed parallel to each other.

- **elongation** – Elongation refers to a type of shape distortion depicted on a radiographic image caused by misalignment of the x-ray tube, body part, and IR. Elongation can be intentionally done to remove superimposition of body parts or to stretch out a body part to better visualize small anatomical structures. For example, angulation of the x-ray tube will cause distortion of an object being imaged. Elongation can occur when the object is parallel to the IR but the central ray is angled, or if the central ray is perpendicular to the object being imaged but the object and IR are not parallel to each other *(see Figure 10–8)*.

- **foreshortening** – Foreshortening occurs when the body part being imaged is not placed parallel to the IR, even though the central ray is perpendicular to the IR. Body parts are typically irregular in shape and often naturally occur at an angle within the body. The appearance of foreshortening on a radiographic image can mask pathological findings and may require tube angulation or special radiographic projections to compensate for this type of shape distortion *(see Figure 10–8)*.

- **spatial distortion** – Spatial distortion is inherent on a radiographic image because of the three-dimensional relationship between the

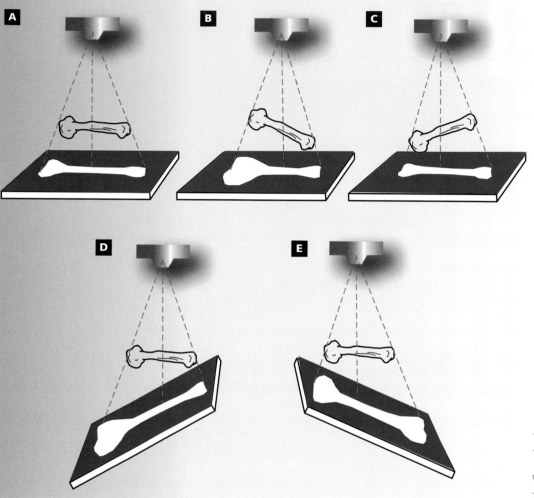

FIGURE 10–8. *A.* Size distortion (magnification). *B* and *C.* Foreshortening. *D* and *E.* Elongation.

Delmar/Cengage Learning.

patient's body parts (as well as the thickness of the patient) and the divergence of the x-ray beam. Body parts farther away from the IR will appear more distorted in comparison to the body parts that lie closer to the IR; therefore, actual space between body parts will be inaccurately depicted on the image. Divergence of the x-ray beam will distort anatomical structures that lie farther away from the most perpendicular portion of the x-ray beam. Angulation of the x-ray tube further compromises the actual space existing between body parts and that which is depicted on the radiographic image *(see Figure 10–9).*

■ **size distortion** – Size distortion, otherwise known as magnification, exists on every radiographic image due to anatomical structures being three dimensional and due to an OID that can never be completely eliminated. The larger the three-dimensional object being imaged, the greater the amount of distortion appearing on the image. The larger the OID, the greater the amount of distortion appearing on the image. Another factor affecting size distortion is the SID (source-to-image distance). The greater the SID, the lesser the amount of distortion appearing on the radiographic image. The rule of thumb

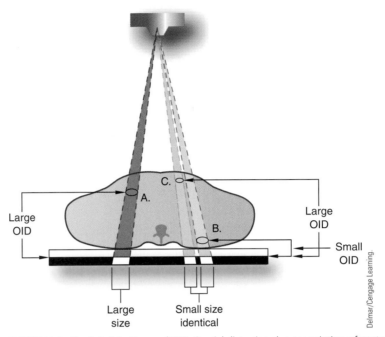

FIGURE 10–9. Spatial distortion and OID. Spatial distortion due to variation of part size and body location relevant to the diverging central ray and the IR. *A.* Large OID and large body part size. *B.* Smallest OID and large body part size. *C.* Largest OID and smallest body part size.

for decreasing size distortion is to increase the SID and decrease the OID (the technologist has no control over the size of the three-dimensional anatomical structure(s) being imaged).

exposure – Exposure can refer to the amount of radiation in the air, the amount of radiation a patient or a population receives, or the amount of radiation an occupational worker encounters within the scope of practice *(see Table 10–7).*

exposure factors/technique – Exposure factors or exposure technique refers to the *four prime factors* (kVp, mA, time, and SID) selected by the technologist to produce a high-quality diagnostic image. The technologist should always adhere to the ALARA principle, which promotes high kVp and low mAs exposure technique selections.

TABLE 10–7   Measuring Units for Radiation Exposure

TRADITIONAL UNIT	MEASURES	TRADITIONAL SYMBOL	SI UNIT (SYMBOL)
roentgen	Radiation in air	R	coulomb per kilogram (C/kg)
rad	Absorbed dose *(patient)*	rad	Gray (Gy)
rem	Effective dose *(occupational worker)*	rem	sievert (Sv)
curie	Radioactivity	Ci	becquerel (Bq)

Data from Carlton, R. R., & Adler, A. M. (2006). *Principles of radiographic imaging: An art and a science* (4th ed.). Clifton Park, NY: Delmar Cengage Learning; Bushong, S. C. (2008). *Radiologic science for technologists: Physics, biology, and protection* (9th ed.). St. Louis, MO: Mosby.

- **kVp** – Kilovoltage peak, or kVp, refers to the thousands of volts necessary to accelerate the electrons produced by thermionic emission across the vacuum x-ray tube (from cathode to anode). kVp determines the penetrability (i.e., quality) of the x-ray beam. The higher the kVp, the more penetrating and energetic the x-ray beam and the lower the patient dose will be. kVp can be referred to as an electromotive force or a potential force. kVp is an *influencing factor* for radiographic density and a *controlling factor* for x-ray beam penetrability and radiographic contrast. In general, it takes a small change in kVp (2–4 kVp) when using a lower kVp range (40–60 kVp) to produce a noticeable change in density, i.e., one that could be detected by the naked eye without the use of any special measuring devices. However, as the range of kVp increases, a greater incremental change in kVp (5–10 kVp) is required to see a noticeable difference in radiographic density. Keep in mind that it takes a 15% increase in kVp to cause a doubling of radiographic density.

  - **kilovolt (kV)** – 1000 volts are equal to 1 kilovolt (1000 volts = 1 kV).

- **mAs** – mAs is the amount of tube current flowing over a given time. It is the product of mA and exposure time, mathematically depicted as: mA × s = mAs.

  - **exposure time** – Exposure times can range between fractions of a second to several seconds (approximate diagnostic range of 0.001–10 seconds) and are chosen accordingly to either hinder involuntary motion naturally occurring within a patient or to create motion as in a breathing technique. Both short and long exposure times can be used to improve the visibility of anatomic structures on image when used correctly. Exposure time combined with a selected mA station results in a specific quantity of mAs.

  - **mA** – Milliamperage is a unit to measure electrical current. A milliampere *(or milliamp)* is 1/1000 of 1 ampere of current. X-ray tube currents have correlating mA stations provided on the control console. Typical mA stations range between 25 mA to 1600 mA (milliamperes) and control heating of the filament, which in turn controls the quantity of electrons and x-ray photons produced.

- **SID (source-to-image distance)** – SID describes the distance between the effective focal spot (point of image production) and the IR. The source-to-image distance for radiographic procedures is typically standardized with recommended distances of 40–44 inches or 72 inches. Keep in mind that the greater the SID, the less magnification and distortion present on an image (this is the premise for doing chest x-rays at a 72-inch SID to reduce magnification of the heart).

exposure index (EI) number – Manufacturers of CR/DR imaging systems provide a range of exposures for producing optimal images. The numeric range will vary depending on the type of imaging system used (e.g., Agfa, GE, Siemens, Kodak, Fuji). The exposure index (EI) number indicates the amount of radiation received by the IR to produce the image. The number provides information relevant to underexposure, overexposure, and noise detected. The EI number is especially valuable in assessing underexposure and overexposure because these factors are not visually apparent on the image but are significant in determining the quality of recorded information and the radiation dose to the patient. Terms similar to the EI number that manufacturers may use include:

- **DEI number** – detector exposure index
- **EXI number** – exposure index
- **LgM number** – log median exposure
- **"S" number** – sensitivity of IR/detector
- **REV number** – reached exposure value
- **exposure rate** – Exposure rate refers to the intensity of the useful beam per milliampere per second (mR/mAs).

exposure maintenance formula – The exposure maintenance formula is a mathematical equation used to calculate the amount of mAs required to maintain radiographic exposure with CR/DR imaging systems after a change in SID has occurred. The formula was previously known as the *density maintenance formula* when the image receptor consisted of a film/screen combination. The formula may also be referred to as the *direct square law* because of the direct relationship between mAs (controlling factor for image receptor exposure/density) and the changing distance (SID). For example, two images taken with the same exposure factors and the same SID will yield two images with the same image receptor exposure/radiographic density. However, with all exposure factors kept constant and SID increased, the resulting radiographic image would appear lighter with less image receptor exposure/radiographic density than the original image with the shorter SID. Therefore, we can say that an increase in SID will require an increase in mAs in order to maintain image receptor exposure/radiographic density between the two images taken at different SIDs. Mathematically this concept is depicted as:

$$\frac{mAs_1}{mAs_1} = \frac{D_1^{(2)}}{D_2^{(2)}}$$

mAs_1 = original mAs

mAs_2 = new mAs (to maintain image receptor exposure/ radiographic density after a change in SID has occurred)

$D_1^{(2)}$ = original distance squared

$D_2^{(2)}$ = new distance squared

fifteen percent (15%) rule – The 15% rule is a mathematical equation used for calculating adjustments in the technical factors of mAs and kVp when a change in image contrast is desired without a change in image density. kVp is the controlling factor for contrast and an influencing factor for radiographic density. Subsequently, a change in kVp will result in a change in both *contrast* and *density*. The 15% rule states that a 15% increase in kVp will result in a decrease in radiographic contrast and a doubling of radiographic density. To only decrease image contrast, a 15% increase in kVp is required along with a halving of the mAs. Halving the mAs is necessary to compensate for the doubling of density that results when the kVp is increased by 15%. The same principle holds true for a 15% decrease in kVp.

TABLE 10–8   The 15% Rule

kVp CHANGE	EFFECT ON CONTRAST	ADJUST mAs TO MAINTAIN DENSITY
Increase kVp by 15%	Decreases	Halve the original mAs (divide by 2).
Decrease kVp by 15%	Increases	Double the original mAs (multiply by 2).

Note: In the diagnostic range of 60–90 kVp, a 15% increase or decrease in kVp is a difference of approximately 10 kVp.

Data from Carlton, R. R., & Adler, A. M. (2006). *Principles of radiographic imaging: An art and a science* (4th ed.); and Wallace, J. (1995). *Radiographic exposure principles & practice.* Philadelphia, PA: F. A. Davis Co.

Decreasing kVp by 15% will result in an increase in image contrast and a halving of radiographic density. To compensate for the reduction in density when kVp has been decreased by 15%, a doubling of mAs is necessary *(see Table 10–8)*. The following three exposure techniques will produce images with the same overall density but with variations in contrast.

> 75 kVp at 40 mAs

> 86 kVp at 20 mAs

■ 15% increase in kVp ($75 \times 0.15 = 11.3$) – Add 11 to 75 to obtain new kVp of 86 and halve the original mAs of 40 to 20 to maintain the density of the original technique.

> 64 kVp at 80 mAs

■ 15% decrease in kVp ($75 \times 0.5 = 11.3$) – Subtract 11 from 75 to obtain new kVp 64 and double the original mAs of 40 to 80 to maintain density of the original technique.

filament – *Refer to Chapter 8: X-ray Tube.*

film – Film is an image-recording medium consisting of a thin flexible polyester base with either a single-emulsion side or a double-emulsion side. An adhesive layer joins the emulsion layer to the film base, and a protective coating or "supercoat" protects the emulsion layer from scratches during handling. The emulsion layer contains silver halide crystals composed of ions of silver (Ag^+), bromine (Br^-), and iodine (I^-). Enhancing film sensitivity are *sensitivity specks* located within the lattice of the of the silver halide crystals. Latent image formation begins at the sensitivity specks *(see Figure 10–10)*. Radiographic film is tinted blue to reduce glare and *crossover*; however, the tint produces an inherent density on the film which must be considered when evaluating *base plus fog* readings.

film type – Radiographic film is being replaced by CR and DR imaging. However, there are still many imaging centers and physician offices that use film to produce diagnostic images. Various types of film include:

■ **direct-exposure film** – Direct-exposure film, also referred to as *nonscreen film*, uses a cardboard or plastic holder that is designed to protect the film from light exposure. With direct-exposure film, the image is created solely by exposure to radiation; there are no intensifying screens present. Direct-exposure film requires a much higher quantity of radiation to produce an image than that required to produce an image using a film/screen combination. For this reason, direct-exposure film is considered obsolete in diagnostic radiography.

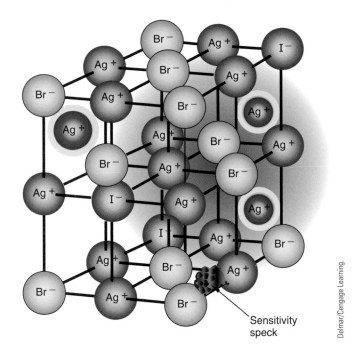

Sensitivity
speck

Delmar/Cengage Learning.

FIGURE 10–10. Film cubic lattice.

- **duplicating film** – Duplicating film, also referred to as copy film, is a single-emulsion film that has undergone *solarization* for the purpose of duplicating a radiographic image.

- **laser film** – Laser film requires a laser printer and an electronic signal from an imaging system to create the image on the film. The laser moves across and down the film (raster pattern), exposing the film to variations of light (dictated by the strength of the electronic signal) until the entire image is formed. The film is sensitive to the complete spectrum of light and therefore must be handled in total darkness.

- **roll film** – Roll film is packaged in a roll and can only be used with imaging systems that are able to accommodate this type of film. Roll film requires a loading container or magazine from which the roll film is advanced as the imaging system operator takes exposures and a second magazine or container into which the exposed roll of film collects. Typically, roll film is used for radiographic studies of organ or system function where a rapid succession of exposures occurs. A special lead device is necessary for feeding and aligning the exposed roll film (collected in the second magazine) through the film processor, thus avoiding damage to the film or processor.

- **screen film** – Screen film is a type of film designed for use with a film cassette containing either one or two intensifying screens. The two types of screen film are:

  - **double-emulsion film** – Double-emulsion film contains a film base with two emulsion sides. Double-emulsion film is designed for use with a film cassette containing two intensifying screens.

  - **single-emulsion film** – Single-emulsion film contains a film base with only one emulsion side. Single-emulsion film is designed for use with a film cassette containing one intensifying screen.

■ **solarized film** – Solarized film has undergone the process of solarization in which the film has been pre-exposed to light, causing maximum density on the film. After further exposure to light, a reverse effect will occur, resulting in a decrease in density.

film cassette – A film cassette is an IR that may contain a single intensifying screen or two intensifying screens along with a radiographic film. The front of the cassette is typically made of a material with a low atomic number, such as carbon fiber or magnesium, to allow x-ray photons to pass through easily for interaction with the intensifying screen and film. The back of the cassette is lead-lined to absorb backscatter. Film cassettes come in various sizes; the most common sizes (in inches) are 5×7, 8×10, 11×14, and 14×17.

film contrast – Film contrast is inherent in the manufacture of film. High-contrast film produces a radiographic image with few shades of gray (short-scale contrast) and a noticeable difference between each shade. Low-contrast film produces a radiographic image with many shades of gray (long-scale contrast) and a less noticeable difference between each shade.

film processor – A film processor or automatic processor is a device that transforms a latent radiographic image into a manifest radiographic image through a series of chemical reactions involving *developer* and *fixer* solutions. Once the film is advanced from the developer to the fixer solution, it goes through a wash (water) compartment to remove any residual chemicals, followed by a drying compartment in which the film emulsion dries and hardens. This process usually takes 30–90 seconds to complete. As CR and DR replace film/screen imaging, the need for film processors will eventually become obsolete. However, film processing and chemicals are mentioned to provide a reference for the evolution of image production within the radiologic profession *(see Table 10–9).*

film/screen combination – Film/screen combination is the use of radiographic film in conjunction with either one intensifying screen cassette or in conjunction with a double intensifying screen cassette. It is estimated that 99% of latent image formation is directly due to light emission from the intensifying screen phosphors when struck by x-ray photons, leaving only 1% of latent image formation attributed to actual x-ray photon interaction. Use of a double intensifying screen cassette (contains two intensifying screens with the radiographic film sandwiched between each intensifying screen) decreases radiation exposure to the patient but also causes a loss of recorded detail on the image as the result of *crossover.*

■ **spectral matching** – Spectral matching refers to matching a film's sensitivity to the color of light emitted from intensifying screen phosphors when stuck by x-ray photons. Proper matching of film sensitivity to light spectrum will provide for the best recording of the object being imaged without causing additional radiation exposure to the patient.

film speed – The speed of a film correlates to its sensitivity to x-ray exposure. Higher film speed means higher sensitive to x-ray exposure. A high-speed film therefore requires less radiation exposure than film with a slower speed to produce an optimal image. The advantage to using a higher-speed film as opposed to a slower-speed film is the decrease in x-ray photons necessary to produce the image; this equates to lower patient dose. The disadvantage of a high-speed film in comparison

TABLE 10–9   Film Processing and Chemicals

AGENT	CHEMICAL	EFFECT
Developer		**Reduce exposed silver halide crystals to black metallic silver**
■ reducing agents	*Hydroquinone*	Develops the black densities
	Phenidone	Develops the gray densities
■ activator	*Sodium carbonate*	Swells emulsion, maintains alkaline pH level
■ restrainer	*Potassium bromide*	Controls fog
■ preservative	*Sodium sulfite*	Extends life of developer
■ hardener	*Glutaraldehyde*	Hardens emulsion
Fixer		**Remove unexposed and undeveloped silver halide crystals**
■ clearing agent	*Ammonium thiosulfate (hypo)*	Removes undeveloped silver halide crystals
■ activator	*Acetic acid*	Stops reducing agents, maintains acid pH level
■ preservative	*Sodium sulfite*	Extends life of fixer
■ hardener	*Potassium alum*	Hardens emulsion
Wash	Water circulates around film	**Removes residual chemicals from film**
Dry	Hot air (120°–150°F) circulates around the film	**Dries and hardens film emulsion**

Data from Carlton, R. R., & Adler, A. M. (2006). *Principles of radiographic imaging: An art and a science* (4th ed.). Clifton Park, NY: Delmar Cengage Learning; Bushong, S. C. (2008). *Radiologic science for technologists: Physics, biology, and protection* (9th ed.). St. Louis, MO: Mosby; Long, B. W., Frank, E. D., & Ehrlich, R. A. (2006). *Radiography essentials for limited practice* (2nd ed.). St. Louis, MO: Mosby; and Wallace, J. (1995). *Radiographic exposure principles & practice.* Philadelphia, PA: F. A. Davis Co.

with a slow-speed film is the loss of detail that high-speed film produces. A film speed of 100 is considered to be par or medium speed; film speed below 100 is considered a slow speed and is used when high detail is required, and film speeds above 100 are considered high-speed films and are used primarily to reduce radiation exposure to patients. Radiographic film is used in conjunction with intensifying screens to further reduce radiation exposure to patients; this is referred to as the film/screen combination.

filtration – *Refer to Chapter 8: X-ray Tube.*

fog – Fog is unwanted radiographic density that hinders the visibility of recorded detail on a radiographic film. Fog can be produced by heat, humidity, automatic processing conditions, chemical fumes, light, and radiation.

four prime factors – There are four prime factors used in the selection of an exposure technique. The four prime factors involved in the production of a radiographic image are: *kVp, mA, time,* and *distance (see exposure factors/technique).*

four radiographic properties – There are four radiographic properties used to judge overall (film) image quality: *contrast, density, recorded detail,* and *distortion.* These four radiographic properties can be further categorized into either *photographic properties* or *geometric properties,* with *density* and *contrast* falling under photographic properties and *detail* and *distortion* falling under geometric properties. It should be noted that, with CR and DR (computed radiography and digital radiography) imaging systems, the term *density* (overall blackness on a radiograph) should not be used as the imaging system does not involve film and "light" to produce an image. Terms used with respect to CR and DR images are *window width* and *window leveling.*

geometric blur – Geometric blur or image blur is the unsharpness of anatomical structures on a radiographic image. Where there is geometric blur, there is a loss of recorded detail. Geometric blur (also referred to as *penumbra*) exists on every radiographic image due to the divergence of the x-ray beam. The highest degree of geometric blur will occur around the periphery of the image as distance increases from the area at which the central ray was directed.

geometric properties – Geometric properties (*detail* and *distortion*) describe the degree of structural sharpness apparent on a radiographic image. Geometric properties in conjunction with *photographic properties* (density and contrast) are considered part of the *four radiographic properties* used to judge overall image quality.

grid – A grid is a device used to hinder secondary (scatter) radiation from reaching the IR. Grids are composed of lead lines (absorbing material) and radiolucent spacing material typically made of plastic or aluminum. Grid use is recommended when body part thickness exceeds 10 cm and/or when the selected kVp exceeds 60.

■ **cross-hatch grid** – A cross-hatch grid is composed of two parallel (linear) grids, one placed on top of the other at a 90° angle. A cross-hatch grid limits the radiographer to using a perpendicular beam (no tube angulation) to avoid producing grid-cut off on the image. The use of a cross-hatch grid is uncommon today in diagnostic imaging *(see Figure 10–11).*

■ **focused (nonlinear) grid** – A focused grid is more commonly used because the grid lines are angled to match the divergence of the x-ray beam. Focused grids are designed to accommodate a specific source-to-image distance in order to have the diverging x-ray beam align with the angled grid lines; this distance range is called the focal range and is listed on the focused grid *(see Figure 10–12).*

■ **parallel (linear) grid** – A parallel grid incorporates grid lines that run parallel to each other. This type of grid is not recommended for large image sizes (11 × 14 inches and 14 × 17 inches) or when a short SID is required, because grid cut-off becomes noticeable at the lateral edges of the image *(see Figure 10–13).*

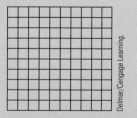

FIGURE 10–11. Cross-hatch grid pattern.

Delmar/Cengage Learning.

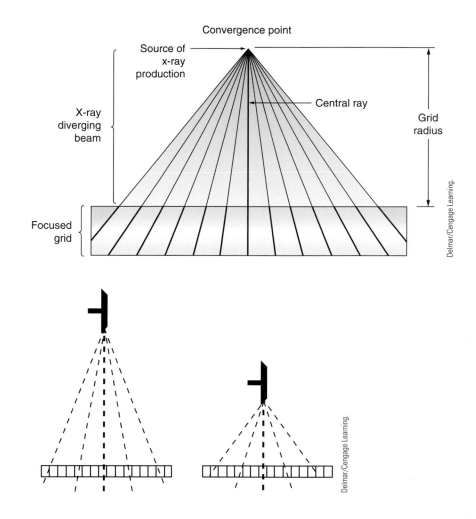

FIGURE 10–12. Focused nonlinear grid.

FIGURE 10–13. Parallel (linear) grid.

grid cut-off – When primary radiation is absorbed by the grid as opposed to absorption of secondary radiation, grid cut-off occurs. This is an undesirable outcome as it causes white lines to obscure the anatomy being imaged. There are five common errors that result in grid cut-off:

1. **off-centering** – Off-centering is also referred to as lateral decentering. This error occurs when the central ray is not centered to the IR, resulting in an overall reduction of radiation reaching the IR.

2. **off-focus** – Off-focus refers to using an incorrect focal distance (source-to-image distance) causing grid cut-off to appear at the lateral margins of the image. Manufacturers indicate on the grid the appropriate focal distal required in order to avoid this type of error.

3. **off-level** – Off-level refers to the central ray not being perpendicular to the IR, either due to the tube being angled or the IR being angled. This typically results in one side of the image demonstrating severe grid cut-off.

4. **incorrect tube angulation** – Incorrect tube angulation refers to angling the x-ray tube perpendicular to the grid lines rather than parallel to the grid lines. This will result in grid cut-off. To avoid grid cut-off when angling the tube, the long axis of the grid must be parallel to the direction of the tube angle.

5. **upside-down** – Upside-down refers to placing the grid upside down. Incorrect grid placement of a focused/nonlinear grid will result in extreme grid cut-off on both lateral sides, with only the center free from grid cut-off. Manufacturers indicate on the grid which side is to face the source of radiation in order to avoid this type of error.

grid frequency – Grid frequency is the number of grid lines per centimeter or per inch. Most grid frequencies range between 60 and 200 lines per inch. The more lines a grid has, the higher the grid frequency and the less noticeable the lines are on an image *(see Figure 10–14).*

grid radius – Grid radius refers to the appropriate SID for a focused grid to provide proper alignment of the diverging x-ray beam and the lead lines of the grid, thus avoiding grid cut-off *(see Figure 10–12).*

grid ratio – Grid ratio refers to the ratio between the height of the lead strips (h) and the distance (D) between the lead strips. The formula **h/D** is used to calculate grid ratio. The higher the grid ratio, the less scatter reaches the IR. However, the disadvantage of using a high grid ratio (16:1) is the increase in exposure factors required to compensate for the removal of radiation by the grid; this would result in higher patient dose *(see Figure 10–15).*

half-value layer – Half-value layer (HVL) is the unit of measure for x-ray beam penetrability. A half-value layer is the amount of absorbing material placed in the path of the x-ray beam to reduce the x-ray beam's intensity to half its original value.

histogram – A histogram is a digital analysis graph depicting the frequencies of pixel values of a radiographic image. With proper positioning of the body

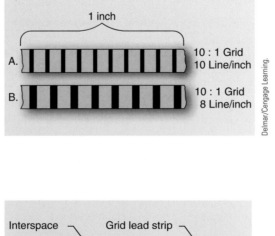

FIGURE 10–14. Grid frequency.

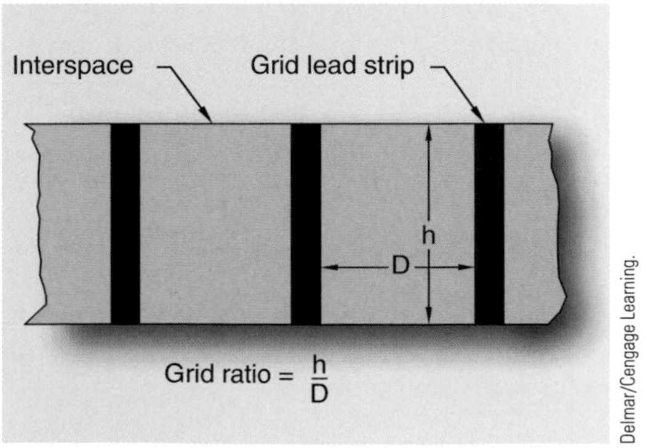

FIGURE 10–15. **III** Grid ratio – lines and space.

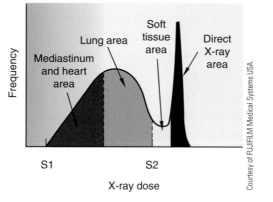

FIGURE 10–16. A histogram.

part and appropriate technical factors set, identical projections are expected to produce similar histograms. A histogram depicting an optimal projection can be stored in the computer system, allowing future projections of the same anatomical area to be rescaled using the pixel values of the optimal histogram (*see Figure 10–16*).

- **look-up table (LUT)** – The LUT provides standardized information regarding the contrast, speed, and latitude for a given projection. This information is provided to allow for a consistent brightness level and a consistent scale of contrast for images of the same anatomical area of interest.

image magnification – Image magnification is a type of size distortion and exists to some degree on all radiographic images because of the inherent distance between the body part and the IR. Because of the three-dimensional shape of the body and the location of the anatomical area of interest within the body, a varying degree of magnification will be present on the radiographic image. Some basic principles must be kept in mind when assessing magnification:

- An increase in OID (object-to-image distance) results in increased magnification.

- A decrease in SID (source-to-image distance) results in increased magnification.

- Image size will always be larger than object size.

To reduce image magnification:

- Position the body part closest to IR.

- Increase SID for any OID that may exist (for 7 inches of SID, correct 1 inch of OID).

Calculating magnification (cross-multiply and solve for missing factor):

$$\frac{\text{image size}}{\text{object size}} = \frac{\text{SID}}{\text{SOD}}$$

Calculating for magnification factor:

$$\frac{\text{image size}}{\text{object size}} \quad \text{or} \quad \frac{\text{SID}}{\text{SOD}}$$

Calculating for percent of magnification:

$$\frac{\text{image size} - \text{object size}}{\text{object size}} \times 100 = \% \text{ of magnification}$$

$$\frac{\text{OID}}{\text{SOD}} \times 100 = \% \text{ of magnification}$$

image receptor (IR) – Image receptors (IR) vary in size and image acquisition method. Image receptors include film/screen cassettes, CR cassettes (containing a PSP imaging plate), and digital detectors (along with a flat panel display monitor) for electronic manipulation as used in DR.

image stitching – Image stitching is a postprocessing enhancement method that allows for the joining of several digital images to create one single image for better visualization of anatomical areas that span distances longer than the size of the largest IR. Image stitching is often used for studies involving the vertebral column and vascular system.

influencing factors – Influencing factors are secondary technical factors that, when adjusted, have an impact on one or on several of the four radiographic properties: radiographic density, contrast, detail, and distortion. There are numerous influencing factors for each of the four radiographic properties, with the most common influencing factors listed separately under each radiographic property.

intensifying screen – An intensifying screen is used with a film-imaging system in which either a single intensifying screen or double intensifying screens are present within the film cassette. Intensifying screens are typically made of a thin, flexible, plastic or cardboard base containing an active layer of rare earth phosphors (replacing calcium tungsten phosphors, which were the phosphor of choice several decades ago, but have been found to be less efficient than rare earth phosphors) that, when struck by x-ray photons, emit light *isotropically*. It is the light emission that forms the *latent image* on the film.

- **afterglow/phosphorescence** – Afterglow or phosphorescence is the continuation of intensifying screen phosphors to emit light after being struck by x-ray photons. This is an undesirable effect.

- **fluorescence** – Fluorescence is the light emitted from intensifying screen phosphors when struck by x-ray photons.

- **relative speed value** – Relative speed value (RSV) describes the various film/screen combination speeds of intensifying screens and radiographic film. Typically film/screen speeds range between 100 and 1200. Slower film/screen speeds (<100) are considered "detail cassettes" and are used when a high degree of detail is required (usually regarding extremities). Because intensifying screens are used with film, it is best to keep in mind that a *spectral matching* between film sensitivity and intensifying screen fluorescence is necessary. The faster the RSV of the intensifying screen/film, the lower the quantity of x-ray photons required to produce a diagnostic image and the lower the patient dose; detail, however, is lessened. The relationship between RSV and mAs is an indirect relationship. The greater the RSV, the less mAs that is required. The following formula can be used when an acceptable technique has been established with a particular intensifying screen speed and mAs, and a change in screen speed is desired requiring the calculation for a new mAs. Remember, when using the formula, (1) represents the original technique and (2) represents what you are changing to.

$$\frac{mAs_1}{mAs_2} = \frac{RSV_2}{RSV_1}$$

intensifying screen phosphors – Intensifying screen phosphors are tiny crystals that emit light *isotropically* when struck by x-ray photons. This *fluorescence* of light will vary in color depending on the type of phosphors used.

- **calcium tungstate phosphors** – These phosphors emit a blue-violet light when struck by x-ray photons. Calcium tungstate phosphors have been replaced by more efficient phosphors, known as rare earth phosphors.

- **rare earth phosphors** – These phosphors are known to emit a yellow-green light when struck by x-ray photons; however, some rare earth phosphors being used today emit a blue-violet or red light. With a wide color spectrum of light possible, it is important for spectral matching to be considered. Rare earth phosphors are the phosphors of choice due to their high conversion efficiency in transforming x-ray photon energy into light energy. The three main rare earth phosphors are gadolinium, lanthanum, and yttrium.

intensity – X-ray beam intensity is measured in the unit roentgen (R) or milliroentgen (mR). Beam intensity and SID have an indirect relationship. This relationship is better known as the *inverse square law* and is used to calculate the increase or decrease in beam intensity when a change in SID has occurred.

inverse square law – The inverse square law is a mathematical equation depicting the inverse relationship between SID and radiation intensity. As the SID increases, radiation intensity decreases. Radiation intensity is measured in the unit roentgen (R) or milliroentgen (mR). SID can be measured in units of centimeters, inches, or feet.

- Increase SID by a factor of 2 *(doubling the SID)* to decrease radiation by a factor of 4, or 1/4 of the original radiation intensity.

- Decrease SID by a factor of 2 *(half the SID)* to increase radiation by a factor of 4, or 4 times the original radiation intensity.

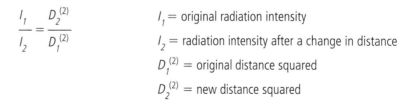

$$\frac{I_1}{I_2} = \frac{D_2^{(2)}}{D_1^{(2)}}$$

I_1 = original radiation intensity

I_2 = radiation intensity after a change in distance

$D_1^{(2)}$ = original distance squared

$D_2^{(2)}$ = new distance squared

isotropic – Isotropic refers to a uniform spreading in all directions from a single point of origin *(see Figure 10–17)*.

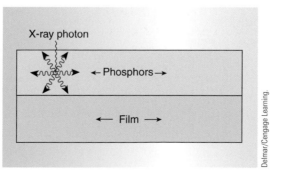

FIGURE 10–17. Light distributed isotropically.

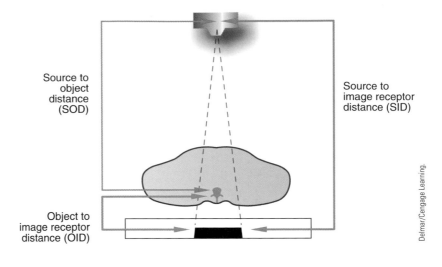

FIGURE 10–18. SOD (tube/patient).

Source to object distance (SOD)

Source to image receptor distance (SID)

Object to image receptor distance (OID)

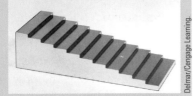

FIGURE 10–19. Penetrometer.

latent image – The latent image is the invisible image produced on a film after x-ray exposure but prior to film processing.

manifest image – The manifest image is the visible image produced after the latent image has undergone film processing.

moiré pattern – A moiré pattern is a digital imaging acquisition artifact associated with computed radiography. This pattern hinders recorded detail of the image and can be attributed to the following factors: use of a stationary grid, grid frequency matching the frequency of the laser scanner as it scans the CR imaging plate, or the laser scanner being parallel to the direction of the grid lines.

non-screen film – *See direct-exposure film.*

object-to-image distance (OID) – Object-to-image distance (OID) is the greatest factor affecting the amount of size distortion present on a radiographic image. The greater the OID, the greater the size distortion present on an image. The rule of thumb for reducing distortion caused by OID is to compensate with an increase in SID *(see Figure 10–18).*

◼   For every 1 inch of OID, increase the SID by 7 inches.

parallax – *See crossover/crosstalk.*

penetrometer – A penetrometer, also referred to as a step wedge, is a device with various steps of aluminum or plastic, with each step representing a doubling of tissue density. When radiographing a penetrometer, one can easily see the density variations, which are measurable with a densitometer and are applicable to the creation of a *characteristic curve (see Figure 10–19).*

penumbra – Penumbra, also referred to as *geometric blur* or *image blur*, describes the loss of detail on anatomical structures being radiographed. The greatest degree of penumbra will occur around the periphery of the image furthest away from the most central part of the x-ray beam. However, the cathode side of the image will always exhibit slightly more penumbra or image blur than the anode side of the image due to greater x-ray beam divergency resulting from the angled anode target. Keep in mind that the greatest degree of recorded detail, known as *umbra*, occurs at the area of anatomical interest to which the central beam is directed. The degree of penumbra on an image can be determined mathematically using the following formula:

$$Penumbra = FSS \times OID/SOD$$

FSS = focal spot size

OID = object-to-image distance

SOD = source-to-object distance

photographic properties – Photographic properties (*density* and *contrast*) affect the visibility of structures apparent on a radiographic image. Photographic properties in conjunction with *geometric properties* (*detail* and *distortion*) are considered part of the *four radiographic properties* used to judge overall image quality.

picture-archiving communication systems (PACS) – A PACS system is a filmless imaging system in which electronic images and relevant patient data from various imaging modalities are digitally transmitted, stored, and easily retrieved for viewing on a display monitor. PACS enables sharing of radiographic images and patient information within various departments of a single medical facility and between multiple medical facilities in a joint effort to provide a collaborative plan of care.

quality – Quality refers to the penetrating ability of the useful x-ray beam determined by kVp, HVL (half-value layer), and the imaging system's degree of filtration. Penetrability of the x-ray beam is measured in *half-value layer (HVL)*.

quantity – Quantity refers to the number of x-ray photons within the useful beam or the intensity of the beam. The units used to measure the intensity of the x-ray beam are the roentgen (R) or the milliroentgen (mR), 0.001 roentgen.

quantum mottle – Quantum mottle is a grainy appearance on a radiographic film (producing a loss of structural detail) resulting from an insufficient quantity of x-ray photons. Quantum mottle is closely associated with high-speed intensifying screens, which require low mAs. Switching to a lower intensifying screen speed will enable the technologist to increase the amount of mAs, thus increasing the quantity of x-ray photons necessary to produce a diagnostic image with little or no quantum mottle.

radiolucent – Radiolucent describes materials that easily allow x-rays photons to transmit through with little or no x-ray absorption. Radiolucent materials do not absorb x-ray photons; therefore, the result is an increase in radiographic density (darkness) on the visible image.

radio-opaque – Radio-opaque describes materials that do not allow x-rays photons to transmit through due to x-ray absorption. Radio-opaque materials absorb x-ray photons; therefore, the result is a decrease in radiographic density (whiteness) on the visible image.

reciprocity law – The reciprocity law refers to variations in mA and time that still produce the same overall mAs. The reciprocity law is used to control motion by either reducing or increasing motion to better visualize anatomical structures. Reducing motion may be necessary when involuntary motion hinders anatomical areas of interest. However, creating motion may be useful when attempting to blur out structures that obscure anatomical areas of interest; this is accomplished through a breathing technique with an exposure time of 3 seconds or more. Each of the following combinations of mA and time yields the same overall mAs, resulting in the same quantity of x-ray photons and the same radiographic density.

$$50 \text{ mA} \times 4 \text{ sec} = \textbf{200 mAs}$$
$$100 \text{ mA} \times 2 \text{ sec} = \textbf{200 mAs}$$
$$200 \text{ mA} \times 1 \text{ sec} = \textbf{200 mAs}$$
$$400 \text{ mA} \times 0.5 \text{ sec} = \textbf{200 mAs}$$
$$800 \text{ mA} \times 0.25 \text{ sec} = \textbf{200 mAs}$$

recorded detail – There are several interchangeable terms (resolution, resolving power, definition, image sharpness, geometric sharpness, and umbra) that relate to the "detail" or "recorded detail" of a radiographic image, all referring to how well defined or sharp the image structures appear. When viewing a radiograph, the more lp/mm (line pairs per millimeter), the sharper the image. When viewing a digital image, the larger the matrix size, the better the detail. Table 10–10 depicts the *controlling factors* and the *influencing factors* for recorded detail.

> ■ **visibility of detail** – Visibility of detail refers to how well you can see the recorded detail on a radiographic image. Density, contrast, and *scatter* greatly affect visibility of detail. Methods for increasing visibility of detail on a radiographic image include utilizing optimal mAs and kVp for the body part being examined, decreasing scatter production, and using methods to reduce scatter from reaching the IR.

resolution – *See recorded detail.*

scatter – Scatter occurs when an x-ray photon interacts with matter and is deflected in a different direction than its intended path. This occurrence results in an unwanted density that hinders visibility of recorded detail on a radiographic image. Scatter is often referred to as fog because of the blanket of gray that it produces on an image. The greatest amount of scatter is produced within the patient; the thicker the patient's body part, the more scatter produced. kVp also contributes to the amount of scatter produced on an image; the greater the kVp, the more scatter produced. *(Refer to Chapter 6: Physics Terms.)*

> ■ Ways to reduce scatter production include:
>
> - decreasing body part thickness
> - increasing collimation (smaller collimation field size)
> - decreasing kVp
>
> ■ Ways to reduce scatter from reaching the IR include:
>
> - reducing scatter production
> - using a grid or an air-gap technique
> - using lead strip absorbers (placed adjacent to body part being imaged) when applicable (e.g., lateral projections of thoracic and lumbar spine)

sensitometer – A sensitometer is a device that places a variation of radiographic densities on a film via exposure to a variation of light rather than from exposure to x-ray photons. A sensitometer is often used for quality control purposes in evaluating automatic processor function relating to density consistency *(see Figure 10–20).*

TABLE 10–10   Controlling and Influencing Factors for Recorded Detail

FACTORS	FACTOR ADJUSTMENT	RESULT OF FACTOR ADJUSTMENT
Controlling factors for recorded detail		
OID	Decrease OID =	Increase in recorded detail
	Increase OID =	Decrease in recorded detail
FSS (focal spot size)	Decrease FSS =	Increase in recorded detail
	Increase FSS =	Decrease in recorded detail
SID	Decrease SID =	Decrease in recorded detail
	Increase SID =	Increase in recorded detail
Influencing factors for recorded detail		
Intensifying screen speed (RSV)	Decrease screen speed =	Increase in recorded detail
	Increase screen speed =	Decrease in recorded detail

Data from Carlton, R. R., & Adler, A. M. (2006). *Principles of radiographic imaging: An art and a science* (4th ed.). Clifton Park, NY: Delmar Cengage Learning; Long, B. W., Frank, E. D., & Ehrlich, R. A. (2006). *Radiography essentials for limited practice* (2nd ed.). St. Louis, MO: Mosby; and Wallace, J. (1995). *Radiographic exposure principles & practice.* Philadelphia, PA: F. A. Davis Co.

source-to-object distance (SOD) – Source-to-object distance describes the distance that lies between the effective focal spot (point of image production at the anode target) and the object being imaged *(see Figure 10–18).*

step wedge – *See penetrometer.*

subject contrast – Subject contrast refers to the variation of body tissue (due to a variation in atomic number) and the degree of x-ray attenuation in accordance to the tissue type and kVp selected.

tube angulation – Angling the x-ray tube changes the SID. When changing the x-ray tube from no angulation at a 40-inch SID to a tube angulation of 20°, an automatic increase in SID occurs, causing distortion and a loss of density on the image. To compensate for the loss of density, the tube must be lowered to maintain a 40-inch

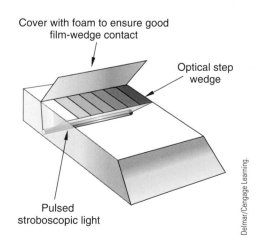

FIGURE 10–20. Sensitometer.

SID. The following rule of thumb is used to maintain density when tube angulation is used:

■ For every 5° of x-ray tube angulation, decrease the SID by 1 inch.

umbra – Umbra refers to the greatest degree of recorded detail on a radiographic image; this area is where the central ray has been directed. Because of the nature of the diverging x-ray beam, a loss of detail *(penumbra)* will occur on the image the further away from the area of interest to which the central ray was directed.

window level – Window level or window leveling is a postprocessing enhancement method for controlling the brightness level of computed or digital radiographic images. Once the image is electronically processed and able to be viewed on the display monitor, the technologist can change the brightness level to make it lighter or darker, similar to changing the density on a radiographic film by adjusting the mAs.

window width – Window width is a postprocessing enhancement method for controlling the scale of contrast on computed or digital radiographic images. Once the image is electronically processed and able to be viewed on the display monitor, the technologist can change the scale of contrast by increasing or decreasing the amount of gray shades, similar to changing the contrast of a radiographic film by adjusting the kVp.

StudyWARE™
CONNECTION

After completing this chapter, complete the Image Labeling exercises or another interactive activity on your StudyWARE™ CD-ROM that will help you learn the content in this chapter.

CONCEPT THINKING QUESTIONS

1. What is the relationship between mAs and density?

2. What is the relationship between mAs and kVp?

3. Differentiate between umbra and penumbra.

4. Explain when a grid should be used and what its purpose is.

5. Identify three ways to reduce the production of scatter.

6. Explain what an air-gap technique is and the effect it has on image contrast.

7. List the controlling factor for image contrast.

8. List the controlling factor for image density.

9. Explain the difference between recorded detail and visibility of detail.

10. Explain when a technologist should use the 15% rule.

11. When is a characteristic curve used and what information does it provide?

12. Explain the differences between CR imaging and DR imaging.

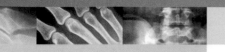

13. Identify three types of shape distortion and explain how they occur.

14. List the controlling factors for increasing or decreasing recorded detail.

15. Explain the difference between widow level and window width.

PRACTICE EXERCISES

1. Using the *reciprocity law*, provide options for mA and time selections that produce the same overall mAs of 400.

2. Draw a typical characteristic curve and label the various sections of the curve with an explanation as to what each section means.

3. Draw a focused grid and a nonfocused grid and explain why a technologist might prefer using a focused grid rather than a nonfocused grid.

4. Define the term *grid cut-off*.

5. Identify the five factors that produce grid cut-off.

6. Draw a grayscale image depicting short-scale contrast and one depicting long-scale contrast.

7. List four ways in which a doubling of radiographic image density can easily be accomplished.

8. Differentiate between fluorescence and phosphorescence and identify which is desirable for an intensifying screen phosphor.

9. Differentiate between a densitometer and a sensitometer.

10. If a given exposure of 20 mAs and 75 kVp produced a radiographic image with optimal density but insufficient contrast, what mathematical formula would need to be used to correct this imaging problem? Show your math and provide the new technical factors for correcting the error.

11. An exposure technique of 12 mAs and 70 kVp was used at a SID of 40 inches to produce an optimal radiographic image. If the SID was increased to 72 inches, what would the new technique need to be to maintain the image receptor exposure/radiographic density of the original image?

12. Explain what you would expect the contrast and density results to be when identical technical factors for mAs and kVp are used to produce two radiographs of the abdomen, one image taken with a low grid ratio focused grid and the other with a high grid ratio focused grid.

MATCHING

Match each term to the appropriate description.

scatter   penumbra   crossover
quantum mottle   lp/mm   target angle <45°
blue tint   voxel   geometric properties
small effective focal spot gadolinium   large effective focal spot
penetrability   toe   sodium sulfite
calcium tungstate   D-max   photographic properties
potassium bromide   mAs   matrix

Description	Term
1. resolution measurement	_____
2. grainy appearance	_____
3. fog	_____
4. geometric unsharpness	_____
5. parallax	_____
6. developer and fixer preservative	_____
7. detail and distortion	_____
8. rare earth phosphor	_____
9. line-focus principle	_____
10. contributes to base plus fog	_____
11. x-ray beam quality	_____
12. increases recorded detail	_____
13. controls photon quantity	_____
14. rows and columns of pixels	_____

RETENTION OF MATERIAL

Retention requires practicing the use of previously learned material. Apply the knowledge you have regarding pharmacology and contrast media to answer the following questions.

1. Explain the inverse square law and write the mathematical formula correlating to it.

2. Explain the direct square law and write the mathematical formula correlating to it.

3. Explain the relationship between the actual focal spot size and the effective focal spot size.

4. How does collimation affect the quantity of x-ray photon production?

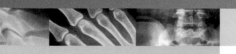

5. Discuss the effect tube angulation has on radiographic density.

6. Discuss how the line-focus principle affects heat dissipation and effective focal spot size.

7. List the components that comprise a radiographic film and those that comprise an intensifying screen.

8. Discuss various methods a technologist might use to reduce scatter from reaching the IR.

9. Explain the effect collimation has on radiographic density and contrast.

10. Explain why magnification exists on every radiographic image.

11. Determine the magnification factor for a body part that measures 3 inches in length with an image size length of 3.5 inches.

12. Determine the amount of penumbra present on a radiographic image that was taken utilizing the following exposure technique: 70kVp, 15 mAs, 1.2 focal spot size, 40-inch SID, and 2-inch OID.

CHAPTER 11

Imaging Principles and Mathematical Equations

OBJECTIVES

Upon completion of this chapter, the reader will be able to:

- Understand mathematical relationships and their use in image production
- Differentiate between a direct and an indirect relationship
- Identify principle concepts related to mathematical formulas and equations
- Correlate units of measure to specific mathematical formulas
- Recognize and apply mathematical formulas appropriately

CONCEPT THINKING

Math as it relates to the imaging profession is often perceived by students as a difficult area of study. Students who have struggled with the subject of math in their formative educational years can be apprehensive about using mathematical formulas related to physics and imaging principles. The perceived notion of "I'm not good at math" or "I can't do complicated math problems" is a very real obstacle to overcome when a negative learning experience has been encountered. To help dismiss any preconceived beliefs about the inability to perform successfully in math, one must remember that behind every mathematical formula lies a basic concept or principle. Once an understanding of the concept or principle is achieved, the application of mathematical equations becomes a natural progression. Math is really about correlating numbers and symbols to established concepts and principles. However, without obtaining a comprehensive knowledge base relevant to the area of study, achieving success in solving associated mathematical problems can be quite challenging.

This chapter offers a compilation of mathematical concepts and equations presented throughout the text as way to distinguish between formulas and recognize the units and relationships involved in each mathematical equation. Concepts and theories previously mentioned in the text are included as a means to support and reinforce the learning and application of math as it relates to the imaging profession. The real key to success in math is to fully understand the underlying concepts or principles from which mathematical formulas are derived. Although there may be mathematical shortcuts, there are no shortcuts to understanding the "why" or "how" of a concept. When presented with a mathematical problem, the first step in the problem-solving process is to identify the units of measure within the question. Second, apply the concept or theory related to the identified units. Finally, write the mathematical formula that correlates to the concept and place known factors into the formula. The mathematical formula, with known factors inserted, provides a visual checkpoint to confirm that (1) the correct formula was chosen, (2) units of measure have been appropriately identified, and (3) the formula depicts an appropriate relationship between known factors. Upon verification that all three checkpoints are correct, the unknown factor can be determined *(see the exposure maintenance formula)*.

RELATED MATHEMATICAL EQUATIONS

Coulomb's law – The electrostatic force existing between two electrical charges is directly proportional to the product of the quantity of charge present and inversely proportional to the square of the distance between the two electrical charges. This phenomenon, known as *Coulomb's law*, is named after 18th-century French physicist Charles-Augustin de Coulomb. Coulomb discovered that creating distance between two electrical charges greatly affected the electrostatic force between the two electrical charges. Coulomb's law is mathematically depicted as follows:

$$F = k \frac{Q_A \times Q_B}{d^2}$$

F = electrostatic force

k = constant of proportionality

Q_A and Q_B = two separate electrostatic charges

d^2 = distance between electrostatic charges squared

density – Density is a term used to describe the overall blackness of a radiographic film or the percentage of light transmitted through a radiographic film when viewed by an illuminator device, most commonly referred to as a viewbox. Optical density (OD) is calculated in a logarithmic manner and can be determined when a given percentage of illuminator light is known.

$$OD = \log_{10} \frac{I_o \text{ (incident light intensity)}}{I_i \text{ (transmitted light intensity)}}$$

> **Note** Density (overall blackness of a radiographic film) cannot exist on an image produced via CR/DR; rather, areas of darkness on a computed/digital image are due to image receptor exposure, with mAs as the controlling factor. Replace the term density with image receptor exposure when referring to the degree of darkness present on an image produced via a CR or DR imaging system.

direct square law – *See exposure maintenance formula.*

exposure maintenance formula – The exposure maintenance formula is a mathematical equation used to calculate for the amount of mAs required to maintain radiographic exposure with CR/DR imaging systems after a change in SID has occurred. The formula was previously known as the *density maintenance formula* when the image receptor consisted of a film/screen combination. The formula may also be referred to as the *direct square law* because of the direct relationship between mAs (controlling factor for image receptor exposure/density) and the changing distance (SID). For example, two images taken with the same exposure factors and the same SID will yield two images with the same image receptor exposure/radiographic density. However, with all exposure factors kept constant and SID increased, the resulting radiographic image would appear lighter with less image receptor exposure/radiographic density than the original image with the shorter SID. Therefore, we can say that an increase in SID will require an increase in mAs in order to maintain image receptor exposure/radiographic density between the two images taken at different SIDs. Mathematically this concept is depicted as follows:

$$\frac{mAs_1}{mAs_2} = \frac{D_1^{(2)}}{D_2^{(2)}}$$

mAs_1 = original mAs

mAs_2 = new mAs (to maintain image receptor exposure/ radiographic density after a change in SID has occurred)

$D_1^{(2)}$ = original distance squared

$D_2^{(2)}$ = new distance squared

Steps involved for determining the new mAs necessary for maintaining image receptor exposure/radiographic density after a change in distance has occurred can be seen in addressing the following problem:

A lateral projection of the cervical spine was taken at a 72-inch SID with 80 kVp and 20 mAs. What would the new mAs need to be to maintain the image receptor exposure/radiographic density of the original image if the SID was changed to 40 inches?

■ **Step 1** – Identify the units of measure in the question: SID is distance (D), kVp is the controlling factor for contrast, and mAs is the the controlling factor for image receptor exposure/radiographic density.

■ **Step 2** – Identify the concept: Maintain exposure/density after a change in distance has occurred.

■ **Step 3** – Apply the formula that matches the concept (exposure maintenance formula) and confirm that a direct relationship between mAs and distance is depicted in the formula.

■ **Step 4** – Add known factors into the formula and solve for the unknown factor.

$$\frac{mAs_1}{mAs_2} = \frac{D_1^{(2)}}{D_2^{(2)}}$$

$$\frac{mAs_1 \, 20}{mAs_2 \, ?} = \frac{D_1^{(2)} \, 5184}{D_2^{(2)} \, 1600}$$

mAs_1 = original mAs = 20 mAs

mAs_2 = new mAs (to maintain image receptor exposure/ radiographic density after a change in SID has occurred)

$D_1^{(2)}$ = original SID squared = 72 inches squared = 5184

$D_2^{(2)}$ = new SID squared = 40 inches squared = 1600

Cross-multiply: $1600 \times 20 = 32{,}000/5184 = $ **6.17, or 6 mAs**

Therefore, **mAs$_2$** (the unknown factor) $=$ **6 mAs**.

The exposure maintenance formula can be used not only to calculate for the new mAs required to maintain image receptor exposure/radiographic density when a change in distance has occurred, but it also can be used to calculate for any portion of mAs such as mA or time. The three exposure maintenance formulas show a direct relationship between mAs and distance, mA and distance, and time and distance.

◼ **Calculation for mA and distance** – When a change in distance has occurred and image receptor exposure/radiographic density is to be maintained through a change in mA stations, the following formula may be used:

$$\frac{mA_1}{mA_2} = \frac{D_1^{(2)}}{D_2^{(2)}}$$

$mA_1 =$ original mA station

$mA_2 =$ new mA station (to maintain image receptor exposure/radiographic density after a change in SID has occurred)

$D_1^{(2)} =$ original SID squared

$D_2^{(2)} =$ new SID squared

◼ **Calculation for time and distance** – Time in seconds or fractions of a second are represented by the lower case (s) or (t) and also share a direct relationship with distance. When a change in distance has occurred and image receptor exposure/radiographic density is to be maintained through a change in time, the following formula may be used:

$$\frac{s_1}{s_2} = \frac{D1^{(2)}}{D2^{(2)}}$$

$s_1 =$ original time (in seconds or fractions of a second)

$s_2 =$ new time in seconds or fractions of a second (to maintain image receptor exposure/radiographic density after a change in SID has occurred)

$D_1^{(2)} =$ original SID squared

$D_2^{(2)} =$ new SID squared

exposure timer test tools – There are two main types of exposure timer test tools: the manual spin top test and the synchronous motor spin test (oscilloscope).

◼ **manual spin top test** – The radiographic image produced using the spin top test will show a specific number of dots for a given exposure time. *(Refer to Figure 13–4.)* The following mathematical formula can be used to determine exposure timer accuracy. The *mathematical triangle* can be used to find the missing component of the formula when two factors are provided. *(Refer to Figure 13–5.)*

• The total number of dots on the radiographic image divided by 120 (the constant variable) = the exposure time.

◼ **synchronous motor spin test** – Because voltage never drops to zero with three-phase equipment, a degree of arc (based on a complete circle or 360°) will appear on the radiographic image rather than a series of dots. The following mathematical formula can be used to determine exposure timer accuracy using a synchronous motor spin test. *(Refer to Figure 13–4.)* The *mathematical triangle* can be used to find the missing component of the formula when two factors are provided. *(Refer to Figure 13–6.)*

- The degree of arc on the radiographic image divided by 360° (the constant variable) = the exposure time.

fifteen percent (15%) rule – The 15% rule is a mathematical equation to be used for calculating adjustments in the technical factors of mAs and kVp when a change in image contrast is desired without a change to image density. kVp is the controlling factor for contrast and an influencing factor for radiographic density. Subsequently, a change in kVp will result in a change in both *contrast* and *density*. The 15% rule states that a 15% increase in kVp will result in a decrease in radiographic contrast and a doubling of radiographic density *(see Table 11–1)*.

grid ratio – Grid ratio refers to the ratio between the height of the lead strips (h) and the distance (D) between the lead strips. The formula **h/D** is used to calculate grid ratio. The higher the grid ratio, the less scatter reaches the image receptor; however, the disadvantage of using a high grid ratio (16:1) is the increase in exposure factors required to compensate for the removal of radiation by the grid; this would result in a greater patient dose. Multiplier factors are necessary to determine the amount of mAs needed to maintain radiographic density between images taken using different grid ratios or between an image taken with no grid and one taken with a grid. The relationship between grid ratios (and their multiplier factors) and mAs required to maintain density is a direct relationship. The greater the grid ratio, the more mAs required to maintain the density of an image produced with a lesser grid ratio *(see Table 11–2)*.

grid ratio/mAs formula – The grid ratio/mAs formula is used to calculate the new mAs required to maintain radiographic density between images taken with different grid ratio multiplier factors.

$$\frac{mAs_1}{mAs_2} = \frac{GMF_1}{GMF_2}$$

mAs_1 = original mAs

mAs_2 = new mAs (to maintain density after a change in grid ratios has occurred)

GMF_1 = original grid ratio multiplier factor

GMF_2 = new grid ratio multiplier factor

heat unit (HU) – A heat unit (HU) is a unit used to measure the amount of thermal heat generated within the x-ray tube during x-ray production. HUs can be

---

TABLE 11-1   The 15% Rule

kVp CHANGE	EFFECT ON CONTRAST	ADJUST mAs TO MAINTAIN DENSITY
Increase kVp by 15%	Decreases	Halve the original mAs (divide by 2).
Decrease kVp by 15%	Increases	Double the original mAs (multiply by 2).

Note: In the diagnostic range of 60–90 kVp, a 15% increase or decrease in kVp is a difference of approximately 10 kVp.

Data from Carlton, R. R., & Adler, A. M. (2006). *Principles of radiographic imaging: An art and a science* (4th ed.). Clifton Park, NY: Delmar Cengage Learning; and Wallace, J. (1995). *Radiographic exposure principles & practice.* Philadelphia, PA: F. A. Davis Co.

TABLE 11–2   Grid Ratios with Multiplier Factors

GRID RATIO	MULTIPLIER FACTOR
No grid	1×
5:1 grid	2×
6:1 grid	3×
8:1 grid*	4×
12:1 grid	5×
16:1 grid	6×

*Most common grid ratio used in diagnostic x-ray.
Data from Carlton, R. R., & Adler, A. M. (2006). *Principles of radiographic imaging: An art and a science* (4th ed.). Clifton Park, NY: Delmar Cengage Learning; and Wallace, J. (1995). *Radiographic exposure principles & practice.* Philadelphia, PA: F. A. Davis Co.

---

calculated for a single x-ray exposure or for multiple x-ray exposures. Formulas for calculating HUs depend upon the type of generator equipment used *(multiplier factors included)*, along with the technical factors selected. Listed are the formulas for calculating heat units based on the type of generator used:

- single-phase generator equipment – kVp × mA × time × **1**
- three-phase; six-pulse generator equipment – kVp × mA × time × **1.35**
- three-phase; 12-pulse generator equipment – kVp × mA × time × **1.41**
- high frequency generator equipment – kVp × mA × time × **1.45**
- fluoroscopic unit – kVp × mA × time × multiplier factor of generator used × **60** *(multiplier factor for fluoroscopy)*

horsepower (hp) – The horsepower (hp) is the British unit to measure electric power.

$$700 \text{ hp} = 1 \text{ watt (W)}$$

image intensifier mathematical equations – The following three mathematical formulas are unique to an image intensifier and are used to determine flux gain, minification gain, and brightness gain.

- **flux gain** – Flux gain refers to the increased amount of light photons from the image intensifier output phosphor in comparison to the number of x-ray photons striking the image intensifier input phosphor. This number can be calculated by using the following mathematical formula:

$$\text{Flux gain} = \frac{\text{\# of output light photons}}{\text{\# of input x-ray photons}}$$

- **minification gain** – Minification gain refers to the ratio of the diameter of the input phosphor squared to the diameter of the output phosphor squared. This number can be calculated by using the following mathematical formula:

$$\text{Minification gain} = \frac{(\text{diameter of input phosphor})^2}{(\text{diameter of output phosphor})^2}$$

- **total brightness gain** – Total brightness gain refers to the increased amount of light or brightness of an image by the use of an image intensifier tube. It is the product of *minification gain* and *flux gain*. Total brightness gain can be calculated by using the following mathematical formula:

$$\text{Brightness gain} = \text{minification gain} \times \text{flux gain}$$

image magnification – Image magnification is a type of size distortion and exists to some degree on all radiographic images because of the inherent distance between the body part to be imaged and the image receptor. Because of the three-dimensional shape of the body and the location of the anatomical area of interest within the body, a varying degree of magnification will be present on the radiographic image. Some basic principles must be kept in mind when assessing magnification:

- an increase in OID (object-to-image distance) results in increased magnification

- a decrease in SID results in increased magnification

- image size will always be larger than object size

To reduce image magnification:

- position body part closest to image receptor

- increase SID for any OID that may exist (7 inches of SID correct 1 inch of OID)

Calculating magnification (cross-multiply and solve for missing factor):

$$\frac{\text{image size}}{\text{object size}} = \frac{\text{SID}}{\text{SOD}}$$

Calculating for magnification factor (MF):

$$\frac{\text{image size}}{\text{object size}} \quad \text{or} \quad \frac{\text{SID}}{\text{SOD}}$$

Calculating for percent of magnification:

$$\frac{\text{image size} - \text{object size}}{\text{object size}} \times 100 = \% \text{ of magnification}$$

or

$$\frac{\text{OID} \times 100}{\text{SOD}} = \% \text{ of magnification}$$

inverse square law – The inverse square law states that the intensity of the x-ray beam will be reduced by a factor of four when the SID is doubled or the intensity of the beam will be increased by a factor of four when the SID is cut in half. There is an inverse relationship between intensity of the beam and the distance of the source to the image receptor. The formula for the inverse square law is:

$$\frac{I_1}{I_2} = \frac{D_2^{(2)}}{D_1^{(2)}}$$

I_1 = original x-ray beam intensity

I_2 = new x-ray beam intensity (after a change in distance)

$D_1^{(2)}$ = original SID squared

$D_2^{(2)}$ = new SID squared

kilovolt (kV) – 1000 volts are equal to 1 kilovolt (1000 volts = 1 kV).

kilovolt heat unit (kHU) – 1000 heat units are equal to 1 kilovolt heat unit (1000 HUs = 1 kHU).

mAs – The total mA (milliamperes) multiplied by the exposure time yields mAs.

$$mA \times s = mAs$$

mechanical energy – Energy resulting from physical exertion by a human or by a machine is known as mechanical energy; there are two types of mechanical energy:

- **kinetic energy** – Kinetic energy is energy in motion.

$$KE = \tfrac{1}{2} (mass \times velocity)^2$$

- **potential energy** – Potential energy is energy that has the potential to be in motion but is not actually in motion.

object-to-image distance (OID) – Object-to-image distance (OID) is the greatest factor affecting the amount of distortion present on a radiographic image. The greater the OID, the greater the distortion present on an image. The rule of thumb for reducing distortion caused by OID is to compensate with an increase in SID.

- For every 1 inch of OID, increase the SID by 7 inches.

ohm (Ω) – The ohm, represented by the symbol Ω, is the unit of measure for resistance within an electrical circuit.

Ohm's law – Ohm's law states that within a given circuit there is voltage (V), current (I), and resistance (R), and that the voltage within the circuit (total voltage or voltage at various points within the circuit) will always be equal to the amount of current flowing through the circuit times the amount of resistance present. Mathematically, Ohm's law can be depicted in any one of three ways:

- $V = I \times R$ V = voltage
- $I = V/R$ I = intensity of current
- $R = V/I$ R = resistance to current flow

> **Note:**   *Current is measured in units of milliamperage (mA) or amperage (A); however, it is represented in Ohm's law as (I) for current intensity.*

orbital shell formula – The orbital shell formula is a mathematical equation utilized to determine the maximum number of electrons that can occupy any orbital shell. $2n^2$ is the formula used to calculate the maximum number of electrons in any orbital shell. (n) Represents the number of the orbital shell as determined by its proximity to the nucleus, starting with the K shell as the number one (*see Table 11–3*).

patient dose – Patient dose is considerably greater with fluoroscopic procedures as opposed to conventional radiographic procedures. To determine an increase in patient dose when employing the magnification mode, the following mathematical formula can be used:

$$\text{patient dose (fluoro)} = \frac{\text{large input phosphor diameter}^2}{\text{small input phosphor diameter}^2}$$

TABLE 11-3   Orbital Shells with Corresponding Electrons

ORBITAL SHELL AND CORRESPONDING #	FORMULA AND MAXIMUM # OF ELECTRONS
K (1)	$2 \times n(1)^2 = 2$
L (2)	$2 \times n(2)^2 = 8$
M (3)	$2 \times n(3)^2 = 18$
N (4)	$2 \times n(4)^2 = 32$
O (5)	$2 \times n(5)^2 = 50$

Data from Carlton, R. R., & Adler, A. M. (2006). *Principles of radiographic imaging: An art and a science.* (4th ed.). Clifton Park, NY: Delmar Cengage Learning; and Wallace, J. (1995). *Radiographic exposure principles & practice.* Philadelphia, PA: F. A. Davis Co.

penumbra formula – The penumbra formula is used to determine the amount of geometric unsharpness present on an image.

$$penumbra = \frac{FSS \times OID}{SOD}$$

FSS = the effective focal spot size

OID = the object to image distance

SOD = the source to object distance

pixel size formula – To determine digital pixel size (measured in millimeters), divide the field of view (FOV) in mm by the matrix size.

$$pixel\ size = \frac{FOV}{matrix\ size}$$

> **Note:**   10 mm = 1 cm.

Planck's constant – Planck's constant refers to the constant proportionality between photon energy and photon frequency; it is assigned a numerical value of $4.15 \times 10^{-15}\,eV^{-s}$. The following mathematical equation depicts the direct relationship between photon energy and photon frequency, and the indirect relationship between photon energy and photon wavelength with the velocity remaining constant *(at the speed of light)*.

■ **Planck's Constant Formula:** **E** (energy) = **h** (Planck's Constant) × **f** (photon frequency)

$$E = h \times f$$

Energy is represented in (eV) electron volts.

Planck's constant is represented by $4.15 \times 10^{-15}\,eV^{-s}$.

f is represented in the unit hertz (Hz).

power – Power as it relates to physics is considered to be the rate of performing work. Units to measure power are the *watt* (W) or the *horsepower* (hp). Mathematically, power is depicted as *power* (P) equals *work* (W) divided by *time* (t).

$$P = W/t$$

■ **total power formula** – Total power (measured in watts) within an electrical circuit is the product of current (measured in amperage) multiplied by the amount of voltage present within the circuit. Mathematically, total power is depicted as $W = I \times V$, where (W) represents total power in watts, (I) represents current in amperage, and (V) represents voltage.

$$\text{total power } (W) = I \times V$$

power loss formula – Power loss is considered to be the amount of current in amperage squared times the amount of resistance in ohms present within the electrical circuit. Mathematically, power loss is depicted as $I^2 \times R$, where I^2 represents current in amperage (squared), and R represents resistance in ohms.

$$\text{power loss} = I^{(2)} \times R$$

reciprocity law – The reciprocity law refers to variations in mA and time to produce the same overall mAs. The reciprocity law is used to control motion by either reducing or increasing motion to better visualize anatomical structures. Reducing motion may be necessary when involuntary motion hinders anatomical areas of interest. However, creating motion may be useful when attempting to blur out structures that obscure anatomical areas of interest; this is accomplished through a breathing technique with an exposure time of 3 seconds or more.

■ 50 mA $\times$ 4 seconds = **200 mAs**

■ 100 mA $\times$ 2 seconds = **200 mAs**

■ 200 mA $\times$ 1 seconds = **200 mAs**

■ 400 mA $\times$ 0.5 seconds = **200 mAs**

■ 800 mA $\times$ 0.25 seconds = **200 mAs**

rectification formula – The rectification formula is a mathematical equation used to calculate a new mAs necessary for maintaining consistent density between two images produced by two different types of rectified x-ray units (e. g., single-phase full-wave rectification versus three-phase, six-pulse rectification). The formula is based upon assigning a multiplier factor or *phase conversion factor (PCF)* to three main types of rectification processes associated with the basic x-ray circuit.

$$\frac{mAs_1}{mAs_2} = \frac{PCF_1}{PCF_2}$$

mAs_1 = original mAs

mAs_2 = new mAs

PCF_1 = original rectified unit

PCF_2 = new rectified unit

■ **phase conversion factor (PCF)** – The PCF represents the reduction in mAs required to maintain radiographic density as you switch to a an x-ray unit with a more efficient type of rectification *(see Table 11-4)*.

relative speed value – Relative speed value (RSV) describes the various film/screen combination speeds of intensifying screens and radiographic film. Typically, film/screen speeds range between 100 and 1200. Slower film/screen speeds (less than

TABLE 11-4 Rectification and PCFs

RECTIFIED UNIT	PCF
Full-wave rectification	1
Three-phase, six-pulse rectification	0.67
Three-phase, 12-pulse rectification	0.5

Source: Delmar/Cengage Learning

100) are considered "detail cassettes" and are used when a high degree of detail is required (usually regarding extremities). Because intensifying screens are used with film, it is best to keep in mind that a *spectral matching* between film sensitivity and intensifying screen phosphorescence is necessary. The faster the RSV of the intensifying screen/film, the lower the quantity of x-ray photons required to produce a diagnostic image and the lower the patient dose; detail, however, is lessened. The relationship between RSV and mAs is an indirect relationship. The greater the RSV, the lower the mAs required. The following formula can be used when an acceptable technique has been established (with a particular intensifying screen speed and mAs) and a change in screen speed is desired, requiring the calculation of a new mAs. Remember that, when using the formula, (1) represents the original technique and (2) represents what you are changing to.

$$\frac{mAs_1}{mAs_2} = \frac{RSV_2}{RSV_1}$$

transformer current law – This mathematical equation depicts the indirect or inverse relationship between the number of turns on the secondary side of a step-up or step-down transformer and the amount of current produced.

$$\frac{N_P}{N_S} = \frac{I_S}{I_P}$$

N_P = number of turns or coil windings on the primary side

N_S = number of turns or coil windings on the secondary side

I_S = current on the secondary side

I_P = current on the primary side

transformer voltage law – This mathematical equation depicts the direct relationship between the number of turns on the secondary side of a step-up or step-down transformer and the amount of voltage produced.

$$\frac{N_P}{N_S} = \frac{V_P}{V_S}$$

N_P = number of turns or coil windings on the primary side

N_S = number of turns or coil windings on the secondary side

V_P = voltage on the primary side

V_S = voltage on the secondary side

tube angulation – Angling the x-ray tube changes the SID. When changing the x-ray tube from no angulation at 40 inches SID to a tube angulation of 20°, an automatic increase in SID occurs, causing distortion and a loss of density on the image. To compensate for the loss of density, the SID must be shortened. The following rule of thumb is used for a perpendicular beam and an angled beam to maintain density when using tube angulation:

- ■ For every 5° of x-ray tube angulation, decrease the SID by 1 inch.

units to measure ionizing radiation – The two units to measure ionizing radiation are the "traditional units" and the "international units," referred to as SI units. The conversion table in Table 11–5 demonstrates ionizing measuring units in traditional units and their equivalent in SI units.

units to measure radioactivity – Radioactivity is measured in curies (Ci) or becquerels (Bq).

- ■ **becquerel (Bq)** – The Bq is the SI unit used to measure radioactive material.
- ■ **curie (Ci)** – The Ci is the traditional unit used to measure radioactive material.

velocity – Velocity refers to the rate of speed an object travels within a certain timeframe.

$$v = d/t$$

v = velocity (speed)

d = distance traveled over a certain time frame

t = time

TABLE 11–5   Conversions of Traditional Radiation Units to SI Units

RADIATION TYPE	TRADITIONAL UNITS	SI UNITS
Radiation absorbed dose (patient)		
	1000 mrad = 1 rad = 100 rad =	0.01 gray (Gy) 1 gray (Gy)
Radiation equivalent dose (occupational exposure)		
	1000 mrem = 1 rem = 100 rem =	0.01 sievert (Sv) 1 sievert (Sv)
Radiation exposure (in air)		
	1000 mR = 1 roentgen (R) =	2.58×10^{-4} coulomb/kilogram (C/kg) in air
Radioactivity		
	1 curie (Ci) =	3.7×10^{10} becquerel (Bq)

Data from Carlton, R. R., & Adler, A. M. (2006). *Principles of radiographic imaging: An art and a science* (4th ed.). Clifton Park, NY: Delmar Cengage Learning.

For radiology purposes, velocity refers to the speed at which a photon travels, which is the speed of light represented by the lowercase letter *(c)*:

velocity *(c)* = frequency (f) × wavelength (λ)

c = velocity (speed of light, 186,000 miles per second)

f = frequency of wavelengths (measured in hertz)

λ = wavelength (measured in angstrom or lambda)

watt (W) – The watt (W) is a unit of measure for electric power. Mathematically, it can be depicted as: 1 W (watt) is equal to 1 A (ampere) of current flowing through an electric potential of 1 V (volt).

$$1W = 1A \times 1V$$

weight – Weight is the force an object possesses as the result of the earth's gravitational pull.

$$Wt = m \times gravity$$

The weight of an object is equal to the object's mass multiplied by the gravitational force of the earth. Gravitational force is noted as 9.8 m/s^2.

work – Work as it relates to physics can be defined as an applied force over a specified distance. Mathematically, it is depicted as *work* (W) is equal to an applied *force* (F) × the *distance* (d) in which the force is applied. The unit to measure work is the joule (J).

$$W = F \times d$$

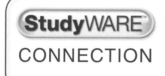

After completing this chapter, complete the interactive activities on your StudyWARE™ CD-ROM that will help you learn the content in this chapter.

CONCEPT THINKING QUESTIONS

1. What is the relationship between mA and radiographic density/image receptor exposure?

2. What is the relationship between time (s) and radiographic density/image receptor exposure?

3. What is the relationship between mAs and radiographic density/image receptor exposure?

4. What is the relationship between mA and time (s)?

5. What formula should be used to change image contrast while maintaining radiographic density/image receptor exposure?

6. What units are used in the formula for the inverse square law?

7. Explain what happens to radiation intensity when changing the SID.

8. Why are the distance factors squared in the direct square law and the inverse square law?

9. Explain how kVp influences radiographic density/image receptor exposure and how much of a kVp change is necessary to double or halve radiographic density/image receptor exposure.

10. Explain how the direct square law and the inverse square law work hand in hand.

11. Why apply a grid ratio multiplier factor when changing from an exam performed with no grid to the same exam performed with a grid?

12. What does a grid multiplier factor of 4 tell you about the grid?

13. Explain why the formula for velocity is different for an object compared with that for electromagnet radiation.

14. Which is the larger measuring unit regarding radiation absorbed dose: 1 rad or 1 gray?

15. Explain what happens to radiographic density/image receptor exposure when you change from a perpendicular beam to a 30° tube angle.

PRACTICE EXERCISES

1. Using the *reciprocity law*, provide three options of mA and time selections that produce 150 mAs.

2. In reviewing the transformer current law and the transformer voltage law, what can you conclude about the relationship between the number of transformer turns and current, and the number of transformer turns and voltage?

3. Identify the traditional unit to measure radioactivity.

4. Identify the traditional unit and the SI unit for measuring radiation absorbed dose.

5. How many mrads are in 1 rad? How many rads are in 1 gray?

6. Using the following technique of 70 kVp at 15 mAs, provide a new technique demonstrating an increase in contrast and a new technique demonstrating a decrease in contrast without altering the radiographic density/image receptor exposure of the original technique.

7. Using the following technique of 75 kVp, 100 mA, 0.05 s, and 1.0-mm FSS, provide three new techniques demonstrating a doubling of radiographic image.

8. If a radiographic image was taken using a technique of 65 kVp, 12 mAs, and 100 RSV, and it is desired to repeat the image using a 400 RSV, what should the new technique be to maintain radiographic density/image receptor exposure?

9. An anteroposterior projection of a knee was taken using 65 kVp at 15 mAs with no grid. A repeat projection of the knee is requested by the physician using an 8:1 grid. What should the new technique be to maintain the radiographic density/image receptor exposure of the original image?

10. An exposure technique of 70 kVp at10 mAs with a 40-inch SID was used with single-phase, full-wave rectification equipment. What should the new technique be when using three-phase, 12-pulse equipment to maintain the radiographic density/image receptor exposure of the image produced with the single-phase equipment?

11. A hand measures 6 inches in length but is 4 inches away from the image receptor because of a nail accidentally driven through it. What would the image size be if a posteroanterior projection were taken using a 40-inch SID?

12. What is the grid ratio for a linear nonfocused grid with lead strips 3 mm high, 1.5 mm wide, and an interspace width of 0.6 mm?

MATCHING

Match each term to the appropriate description.

mrad	1A × 1V	F × d
2n²	PCF 0.67	mR
inverse square law	8 electrons	I²R
4 electrons	W/t	Ohm's law
OID	object size	PCF 0.5
8:1 grid	12:1 grid	direct square law
1/1000 V	1000 V	watt

Description	Term
1. work	_____
2. radiation exposure unit	_____
3. three-phase, six-pulse rectification	_____
4. x-ray beam intensity formula	_____
5. L orbital shell	_____
6. orbital shell formula	_____
7. power	_____
8. $V = I \times R$	_____
9. SID − SOD =	_____
10. GMF of 5	_____
11. absorbed dose unit	_____
12. 1 kilovolt	_____

RETENTION OF MATERIAL

Retention requires practicing the use of previously learned material. Apply the knowledge you have learned regarding imaging principles to answer the following questions.

1. Identify the units of measure correlating to the inverse square law and explain the relationship between the two types of units.

2. Identify the units of measure correlating to the direct square law (exposure maintenance law) and explain the relationship between the two types of units.

3. Explain Ohm's law and write the three mathematical equations depicting it.

4. Explain what occurs to beam intensity when increasing the SID from 40 inches to 72 inches, keeping all other factors constant (80 kVp at 25 mAs).

5. Using question #4, explain how the technologist will compensate for what occurred when the SID was changed from 40 inches to 72 inches.

6. If a radiograph is taken using 80 kVp at 40 mAs with a 40-inch SID and a repeat radiograph is taken at 80 inches SID, what should the new mAs be to maintain image receptor exposure/density? Try to determine the answer without the aid of calculator and rely on applying the concept. *If you are not sure of the concept, first identify the units within the question.*

7. Increasing kVp has what effect on contrast and what effect on scale of contrast?

8. When using a step-up transformer, we know the number of turns or coils will be greater on the secondary side; therefore, what can we anticipate about the voltage on the secondary side of the transformer?

9. Write the mathematical formula depicting the concept determined in question #8.

10. What is the relationship between voltage and current? Apply this knowledge to question #8 and explain what occurs on the secondary side of a step-up transformer regarding voltage and current.

11. Determine the digital image pixel size from a matrix size of 2500 $\times$ 2500 with a FOV (field of view) of 50 cm.

12. Determine the percentage of magnification present on a radiographic image when the object size measures 3 inches and the image size measures 3.5 inches.

IV

Radiation Effects and Protective Measures

CHAPTER 12

Radiation Biology

OBJECTIVES

Upon completion of this chapter, the reader will be able to:

- Describe acute radiation syndrome
- Discuss long-term and short-term effects of radiation
- Identify cellular components and their function
- Differentiate between somatic effects and genetic effects
- Discuss the law of Bergonié and Tribondeau
- Discuss dose-response relationships and what they represent
- Differentiate between stochastic and nonstochastic effects
- Explain the relationship between linear energy transfer and relative biological effect

CONCEPT THINKING

Radiation biology is the study of radiation effects on living organisms. One must first have an understanding of normal biological structures and functions of the human body before investigating the effects of ionizing radiation as it relates to cellular damage. Ionization, or the removal of electrons from an atom, results in an unstable atom. Unstable atoms look to become stable by joining with another atom, not necessarily a good or healthy pairing. Ionization can also cause a break in a molecular bond affecting the function, reproduction, and life span of the cells involved. The interaction of an ionizing photon with cellular cytoplasm or the nuclei can cause no biological damage or a variation of biological damage. Energy transferred from ionizing radiation to a cell's cytoplasm can produce free radicals (carcinogens), whereas the effect of ionizing radiation on the master molecule (DNA) can effect in chromosome damage, resulting in cell mutations and even cell death. However, the human body has the perfect design in that cellular composition is predominately empty space, allowing ionizing radiation to pass through with only a small chance of interaction with cell components. Even when interaction does occur, causing a direct or indirect effect on the cell, there is a high probability of cellular repair. However, because of the potential of radiation causing biological damage, no amount of radiation is considered to be safe. This is the premise for the ALARA principle (*as low as reasonably achievable*), embraced in the profession's code of ethics.

RELATED TERMS

absorbed dose equivalent – The absorbed dose equivalent is a measurement of the biological effect of different types of radiation, measured in the unit of rem (or sievert). The following mathematical equation is used to determine absorbed dose equivalent:

$$\text{absorbed dose equivalent (rem)} = \text{absorbed dose (rad)} \times \text{radiation weighting factor } (W_R)$$

W_R (radiation weighting factors) for different types of ionizing radiation are based upon the ability for biologic damage to occur:

- x-ray, gamma rays = W_R of 1
- beta particles = W_R of 1
- alpha particles = W_R of 20
- neutrons = W_R of 20

The greater the W_R, the greater the absorbed dose equivalent, resulting in more biological damage as the absorbed dose (rad) is kept at a constant. It should be noted that the terms W_R and *quality factor* (QF) are interchangeable.

acute – Acute refers to rapid onset of illness, i.e., within a short period of time.

acute radiation dose – An acute radiation dose describes a high dose of radiation (10 rad or more) delivered to the whole body at once.

acute radiation symptoms – Acute radiation symptoms, otherwise referred to as radiation sickness, occurs after an individual has received an acute radiation dose. Symptoms are directly related to amount of radiation delivered *(see Table 12–1).*

acute radiation syndrome – Acute radiation syndrome describes the effects (classified by three syndromes) of a whole-body dose of radiation in which 100 rad or more are delivered to an individual within a short period of time (minutes to hours). The three syndromes of acute radiation exposure correlate to an approximate range of radiation necessary to cause the effect. Each of the following three syndromes have four distinct stages that present at different time intervals due to the amount of whole-body radiation delivered to the individual *(see acute radiation syndrome staging).*

- **hematologic syndrome** – The hematologic syndrome, also referred to as the hematopoietic syndrome, is caused by an acute whole-body radiation dose of approximately 100–1000 rad. Radiation exposure at this level will have an immediate effect on blood-forming organs, causing a significant decrease in the production of erythrocytes (red blood cells) and leukocytes (white blood cells). Depending on the dose of radiation an individual receives, life expectancy is approximately 2–8 weeks after exposure.

■ **gastrointestinal syndrome** – The gastrointestinal syndrome is caused by an acute whole-body radiation dose of approximately 1000–5000 rad. Radiation exposure at this level will have initiated the hematologic syndrome; however, because of the high level of radiation exposure, the gastrointestinal tract will be immediately effected, causing deterioration of the mucosa (lining) of the stomach and intestines. Depending on the dose of radiation an individual receives, life expectancy is approximately 3–10 days after exposure.

■ **central nervous syndrome** – The central nervous syndrome is caused by an acute whole-body radiation dose of approximately 5000 rad or greater. Radiation exposure at this level will have initiated both the hematologic syndrome and the gastrointestinal syndrome; however, because of the extremely high level of radiation exposure, death will occur before symptoms of either syndrome become evident. Life expectancy for an individual exposed to this amount of radiation is approximately several hours to a few days.

TABLE 12–1   Acute Radiation Symptoms

WHOLE-BODY RADIATION DOSE	EFFECT OF WHOLE-BODY DOSE
25–100 rad	Damage to blood cells (RBC and WBC)* Decrease in blood cell production Increase susceptibility to infection
>100 rad	Acute radiation syndrome–hematologic syndrome
150 rad	Nausea Vomiting Diarrhea Acute radiation syndrome–hematologic syndrome
200–300 rad	Alopecia Erythema Desquamation Temporary sterility Acute radiation syndrome–hematologic syndrome
600–1000 rad	Acute radiation syndrome–hematologic syndrome Gastrointestinal syndrome Permanent sterility
>1000 rad	Acute radiation syndrome–central nervous syndrome Death

*RBC, red blood cell; WBC, white blood cell.

Based on data from: Bushong, S. C. (2008). *Radiologic science for technologists: Physics, biology, and protection* (9th ed.). St. Louis, MO: Mosby; Dowd, S. B., & Tilson, E. R. (1999). *Practical radiation protection and applied radiobiology* (2nd ed.). Philadelphia, PA: Saunders; Forshier, S. (2009). *Essentials of radiation biology and protection* (2nd ed.). Clifton Park, NY: Delmar Cengage Learning.

acute radiation syndrome staging – Acute radiation syndrome staging defines the four distinct stages associated with each of the three acute radiation syndromes. These stages are as follows and are consistent with each syndrome:

- ■ **prodromal stage** – The prodromal stage is the first stage of acute radiation syndrome, in which the onset of symptoms occur.

- ■ **latent stage** – The latent stage can be considered a dormant period in which no visible symptoms appear, even though biologic damage has occurred.

- ■ **manifest stage** – The manifest stage is the stage in which symptoms become visibly noticeable.

- ■ **recovery or death stage** – The recovery or death stage is dependent on the radiation dose; either the body will begin to recover (generally doses lower than 600 rad) or death will result. Death is inevitable at a whole-body radiation dose of 1000 rad or more.

alopecia – Alopecia is a medical condition in which an individual experiences hair loss. An acute radiation dose of 200–300 rad is known to cause alopecia.

anabolic – Anabolic describes a metabolic process in which the production of a substance or material occurs.

biological effect – Ionizing radiation can cause biological damage to a cell. The extent of damage depends on the type of interaction (direct or indirect hit) between x-ray photon and cell. Possible biological effects from ionizing radiation include:

- ■ no damage to the cell

- ■ damage to the cell with cell recovery and normal functional ability

- ■ damage to the cell with cell recovery and abnormal functional ability

- ■ damage to the cell resulting in death

biology – Biology is the study of living organisms.

carcinogen – A carcinogen is a substance or agent that is harmful to normal cell production and results in cancer.

catabolic – Catabolic describes a metabolic process in which the breakdown of a substance or material occurs.

cell – A cell is considered to be the smallest unit of a living organism. There are various cell types (e.g., epithelial cells, connective tissue cells, muscle cells, nerve cells), each designed to perform a specific function with the commonality of having a plasma membrane and two main components: cytoplasm and a nucleus. A cell is able to function independently, maintain homeostasis, and, for the majority of human cells, reproduce. The reproductive rate or mitotic rate (cell division) varies with cell type and degree of maturity. The neuron, for example, cannot reproduce or regenerate without medical intervention. The typical cell, along with its components and associated functions, are provided for further review (*see Figure 12-1 and Table 12-2*).

chromosome – A chromosome is a tiny strand-like structure located within the nucleus of a cell and containing genetic information in the form of DNA

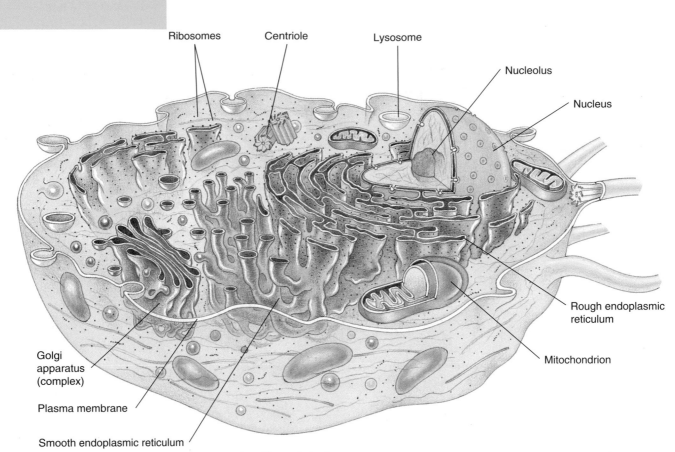

Ribosomes   Centriole   Lysosome

Nucleolus

Nucleus

Rough endoplasmic reticulum

Mitochondrion

Golgi apparatus (complex)

Plasma membrane

Smooth endoplasmic reticulum

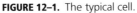

FIGURE 12–1. The typical cell.

Delmar/Cengage Learning.

(deoxyribonucleic acid). There are 23 pairs of chromosomes; half of each pair is from the mother, the other half is from the father.

chronic – Chronic refers to slow progression of an illness that lasts over an extended period of time.

chronic radiation dose – A chronic radiation dose describes a small dose of radiation delivered to the whole body over an extended period of time.

congenital effect – A congenital effect is a genetic anomaly present at birth.

cumulative exposure – Cumulative exposure is the amount of radiation an occupational worker receives throughout the scope of practice performance. The National Council on Radiation Protection and Measurements (NCRP) recommends an occupational worker not exceed the annual effective dose equivalent limit of 5 rem and to not exceed the annual effective cumulative dose equivalent limit of the sum of the worker's age in years $\times$ 1 rem.

desquamation – Desquamation describes a sloughing off or peeling of the skin. An acute radiation dose of approximately 300 rad is known to cause desquamation.

differentiated cell – Mature cells that are specialized to perform a specific function are referred to as differentiated cells.

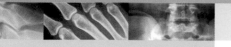

TABLE 12–2   Cell Components and Functions

CELL COMPONENTS	FUNCTION
Cell membrane	Semipermeable barrier designed to protect cell components and permit selected materials to pass through
Cytoplasm	Cell contents: consists of proteins, carbohydrates, lipids, nucleic acids (RNA and DNA), electrolytes, and water
▬ cytosol	Fluid substance within the cell
▬ organelles	Components of cell consisting of *nonmembranous organelles* and *membranous organelles*
Organelles	
▬ *Nonmembranous*	Organelle containing no membrane
• *cilia*	Finger-like projections on the surface of the cell permit cell movement and movement of extracelluar material along the cell membrane
• *microvilli*	Small finger-like projections on the surface of the cell increase surface area for cellular absorption
• *centrioles*	Two centrioles positioned 90° to each other assist in moving chromosomes
• *ribosomes*	Production of proteins
▬ *Membranous*	Organelle containing a membrane
• smooth and rough endoplasmic reticulum (ER)	Smooth ER: produces carbohydrates and lipid (contains no ribosomes) Rough ER: produces proteins (contains ribosomes)
• golgi apparatus	Produces lysosomes and stores secretory materials
• lysosome	Contains enzymes for digesting old or damaged organelles
• mitochondria	Provide energy for cellular activity
• nucleus	Regulates production of cellular material, contains DNA (genetic information), and serves as the cell's control center

Data from: Rizzo, D. C. (2010). *Fundamentals of anatomy physiology* (3rd ed.). Clifton Park, NY: Delmar Cengage Learning; Forshier, S. (2009). *Essentials of radiation biology and protection* (2nd ed.). Clifton Park, NY: Delmar Cengage Learning.

■ **undifferentiated cell** – An undifferentiated cell (or stem cell) is a very young, immature cell that has not yet become specialized to perform a specific function.

DNA – DNA, or deoxyribonucleic acid, is a nucleic acid found within the nucleus of a cell. DNA is often referred to as the "master molecule" of the cell because it contains the genetic coding for all cellular function. DNA takes the shape of a double helix with deoxyribose and phosphoric acid forming the foundation of what appears to be a twisting ladder, with the four organic nitrogenous bases as steps within the ladder. These nitrogenous bases house the genetic codes for all cellular function and are bound in a unique pairing of purine to purine (adenine and guanine) and pyrimidine to pyrimidine (thymine and cytosine) *(see Figure 12-2)*.

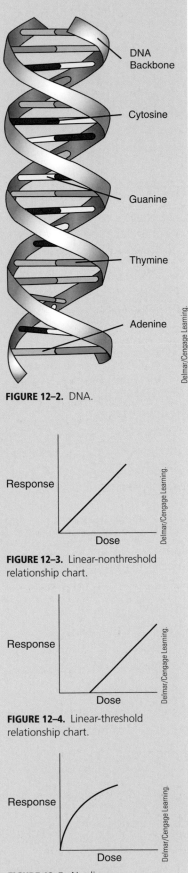

FIGURE 12–2. DNA.

DNA Backbone

Cytosine

Guanine

Thymine

Adenine

Response

Dose

FIGURE 12–3. Linear-nonthreshold relationship chart.

Response

Dose

FIGURE 12–4. Linear-threshold relationship chart.

Response

Dose

FIGURE 12–5. Nonlinear-nonthreshold relationship chart.

dose-effect relationships – There are four dose-effect relationships or dose-response curves that signify a specific relationship between radiation exposure (dose) and a biological response (effect). The dose-effect relationship associated with occupational workers is the *linear-nonthreshold* relationship. It demonstrates the smallest quantity of radiation as unsafe (nonthreshold) and further demonstrates a proportional relationship between an increase in radiation dose and an increase in the body's biological response.

- **linear-nonthreshold relationship** – The linear aspect of the dose-effect relationship graph seen as a straight diagonal line demonstrates a proportional relationship between dose and biological response. Increasing the radiation dose will increase the biological response. The nonthreshold (meaning there is no quantity of radiation considered safe) aspect of the dose-effect relationship graph is depicted by the diagonal line originating at the intersection of the *x*- and *y*-axes *(see Figure 12–3)*.

- **linear-threshold relationship** – The linear aspect of the dose-effect relationship graph seen as a straight diagonal line demonstrates a proportional relationship between dose and biological response. Increasing the radiation dose will increase the biological response. The threshold (meaning there is an established quantity of radiation considered to be safe, causing no biological response) aspect of the dose-effect relationship graph is depicted by the diagonal line originating along the *x*-axis and not at the intersection point of the *x*- and *y*-axes *(see Figure 12–4)*.

- **nonlinear-nonthreshold relationship** – The nonlinear aspect of the dose-effect relationship graph seen as a sigmoid (s-curve) line demonstrates a nonproportional relationship between dose and biological response. Increasing the radiation dose will not necessarily increase the biological response. The nonthreshold (meaning there is no quantity of radiation considered safe) aspect of the dose-effect relationship graph is depicted by the sigmoid line originating at the intersection of the *x*- and *y*-axes *(see Figure 12–5)*.

- **nonlinear-threshold relationship** – The nonlinear aspect of the dose-effect relationship graph seen as a sigmoid (s-curve) line demonstrates a non-proportional relationship between dose and biological response. Increasing the radiation dose will not necessarily increase the biological response. The threshold (meaning there is an established quantity of radiation considered to be safe, causing no biological response) aspect of the dose-effect relationship graph is depicted by the sigmoid line originating along the *x*-axis and not at the intersection point of the *x*- and *y*-axes *(see Figure 12–6)*.

dose-response curves – *See dose-effect relationships.*

doubling dose – The doubling dose refers to the quantity of radiation necessary to double the amount of genetic mutations within a population. The estimated doubling dose for the human population is 50–250 rad.

effects of radiation – Effects of radiation can either manifest within the individual who has been exposed to radiation or to the offspring of the

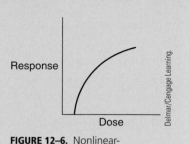

FIGURE 12–6. Nonlinear-threshold relationship chart.

individual exposed to radiation. Not all radiation exposure produces biological effects (*see stochastic and non-stochastic effects*). However, even the smallest amount of radiation exposure has the potential to cause a biological response (linear-nonthreshold).

- **genetic effect** – A genetic effect of radiation exposure manifests in the offspring (future generations) of the individual who has been exposed to radiation.

- **somatic effect** – A somatic effect of radiation exposure manifests within the individual who has been exposed to radiation.

entrance skin exposure (ESE) – Entrance skin exposure is an estimated exposure dose to a patient based on the amount of radiation entering at the level of the skin (source to object distance) as opposed to the amount of radiation that will transverse to deeper levels of the body. ESE takes into account mR/mAs, amount of total filtration, source-to-image distance, and kVp used for a given radiographic exposure. ESE can be determined through the use of a *nomogram*, where total filtration is indicated on the *x*-axis, x-ray intensity (mR/mAs) is indicated along the *y*-axis, and kVp ranges (typically in increments of 10 kVp) are curved lines that lie in the center of the graph between the *x*- and *y*-axes. Plotting the intersection of the x-ray unit's total filtration and the kVp selected for the radiographic exposure will provide an additional plot point, which, when followed in a straight horizontal line to the *y*-axis, will demonstrate the x-ray intensity of the selected exposure. Multiplying the x-ray intensity (mR/mAs) by the mAs selected for the radiographic exposure will yield an estimated ESE.

epilation – *See alopecia.*

erythema – Erythema describes reddening of the skin. An acute radiation dose of approximately 300 rad is known to cause erythema.

fractionation – Fractionation is a therapeutic term related to radiation therapy in which a prescribed dose of radiation is delivered to a patient in small doses over a specified period of time. Distributing a large dose of radiation through small incremental doses over a period of time allows normal cells a chance to recover or repopulate while allowing abnormal or cancerous cells to die.

free radical – A free radical is a molecule or atom that has that has been ionized (missing an electron). A free radical can be described as an unstable molecule or atom, which has the potential to cause biological damage. Free radicals can occur via *radiolysis*.

gene – A gene is the unit of heredity that resides within the chromosome of a cell. Genes come in pairs and carry the DNA for genetic coding of future offspring.

genetics – Genetics involves the transference of DNA coding from germ cells to future generations upon the union of ova and spermatozoa.

genetic significant dose (GSD) – The genetic significant dose (GSD) is the equivalent dose received by a whole population, resulting in the same genetic effect on the entire population as the sum of individual doses. GSD is an estimated annual weighted average gonadal dose of radiation within a given population of persons within the childbearing years. The total GSD for the U.S. population is estimated at 120 mrad/yr when one takes into account natural background radiation (100 mrad/yr) and radiation exposure through medical procedures (20 mrad/yr). Populations are typically categorized by geographic location and consider age, gender, and the expected number of offspring for the given population.

germ cell – A germ cell is a reproductive cell; either a spermatozoa or an ova. Germ cells reproduce through a process of division known as meiosis.

gonads – Gonads refer to both male and female reproductive organs. Gonadal protective shielding is required during radiographic procedures when the primary beam is within 5 cm of the gonads unless the protective shielding hinders the anatomical area of interest being imaged.

heredity – Heredity is the genetic information (DNA) passed along to future generations during meiosis.

law of Bergonié and Tribondeau – The law of Bergonié and Tribondeau originated from two scientists who studied the biological effects of radiation in the early 1900s. Their studies revealed a direct relationship between cell sensitivity and biological response. Cells that are most sensitive to radiation are:

- immature (young)
- undifferentiated (not specialized in function)
- possess a high metabolic rate (divide rapidly)

LD$_{50/60}$ – The LD$_{50/60}$ signifies an acute whole-body radiation dose resulting in 50% of the population dying within 60 days after exposure. The LD$_{50/60}$ for humans is approximately 320–520 rad depending on medical treatment received.

LD$_{100}$ – The LD$_{100}$ signifies a whole-body radiation dose of 1000 rad or more in which 100% of the population will die.

linear energy transfer (LET) – Linear energy transfer (LET) is the amount of energy transferred from ionizing radiation to tissue. Highly ionizing radiation will deposit more energy in tissue as it passes through it than will a lower ionizing radiation. Low ionizing radiation, such as x-rays or gamma rays, is considered highly penetrating and therefore can more readily pass through tissue, depositing little energy. Highly ionizing radiation such as alpha particles or fast neutrons is less penetrating, unable to pass through tissue easily and resulting in a large transference of energy. Subsequently, LET shares a direct relationship with relative biological effect (RBE). The greater the LET, the greater the RBE.

lethal – The term "lethal" means deadly, i.e., able to cause death (*see LD$_{50/60}$*).

mean marrow dose – Mean marrow dose refers to the average dose of radiation delivered to anatomic areas that contain active bone marrow.

meiosis – Meiosis is the process of cell division involving germ cells or reproductive cells in which half the total number of chromosomes (23) occurs in the formation of a spermatozoa or ova. This cellular division allows for a union of sperm and ovum in the creation of a zygote, which will contain chromosomes from each germ cell for a total of 46 chromosomes.

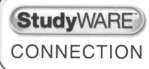

StudyWARE™
CONNECTION

View the Meiosis animation on your StudyWARE™ CD-ROM.

mitosis – Mitosis is the process of cell division involving somatic cells (non-reproductive cells) in which the number of chromosomes for a human somatic cell (23 pairs of chromosomes or 46 chromosomes) is maintained in each subsequent somatic cell. The somatic cellular cycle begins with *interphase*. Interphase is the where cell growth occurs; this phase can be further classified by three subphases: G_1 (cell growth), S (production of DNA), and G_2 (chromosomes double). After interphase, which is the longest part of the cellular cycle, are the four stages of mitosis.

■ **prophase** – Prophase is the first stage of mitosis; chromatin forms chromosomes and spindle formation occurs at opposite poles of the cell.

■ **metaphase** – Metaphase is the second stage of mitosis; chromosomes align along the metaphase plate (center of the cell).

■ **anaphase** – Anaphase is the third stage of mitosis; paired chromosomes move to opposite poles of the cell.

■ **telophase** – Telophase is the final stage of mitosis; cell division occurs and produces two daughter cells each containing a nucleus.

StudyWARE™
CONNECTION

View the Mitosis animation on your StudyWARE™ CD-ROM.

molecule – A molecule is produced when two or more atoms of either the same element or different elements combine.

mutation – A mutation is a genetic deviation resulting from an alteration (or damage) in the DNA of a germ (reproductive) cell.

nomogram – A nomogram is a chart or graph from which approximate entrance skin exposure (ESE) can be determined. The following steps are used to calculate ESE *(see Figure 12–7).*

1. Identify the x-ray unit's total filtration on the *x*-axis and follow it vertically until it intersects with the appropriate kVp curve (selected kVp for exposure).

2. At the point of intersection between total filtration and the selected kVp, draw an imaginary line horizontally until it intersects with the *y*-axis of skin exposure (mR/mAs).

3. Identify the number on the *y*-axis that represents skin exposure (mR/mAs) and multiply it by the mAs used in the exposure to determine the approximate entrance skin exposure (ESE) to the patient.

oxygen enhancement ratio (OER) – Oxygen enhancement ratio is the ratio of biological effects of radiation resulting from conditions in which oxygen is

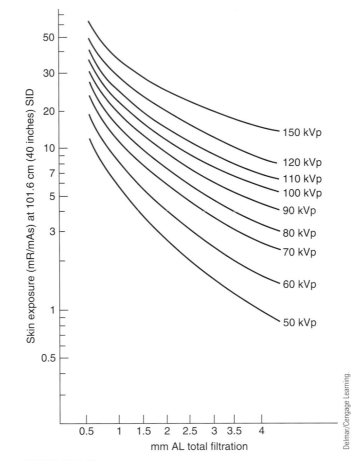

Skin exposure (mR/mAs) at 101.6 cm (40 inches) SID

mm AL total filtration

Delmar/Cengage Learning.

FIGURE 12–7. Nomogram.

present versus biological effects of radiation resulting from conditions in which oxygen is not present.

proliferate – Proliferate is to multiply, grow, or produce new cells.

quality factor – *See radiation-weighting factor (W_R).*

radiation-weighting factor (W_R) – The radiation-weighting factor (W_R) or quality factor *(QF)* is a numerical assignment given to various types of radiation based on the amount of radiation absorbed dose required to cause the same biological effect.

- ▪ x-rays, gamma rays, and beta particles = W_R or *QF* of 1
- ▪ alpha particles and neutrons = W_R or *QF* of 20

radiolysis – Radiolysis is the breakdown of a water molecule within a cell as a result of ionizing radiation. This process can cause free radicals to arise, resulting in biological damage to the cell. This type of damage is considered to be an *indirect effect* of ionizing radiation.

radioresistant cells – Radioresistant cells are considered to be less sensitive to the effects of radiation. Mature cells are more radioresistant than young undifferentiated stem cells. The following cell types are considered radioresistant:

- ▪ muscle cells (myocytes)
- ▪ nerve cells (neurons)

    (see law of Bergonié and Tribondeau)

radiosensitive cells – Radiosensitive cells are considered to be highly sensitive to the effects of radiation. Stem cells are more radiosensitive than differentiated mature cells. The following cell types are considered radiosensitive:

- lymphocytes (white blood cells)
- erthyocytes (red blood cells)
- germ cells (reproductive cells)
- intestinal crypt cells (small intestine cells – referred to as "Crypts of Lieberkühn) *(see law of Bergonié and Tribondeau)*

radiosensitive organs – The radiosensitive organs of the body are the blood-forming organs, which include: bone marrow, lymph nodes, thymus, and spleen.

relative biological effect (RBE) – RBE is a comparison between x-rays (using a standard of 250 keV) and other types of ionizing radiation producing the same biological damage.

restitution – Restitution refers to the ability of DNA to repair itself.

RNA – RNA or ribonucleic acid is a nucleic acid produced in the cells nucleolus. RNA can be found in ribosomes.

somatic cell – Somatic cells are found throughout the body and proliferate through the process of mitosis. Somatic cells are considered nonreproduction cells.

stem cell – Stem cells can be categorized into two main types, *embryonic stem cells* and *adult stem cells*. Embryonic stem cells are found in embryos; they are young immature cells unspecialized (or undifferentiated) in their function. Adult stem cells are undifferentiated cells that provide the body with the mechanism to repair and maintain differentiated cells within a tissue type.

stochastic effect – A stochastic effect or nondeterministic effect is a biological effect of radiation exposure that is considered random and unpredictable. Stochastic effects are associated with low levels of radiation exposure over an extended period of time. Because of the unpredictability of a stochastic effect, no amount of radiation is considered safe; therefore, radiation protective measures are employed for both patients and occupational workers. Common stochastic effects include cancer, leukemia, cataracts, and genetic anomalies.

- **nonstochastic effect** – A nonstochastic effect or a deterministic effect is a biological effect of radiation exposure that is considered predictable and measurable. Nonstochastic effects are associated with high levels of radiation exposure over a short period of time. Nonstochastic effects have a threshold at which expected effects begin to occur; radiation levels below the threshold do not produce the expected effect. Common nonstochastic effects include a decrease in RBC and WBC formation, nausea, vomiting, and diarrhea (NVD), erythema, alopecia, sterility, cataracts, and radiation sickness (acute radiation syndrome).

symptom – A symptom is a manifestation or indication of a disease or illness. A fever is considered a symptom of an infection within the body.

target theory – Target theory is the principle by which radiation damage to a cell can be classified as either resulting from a direct effect or an indirect effect.

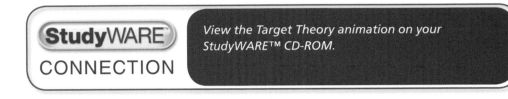

■ **direct effect** – A direct effect of ionizing radiation occurs when the master molecule of the cell (DNA) is damaged. DNA damage can cause severe alterations to the transference of genetic information and/or cellular death.

■ **indirect effect** – An indirect effect of ionizing radiation occurs when the cytoplasm of the cell, which contains water molecules, is affected, causing the formation of free radicals. Free radicals can cause damage or cellular death.

StudyWARE CONNECTION

View the Target Theory animation on your StudyWARE™ CD-ROM.

threshold – A threshold is an established point at which an effect or specified outcome presents.

StudyWARE CONNECTION

After completing this chapter, complete the Championship game or another interactive game on your StudyWARE™ CD-ROM that will help you learn the content in this chapter.

CONCEPT THINKING QUESTIONS

1. What is linear energy transfer (LET) and what relationship does it have with relative biological effect (RBE)?

2. Identify the three syndromes classified as an acute radiation syndrome.

3. Differentiate between a stochastic effect and a nonstochastic effect.

4. What is a congenital effect?

5. Identify the master molecule of a cell.

6. Differentiate between a somatic cell and a germ cell.

7. Explain the possible biological effects of ionizing radiation on a somatic cell.

8. Explain what radiolysis is and the biological effect it can produce.

9. Name the four dose-response relationships and identify the one that is considered standard for diagnostic imaging procedures.

10. Identify the two categories of a stem cell.

11. What is the $LD_{50/60}$ for humans?

12. What cells within the human body are considered the most radioresistant?

PRACTICE EXERCISES

1. List the four phases of mitosis.

2. Which cell types undergo cell reproduction through the process of meiosis?

3. Provide two examples of a stochastic effect.

4. Provide two examples of a non-stochastic effect.

5. Draw the dose-response relationship that correlates to radiation exposure through diagnostic imaging procedures.

6. Explain what the term "doubling dose" means.

7. List two types of ionizing radiation yielding a high LET.

8. List two types of ionizing radiation yielding a low LET.

9. Identify the three classifications of acute radiation syndrome along with their associated exposure dosages.

10. Name the two main components of a typical cell, and explain the function of the semipermeable membrane.

11. Identify the cell's membranous organelles and nonmembranous organelles.

12. Determine the maximum annual cumulative exposure dose for a 37-year-old occupational worker in accordance with recommendations by the National Council on Radiation Protection (NCRP).

MATCHING

Match each term to the appropriate description.

undifferentiated	age in yrs. × 1 rem	desquamation
nomogram	restitution	radioresistant
radiosensitive	mitochondria	lysosome
gene	epilation	urticaria
fractionation	pronation	golgi apparatus
radiolysis	NVD	temporary sterility
mutation	OER	RBE

Description	Term
1. provides cellular energy	_____
2. DNA repair	_____
3. immature cell	_____
4. neurons	_____
5. oxygen and biological effects	_____

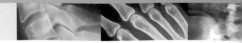

6. destruction of H$_2$O molecule   _____

7. germ cell   _____

8. hair loss   _____

9. unit of heredity   _____

10. peeling of skin   _____

11. genetic deviation   _____

12. small doses of radiation over long time   _____

RETENTION OF MATERIAL

Retention requires practicing the use of previously learned material. Apply the knowledge you have regarding radiation biology principles to answer the following questions.

1. Identify the four stages of acute radiation syndrome and explain what occurs during each stage.

2. What level of radiation exposure to an individual qualifies as an acute radiation dose?

3. Explain the law of Bergonié and Tribondeau and relate its significance to understanding biological responses to radiation exposure.

4. Identify the components that constitute a DNA double helix.

5. Explain the function of lysosomes within the cell.

6. Name the two types of nucleic acids found within a cell.

7. Differentiate between the functions of rough and smooth endoplasmic reticulum (ER).

8. Differentiate between an anabolic and catabolic process; provide an example of each.

9. Identify the four chemical components found within a typical cell.

10. Identify the components of a typical cell along with their main function.

CHAPTER 13

Radiation Protection

OBJECTIVES

Upon completion of this chapter, the reader will be able to:

- Discuss the ALARA principle
- Distinguish between primary and secondary barriers
- List types of radiation protection devices and their usage
- Identify NCRP dose-limit recommendations
- Identify traditional and SI units for radiation measurement
- Discuss the three cardinal rules of radiation protection
- Describe types of radiation personnel monitors and radiation detectors
- Explain methods to minimize patient exposure
- Discuss protective measures used for fluoroscopic procedures and mobile radiography
- Discuss personal protection of a pregnant radiographer

CONCEPT THINKING

Radiation protection involves radiation safety practices used within the imaging profession to protect both the public and occupational workers from unnecessary exposure to ionizing radiation. Effects of low-dose radiation are considered to be stochastic (random) in nature; therefore, precautions are taken to minimize radiation exposure occurring from diagnostic medical procedures. The standard practice that radiologic technologists adhere to regarding patient safety and the use of ionizing radiation is the ALARA principle. ALARA is the acronym for *as low as reasonably achievable*. To ensure that patients are receiving minimum amounts of radiation in the production of diagnostic images, technologists use optimal exposure techniques, including high kVp within the acceptable range for appropriate penetration, low mAs (shortest amount of time, when a breathing technique is not desired), four-sided collimation, and protective shielding. Technologists must also protect themselves from exposure to secondary radiation (scatter) because radiographic procedures often require technologists to be in the same room as the patient undergoing the diagnostic imaging procedure. These types of procedures typically involve fluoroscopy and mobile radiography, which require technologists to use the following cardinal rule for minimizing exposure to ionizing radiation: *time*, *distance*, and *shielding*. Reducing the *time* exposed to ionizing radiation reduces the dose received. Doubling *distance*, which is considered the best form of radiation protection as evidenced in the inverse square law, from the radiation source reduces beam intensity by a factor of four. Reducing beam intensity by a factor of four equates to one-quarter of the original dose. The use of protective *shielding* (e.g., lead apparel, such as aprons, goggles, gloves, and thyroid shields) greatly minimizes the exposure dose of occupational workers. Occupational workers are required to wear a radiation personnel monitoring device *(dosimeter)* to monitor the amount of radiation exposure received on a monthly, quarterly, or annual basis via occupational exposure. Employers and the designated Radiation Safety Officer maintain and monitor all employee dosimetry reports, providing employees with a dose record indicating current exposure dose (quarterly), year-to-date dose, and cumulative exposure dose. Radiation exposure is cumulative, requiring future employers of an occupational worker to request the most current dosimetry report readings from the previous employer. This transfer of information ensures that a continuous and accurate record of occupational exposure is maintained for each employee regardless of a change in employers.

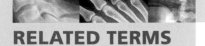

RELATED TERMS

ALARA – ALARA is the radiation safety acronym for *as low as reasonably achievable*, meaning to set exposure techniques for optimal images while using minimum radiation as a means of protecting the patient from unnecessary radiation exposure.

automatic exposure control devices (AEC) – Automatic exposure control devices, often referred to as AEC devices, are x-ray imaging systems that use mechanisms designed to reduce repeat radiation exposure to patients while producing consistent radiographic images. The two types of AEC imaging systems common to diagnostic radiography are the *ionization chamber* and the *photomultiplier tube*; each operates differently, yet both produce quality standard images. AEC selectors are located on the x-ray control console and permit technologists to choose from an array of radiographic procedures in which the appropriate detection chamber (or photocell arrangement), mA station, and kVp value has been pre-set. *(Refer to Chapter 7: Circuitry.)*

dosimeter – A dosimeter is a device that detects and measures ionizing radiation. Two main types of dosimeters are *personnel monitoring devices* and *field survey instruments*.

■ **personnel monitoring devices** – A radiation personnel monitoring device is worn by an occupational worker (e.g., radiographers, radiologists, special procedure nurses), usually at the level of one's collar (and outside the lead apron during fluoroscopic procedures or mobile radiography), to measure exposure to ionizing radiation. Dosimeter rings are also available for occupational workers whose extremities may be close to the radiation source. Depending on the health care facility, these monitors may be measured monthly or quarterly with dosimetry reports maintained on record by the Radiation Safety Officer (RSO). The four types of personnel monitoring devices are described in *Table 13–1*.

TABLE 13–1   Personnel Monitoring Devices

TYPE OF DEVICE	HOW IT WORKS	ADVANTAGES	DISADVANTAGES
Film badge dosimeter *(see Figure 13–1)*	Plastic clip-on case houses radiographic film and aluminum and copper filters (possess different atomic numbers that determine the quality or type of ionizing radiation). A densitometer is required to read the film density; density is proportional to the radiation detected.	▪ inexpensive ▪ distinguishes types of ionizing radiation ▪ permanent legal record	▪ fogging of film contributes to exposure reading ▪ can only be worn one month ▪ cannot detect radiation levels lower than 10 mrem
Optically stimulated luminescence dosimeter (OSL)* *(see Figure 13–2)*	Plastic clip-on case houses aluminum oxide crystals that, when stimulated by a laser light, release energy in the form of light. The light is directly proportional to the radiation detected and is measured by a photomultiplier tube.	▪ can detect radiation levels as low as 1 mrem ▪ reliable readings ▪ provides additional information on quality of ionizing radiation	▪ expensive
Pocket dosimeter	Ionization chamber contains air and two electrodes. Electrodes are charged, causing ions to form when radiation is detected. Requires a light source to read the exposure scale.	▪ immediate readout ▪ can detect radiation levels as low as 1 mrem	▪ very expensive ▪ provides no legal record ▪ must be reset to zero after each reading ▪ electrodes not charged properly can cause inaccurate readings ▪ not recommended for routine use
Thermoluminescent dosimeter (TLD) *(see Figure 13–3)*	Plastic clip-on case houses lithium fluoride crystals that, when heated, release energy in the form of light. The light is directly proportional to the radiation	▪ worn for a 3-month period ▪ available in a ring to be worn on finger ▪ can be reused up to 1 year	▪ expensive ▪ provides no permanent record

(Continued)

TABLE 13–1   Personnel Monitoring Devices *(Continued)*

TYPE OF DEVICE	HOW IT WORKS	ADVANTAGES	DISADVANTAGES
	detected by the TLD and is measured by a photomultiplier tube.	■ can detect radiation levels as low as 5 mrem ■ not affected by environmental conditions	

*Most popular dosimeter.

Data from Carlton, R. R., & Adler, A. M. (2006). *Principles of radiographic imaging: An art and a science* (4th ed.). Clifton Park, NY: Delmar Cengage Learning; Bushong, S. C. (2008). *Radiologic science for technologists: Physics, biology, and protection* (9th ed.). St. Louis, MO: Elsevier. Copyright © Elsevier; and Forshier, S. (2009). *Essentials of radiation biology and protection* (2nd ed.). Clifton Park, NY: Delmar Cengage Learning.

■ **field survey instruments** – Field survey instruments are radiation detection devices used to measure ionizing radiation in the air. There are three types of field survey instruments: ionzation chamber, Geiger-Muller counter, and scintillation counter *(see Table 13–2)*.

effective dose limit recommendations – The National Council on Radiation Protection and Measurements (NCRP) makes recommendations for dose limits for occupational workers and the general public (including recommendations for embryo/fetus and trainees/radiography students; *see Table 13–3)*. Reports published by the NCRP can be accessed via the NCRP website: http://www.ncrp.com.

TABLE 13–2   Field Survey Instruments

TYPE OF DEVICE	HOW IT WORKS
Ionization chamber *(Cutie Pie)*	Ionization chamber (typically referred to as the *Cutie Pie*) contains air (gas) and 2 electrodes, one positive (+) and one negative (−). Electrodes are charged, causing ions to form when radiation is detected. The amount of negative ions formed is in direct relationship to the amount of radiation detected. The ionization chamber is perhaps the most popular field survey instrument for reasons of easy portability, wide detection range (>1 mR/hr), and high accuracy. Best for use where fluoroscopic procedures are conducted.
Geiger-Muller counter	The Geiger-Muller counter uses a gas detection chamber and provides a progressing audible sound with the detection of increasing amounts of alpha particles, beta particles, and gamma rays. Used in areas in which radioactive materials are found (e.g., nuclear medicine labs, research labs).
Scintillation counter	The scintillation counter houses specialized crystals that, when struck by radiation (x-ray and gamma), emit light. The amount of light emitted is directly related to the amount of radiation detected. A photomultiplier tube measures the light. Scintillation counters are very sensitive and are more commonly associated with nuclear medicine facilities.

Data from: Carlton, R. R., & Adler, A. M. (2006). *Principles of radiographic imaging: An art and a science* (4th ed.). Clifton Park, NY: Delmar Cengage Learning; Bushong, S. C. (2008). *Radiologic science for technologists: Physics, biology, and protection* (9th ed.). St. Louis, MO: Elsevier. Copyright © Elsevier; and Forshier, S. (2009). *Essentials of radiation biology and protection* (2nd ed.). Clifton Park, NY: Delmar Cengage Learning.

TABLE 13-3   NCRP Effective Dose Limit Recommendations

	TRADITIONAL UNITS	SI UNITS
Occupational exposures		
■ Effective dose limits:		
• Annual	5 rem	50 mSv
• Cumulative	1 rem × age	10 mSv × age
■ Dose equivalent annual limits for tissues and organs		
• Lens of eye	15 rem	150 mSv
• Skin, hands, and feet	50 rem	500 mSv
Public annual exposures		
■ Effective dose limits:		
• Continuous or frequent exposure	0.1 rem	1 mSv
• Infrequent exposure	0.5 rem	5 mSv
■ Effective dose limits for tissues and organs		
• Lens of eye	1.5 rem	15 mSv
• Skin, hands, and feet	5 rem	50 mSv
Embryo-fetus monthly exposures		
■ Equivalent dose limit	0.05 rem	0.5 mSv
Education/training annual exposures		
■ Effective dose limit	0.1 rem	1 mSv
■ Dose equivalent limit for tissues and organs		
• Lens of eye	1.5 rem	15 mSv
• Skin, hands, and feet	5 rem	50 mSv
Negligible individual annual dose	0.001 rem	0.01 mSv

Adapted with permission of the National Council on Radiation Protection and Measurements, *NCRP Report No. 116: Limitations of exposure to ionizing radiation*; Table 19–1; Summary of Recommendations, http://www.ncrp.com.

entrance skin exposure (ESE) for fluoroscopic procedures – The entrance skin exposure rate is greater for fluoroscopic procedures than for diagnostic radiographic procedures. To protect patients from excess exposure to ionizing radiation, state and federal agencies mandate the ESE for fluoroscopic procedures to not exceed 10 R/min. The average ESE for fluoroscopic procedures is between 3 and 5 R/min.

exposure linearity – Exposure linearity refers to various combinations of mA stations and exposure times to produce the same overall mAs without exceeding a ±10% variation of radiation intensity for adjacent mA stations. To accurately test for exposure linearity, a series of radiographic exposures using combinations of mA and exposure time to yield the same overall mAs must be taken.

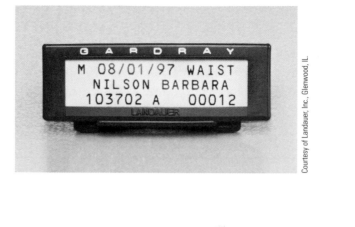

G A R D R A Y
M 08/01/97 WAIST
NILSON BARBARA
103702 A 00012
LANDAUER

FIGURE 13–1. Film badge.

Courtesy of Landauer, Inc., Glenwood, IL.

Open Window
Aluminum Oxide Detector Film
Copper Filter
Tin Filter
Imaging Filter
LAURA SUMMERS
RADIOLOGY
UNIVERSITY MEDICAL CENTER
luxel+
LANDAUER
N-144

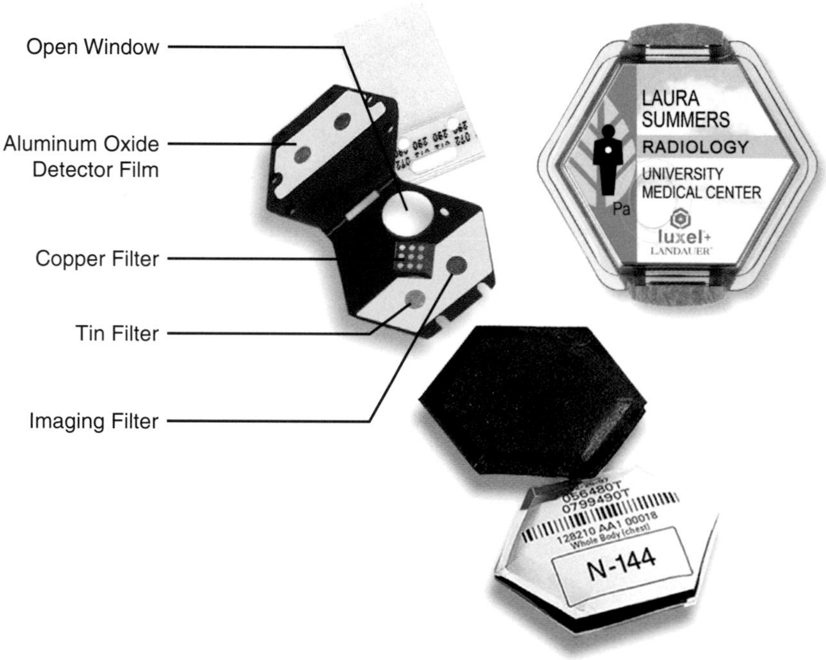

FIGURE 13–2. OSL dosimeter.

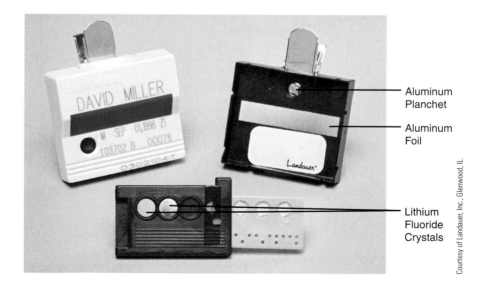

Courtesy of Landauer, Inc., Glenwood, IL.

DAVID MILLER
M SEP 01,1998 Z1
103702 B 00078
Landauer
Aluminum Planchet
Aluminum Foil
Lithium Fluoride Crystals

FIGURE 13–3. TLD.

Courtesy of Landauer, Inc., Glenwood, IL.

■ Exposure linearity testing requires a dosimeter to accurately measure radiation intensity for each exposure taken yielding the same mAs while varying the mA and exposure time. These readings should not exceed a ±10% variation for adjacent mA stations.

exposure reproducibility – Exposure reproducibility refers to taking a series of radiation exposures utilizing the same exposure settings (mA, kvp, and time), with changes to the settings made between the exposures, to produce the same radiation intensity for each exposure without exceeding a ±5% variation.

■ Exposure reproducibility testing requires a dosimeter to accurately measure radiation intensity for each exposure in the series.

exposure timer accuracy – Exposure timer accuracy is tested annually or when a change to the x-ray tube has occurred. Single-phase full-wave rectified equipment requires a *manual spin top test* to measure timer accuracy. A predetermined number of dots should appear on a radiographic image to confirm an accurate exposure time within ±5% > 10 ms exposures or within ±20% < 10 ms exposures. *(Refer to manual spin top test.)* Three-phase rectified equipment requires a synchronous motor spin test or an oscilloscope to measure timer accuracy. A predetermined degree of arc should appear on a radiographic image confirming an accurate exposure time.

exposure timer test tools – There are two main types of exposure timer test tools: the manual spin top test and the synchronous motor spin test (oscilloscope).

■ **manual spin top test** – This timer test tool must be manually spun on top of an image receptor (IR) while an exposure is taken *(see Figure 13-4)*. Because current in the United States is a 60-hertz cycle, we can anticipate a full-wave rectified unit will produce 120 impulses (60 hertz cycle = two positive impulses within one hertz cycle or 120 impulses). The 120 impulses remain a constant variable, with exposure time being the changing variable. The radiographic image produced using the spin top test will show a specific number of dots for a given exposure time. The following mathematical formula can be used to determine exposure timer accuracy. The *mathematical triangle* can be used to find the missing component of the formula when two factors are provided *(see Figure 13-5)*.

● The total number of dots on the radiographic image divided by 120 (the constant variable) = the exposure time *(see Figure 13-5)*.

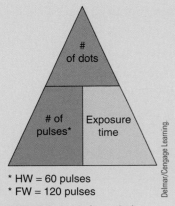

* HW = 60 pulses
* FW = 120 pulses

FIGURE 13–5. Mathematical triangle for manual spin top test.

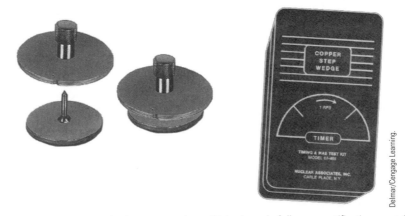

FIGURE 13–4. Manual spin top test using a 60-hertz cycle full-wave rectification wave form *(left)* and a synchronous motor spin tester *(right)*.

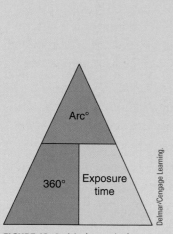

FIGURE 13–6. Mathematical triangle for synchronous motor spin test.

- **synchronous motor spin test** – This timer test tool has a synchronous motor, which is placed on top of an IR while an exposure is taken. Because current in the United States is a 60-hertz cycle, we can anticipate a full-wave rectified unit will produce 120 phases per one-hertz cycle and three-phase equipment will produce an overlap of three voltage waveforms synchronized 120° apart from one another. Because voltage never drops to zero with three-phase equipment, a degree of arc (based on a complete circle or 360°) will appear on the radiographic image rather than a series of dots. The following mathematical formula can be used to determine exposure timer accuracy using a synchronous motor spin test. The *mathematical triangle* can be used to find the missing component of the formula when two factors are provided *(see Figure 13–4)*.

  - The degree of arc on the radiographic image divided by 360° (the constant variable) = the exposure time *(see Figure 13-6)*.

flat contact shield – A flat contact shield is commonly used for recumbent patients. It is easily placed either over the gonads for general diagnostic radiographic procedures or under the patient for fluoroscopic procedures in which the radiation source originates underneath the patient.

focal spot testing – Focal spot testing is performed annually or when a change to the x-ray tube has occurred. The purpose of the testing is to measure the size of the effective focal spot and confirm that it is within the tolerance range of the manufacturer's specifications. Testing tools that can be used to measure focal spot size are the pinhole camera, star pattern, slit camera, and line pair resolution tool.

gonadal shield – A gonadal shield is a type of lead-impregnated shielding used to protect the patient's gonads (ovaries and testes). Gonadal shielding should possess a minimum of 0.5 mm of lead equivalent and be used when the primary beam is within 5 cm of the reproductive organs and not interfere with the anatomy of interest. Types of gonadal shields include flat contact shields, shadow shields, and shaped contact shields.

- **shadow shield** – The shadow shield is connected to the tube housing where the collimator box is located, allowing for an attached shape of lead (e.g., square, oval, round) to be positioned within the light field to cast a shadow over the patient's gonads. This type of shield is recommended for sterile procedures to prevent the technologist from contaminating the sterile field when attempting to shield patient.

- **shaped contact shield** – A shaped contact shield is cup-shaped and provides the best protection for the male gonads as the patient is able to move into various radiographic positions and maintain protection.

half-value layer (HVL) – A half-value layer is the amount of absorbing material placed in the path of the x-ray beam to reduce the x-ray beam's intensity to half its original value.

incident report – An incident report is a document detailing the occurrence of an accident typically involving injury to an individual while on the premises of a health care facility (i.e., employee, patient, trainee, visitor, volunteer). The immediate supervisor should complete an incident report directly after the incident to accurately document the circumstances surrounding the occurrence. Health care facilities maintain a record of all incident reports for a predetermined amount of time for liability reasons should the incident become a legal matter. *(Refer Appendix H: Radiation Dosimetry Report.)*

leakage radiation – Leakage radiation is the radiation that exits through the protective metal tube housing. Leakage radiation cannot exceed 100 mR/hr at a distance of 1 meter from the source.

National Council on Radiation Protection and Measurements (NCRP) – The NCRP is an advisory organization within the United States that serves to establish guidelines and recommendations for the development of policies and procedures regarding radiation protection.

Nuclear Regulatory Commission (NRC) – The NRC is a U.S. federal regulatory agency that oversees licensure for facilities using ionizing radiation and radioactive material and enforces radiation protection recommendations as established by the NCRP to protect the public from unnecessary and potentially harmful radiation exposure.

positive beam limitation (PBL) – Positive beam limitation is a safety feature of all modern x-ray imaging systems in which an automatic collimated x-ray beam field size is created to match the size of the IR when using a Bucky grid. The PBL must be within 2% of the source-to-image distance (SID). Even with the use of PBL, technologists are expected to collimate further (manually adjust the collimator shutters) to reduce the x-ray beam field size and reduce excess radiation exposure to the patient when it does not interfere with the anatomy of interest.

- increase collimation = smaller x-ray beam field size = less radiation exposure to patient

- increase collimation = less scatter radiation reaching IR = increase in image quality

pregnant radiographer/trainee – A pregnant radiographer or trainee is a radiologic technologist or student who has voluntarily declared her pregnancy to the medical facility or to the educational institution she attends. A second dosimeter will be ordered by the RSO for the pregnant radiographer/student to wear at waist level to monitor fetal exposure to ionizing radiation.

- **fetal personnel monitoring device** – A fetal dosimeter monitor is required for pregnant workers and pregnant radiography students who have declared their pregnancy either to their supervisor, education director, or RSO. A second dosimeter is provided to the pregnant worker/student to wear at waist level and under the lead apron during fluoroscopic procedures or mobile radiography to detect fetal exposure to ionizing radiation.

protective barrier – A protective barrier is barrier designed to protect individuals from exposure to ionizing radiation. Primary and secondary radiation (scatter radiation and leakage radiation) are taken into consideration when determining the amount of lead or lead equivalent necessary for a protective barrier.

■ **protective barrier considerations** – Protective barrier considerations are those variables considered in establishing appropriate amounts of lead (or lead equivalent) for protective barriers within medical facilities using ionizing radiation. These barriers are designed to protect both the public and occupational workers from unnecessary radiation exposure.

- **distance (D)** – Distance between the radiation source (x-ray tube) and the barrier.

- **occupancy (T)** – Occupied area on other side of the barrier; classified as either a controlled area or an uncontrolled area. Time of occupancy (frequent or infrequent) is also considered in determining the appropriate thickness of lead (or lead equivalent) for protective barriers.

  - **controlled area** – Occupational workers wearing a dosimeter badge and who have been training in radiation safety occupy what is considered a controlled area. This area is shielded so as to not exceed the annual effective absorbed dose limit of 5 rem per year.

  - **uncontrolled area** – The general public occupy uncontrolled areas such as hallways, stairways, waiting rooms, and restrooms. This area is shielded so as to not exceed the annual effective absorbed dose limit of 0.5 rem for infrequent exposure.

- **use factor (U)** – Use factor indicates the amount of time the primary beam is energized and pointing towards the barrier.

- **workload (W)** – Workload is measured in mA minutes per week. (mA min/wk) and factors in the radiographic volume and workload.

■ **primary protective barrier** – A primary protective barrier is a barrier toward which the primary beam can be directed. For these walls (and floor, if radiation source is located above the first level) where adjacent areas are occupied by either the general public (uncontrolled) or occupational workers (controlled area), a minimum of 1/16 inch of lead shielding or a lead equivalent (4 inches of masonry) is required. Primary barrier walls must extend 7 feet up from the floor.

■ **secondary protective barrier** – A secondary protective barrier is a barrier toward which the primary beam cannot be directed. For these walls, and for the walls that separate adjacent areas where the general public (uncontrolled) or occupational workers (controlled area) may be located, a minimum of 1/32 inch of lead shielding or a lead equivalent (2 inches of masonry) is required. Secondary barriers must overlap primary barriers by 1/2 inch. Lead equivalent materials considered for secondary barriers include concrete (masonry), glass, gypsum, wood, and steel.

protective devices – Protective devices are lead-impregnated vinyl shielding apparel designed to absorb scatter radiation and reduce radiation exposure to the patient and/or occupational worker (*see Table 13–4*).

TABLE 13–4 Protective Devices and Recommended Minimum Lead Requirements

PROTECTIVE DEVICE	MINIMUM LEAD (Pb) REQUIRED (OR EQUIVALENT)
Contact shields	0.25 mm
▬ Thyroid shield	0.50 mm
Aprons	0.25 mm
▬ Fluoroscopy aprons	0.50 mm
Gloves	0.25 mm
Eyeglasses/goggles	0.35 mm
Bucky slot cover	0.25 mm
Fluoro curtain/drape	0.25 mm
X-ray tube housing	Sufficient lead equivalent to prevent leakage radiation from exceeding 100 mr/hr at 1 meter from the source

Data from: Carlton, R. R., & Adler, A. M. (2006). *Principles of radiographic imaging: An art and a science* (4th ed.). Clifton Park, NY: Delmar Cengage Learning; and Bushong, S. C. (2008). *Radiologic science for technologists: Physics, biology, and protection* (9th ed.). St. Louis, MO: Elsevier. Copyright © Elsevier.

quality management – Quality management encompasses both *quality assurance* and *quality control* to ensure the public receives high-quality medical care.

▬ **quality assurance (QA)** – Quality assurance or continuous quality improvement (CQI) pertains to the service aspect of patient care. This involves patient scheduling, reception, procedure wait time, and the efficiency of general services provided to the patient during their medical stay.

• **The Joint Commission (TJC), previously known as the Joint Commission on Accreditation of Healthcare Organizations (JCAHO)** – The TJC promotes health care organizations to establish their own quality improvement plan with defining goals and expected outcomes. A quality improvement plan involves a process in which relevant health care data are collected, evaluated, and areas in need of improvement are identified. Plans for quality improvement are developed, implemented, and assessed (within a specified timeframe) regarding the ability to improve overall quality of patient care delivery. The TJC provides organizations with established standards that serve as a guide for providing consistent, quality patient care. The TJC evaluates and grant accreditation to various medical facilities demonstrating compliance with the accrediting agency's standards. The 2010 National Patient Safety Goals from the TJC include the following medical care facilities (http://www.jointcommission.org):

• ambulatory

• behavioral health care

• critical access hospital

- home care
- hospital
- laboratory
- long-term care
- office-based surgery

■ **quality control (QC)** – Quality control pertains to the diagnostic aspect of patient care, in which diagnostic imaging equipment is optimally maintained (tested and inspected) to produce quality images for interpretation by a radiologist, with minimal radiation exposure to the patient. Quality control includes routine performance monitoring (scheduled testing), preventive maintenance (replacing parts before equipment failure), and acceptance testing (testing new equipment and/or equipment with replaced parts prior to clinical use) *(see Table 13–5 and Table 13–6)*.

TABLE 13–5 Quality Assurance for Diagnostic Imaging Equipment

Filtration (HVL)	Minimum HVL (mm of Al)
	■ 50 kVp – 1.2
	■ 60 kVp – 1.3
	■ 70 kVp – 1.5
	■ 80 kVp – 2.3
	■ 90 kVp – 2.5
Light field and x-ray field alignment	±2% of SID
Focal spot size	±50%
kVp calibration	±5% Less over limited range, e.g., ±2 kVp for 60–100 kVp
mR/mAs	±10%
Exposure timers	Three-phase generator ±5% Single-phase generator (*see Table 13–7*)
Exposure linearity	±10% over clinical range
Exposure reproducibility	±5%

Testing is performed on new x-ray equipment, when a change to the x-ray tube unit has occurred, and annually (with the exception of light field/x-ray field alignment, which is tested semi-annually).

Adapted with permission of the National Council on Radiation Protection and Measurements, *NCRP Report No. 99: Quality assurance for diagnostic imaging*; Table A.2: Radiographic quality control (Section 7), and Table 7-1: Minimum half-value layers (FDA, 1986), www.ncrp.com.

TABLE 13–6   **Exposure Time Control Limits for Single-Phase Full-Wave Rectified Generators**

EXPOSURE TIME (sec)	ACCEPTANCE LIMITS
1/5	24 ± 1 dot
1/10	12 ± 1 dot
1/20	6 ± 0 dots
1/30	4 ± 0 dots

Adapted with permission of the National Council on Radiation Protection and Measurements, *NCRP Report No. 99: Quality assurance for diagnostic imaging*; Table 7–3: Exposure time control limits for shingle phase full-wave rectified generators, www.ncrp.com.

radiation dosimetry report – A radiation dosimetry report is a report provided to a medical facility and/or educational institution's department head or RSO. This report details radiation exposure for occupational workers or trainees by type of radiation exposure, tissue level of radiation exposure (deep or shallow), monthly or quarterly radiation exposure, year-to-date exposure, and cumulative exposure. The RSO is responsible for reviewing these reports and taking appropriate action with any individual who may be in danger of exceeding acceptable NCRP-recommended dose limits. The RSO is also required to protect occupational workers' (and trainees') identifying information while providing dosimeter readings to each individual. Reports are to be maintained on record by the facility or educational institution. (*Refer to Appendix H*: Radiation Dosimetry Report.)

radiation safety officer (RSO) – The radiation safety officer (RSO) is the designated individual at a medical facility or education institution where ionizing radiation is used for diagnostic or therapeutic procedures who is responsible for ensuring radiation safety measures are established and enforced. The RSO oversees radiation dosimetry reports, maintains a current record for all occupation workers, counsels occupational workers who may be close to exceeding the NCRP-recommended dose limits, and orders fetal dosimeters for female technologists who have declared their pregnancy.

risk management – Risk management is an institution's or facility's method for safeguarding the health of individuals associated with the institution either through employment, training, volunteerism, receiving services, or visitation. Safety policies and procedures/protocols are followed as a means of ensuring the health and well being of those within the institution or facility. Medical facilities in which ionization radiation is used to diagnose and/or treat patients must demonstrate compliance with federal and state regulatory agencies. The RSO is responsible for ensuring that ALARA principles are maintained, radiation exposure for occupational workers are monitored (monthly or quarterly) and records maintained, dosimetry readings are disclosed privately to employees, and equipment operations are in compliance with the Nuclear Regulatory Commission and state laws.

units of ionizing radiation – The International Commission on Radiologic Units (ICRU) provides standardized units of measurement regarding ionizing

TABLE 13–7 Conversions Between Conventional Units and SI Units

CONVENTIONAL UNIT (COLUMN A)	CONVERSION FACTOR (COLUMN B)	SI UNIT (COLUMN C)
roentgen	2.58×10^{-4}	coulomb/kilogram
rad	0.01	Gray
rem	0.01	sievert
curie	3.7×10^{10}	becquerel

- Column A amount multiplied by Column B equals Column C amount.
- Column C amount divided by Column B equals Column A amount.

Adapted with permission of the National Council on Radiation Protection and Measurements, NCRP Report No. 93: *Ionizing radiation exposure of the population of the United States,* www.ncrp.com.

radiation; they are known as traditional units as opposed to *SI units*, which are the French units of measurement for ionizing radiation derived from the Système international d'unités. Traditional units for measuring radiation are the rad, for radiation absorbed dose; the rem, for radiation equivalent in humans; and the roentgen, for radiation in air. Remember that a millirad, millirem, or milliroentgen is 1/1000 of the unit rad, rem, or roentgen; and a milligray (mGy) or millisievert (mSv) is 1/1000 of the unit gray or sievert. (*Refer to Chapter 6: Physics Terms, Table 6-3: Conversions of Traditional Radiation Units to SI Units; see Table 13-7.*)

wire mesh test – A wire mesh test is used to check for warping of an intensification screen (used in conjunction with film). A warped screen will cause poor film/ screen contact and will produce a radiographic image with increased density and poor resolution. Imaging a wire mesh screen on top of a film/screen cassette should produce a radiographic image with symmetrical rows and columns. An image of a wire mesh screen with asymmetrical rows and columns would reveal a poor film/ screen contact usually caused by a warped or damaged film/screen cassette.

StudyWARE™ CONNECTION

After completing this chapter, listen to audio pronunciations in the audio library or play an interactive game that will help you learn the content in this chapter.

CONCEPT THINKING QUESTIONS

1. In keeping with the ALARA principle, what actions should radiologic technologists be taking?

2. What does a *quality management* program encompass?

3. What is the role of The Joint Commission regarding medical facilities?

4. What is the SI unit equivalent for 1 rem?

5. What testing tool is required to check timer accuracy on a three-phase x-ray unit?

6. Identify the two main types of radiation detection devices.

7. Identify four acceptable lead equivalent materials used for constructing primary or secondary barriers.

8. Explain the cardinal rule of *time*, *distance*, and *shielding*.

9. Why is PBL considered a safety feature?

10. Identify the agency that provides effective dose limit recommendations for occupational workers and the general public.

PRACTICE EXERCISES

1. Explain the difference between a primary barrier and a secondary barrier.

2. Differentiate between a "controlled area" and an "uncontrolled area."

3. What would be the acceptable tolerance range denoting kVp accuracy with a setting of 80 kVp?

4. Identify the responsibilities of a RSO.

5. Explain what is meant by exposure linearity.

6. Identify types of testing tools used for determining focal spot accuracy.

7. Which personnel-monitoring device uses aluminum oxide crystals?

8. List two advantages of using a film badge dosimeter.

9. List two disadvantages of using a film badge dosimeter.

10. Identify the three types of field survey instruments for detecting and measuring ionizing radiation.

MATCHING

Match each term to the appropriate description.

HVL	fogging	RSO
QA	TLD	primary barrier
beam/light congruency	shadow shield	accident leakage
5 rem	QC	radiation
secondary barrier	0.25 mm Pb	contact shield
5 mSv	mA min/wk	0.5 mm Pb

Description	Term
1. utilizes lithium fluoride crystals	_____
2. 100 mR/hr at 1 meter from the source	_____
3. reduces beam intensity by half	_____
4. service aspect of quality management	_____
5. incident report	_____
6. workload (W)	_____
7. ±2% of SID	_____
8. recommended for sterile procedures	_____
9. annual occupational effective dose limit	_____
10. Bucky slot cover	_____
11. public annual effective dose limit	_____
12. extends 7 feet from floor	_____

RETENTION OF MATERIAL

Retention requires practicing the use of previously learned material. Apply the knowledge you have regarding radiation protection principles to answer the following questions.

1. Identify methods for reducing radiation exposure to the patient.

2. Explain the purpose of the Bucky slot cover and the fluoro curtain/drape.

3. Describe a scenario at a medical facility that would require the completion of an incident report.

4. Identify the four main variables considered for determining the proper amount of shielding for protective barriers.

5. Why do dosimetry reports include a cumulative reading, and how does one determine their cumulative effective dose limit?

6. Explain how patient dose is affected when collimation is increased.

7. Does a pregnant technologist or radiography student have to declare her pregnancy?

8. Which field survey instruments are primarily used for detecting radioactive material?

9. Identify the most common type of protective shielding used for recumbent patients.

10. How many dots should appear when testing for timer accuracy on a full-wave rectified x-ray unit with an exposure time of 0.15 seconds?

V

Anatomy and Imaging Procedures

CHAPTER 14

Organ System Anatomy

OBJECTIVES

Upon completion of this chapter, the reader will be able to:

- List all 11 organ systems and their physiologic role
- Identify organ systems commonly imaged in general radiography
- Describe blood flow through the cardiovascular system
- Describe structures of the digestive tract in terms of being proximal or distal to one another
- Identify the three accessory organs of the digestive system and explain their function
- Describe the order of air flow through the respiratory system
- Describe the series of events that take place in the production of urine

CONCEPT THINKING

Each of the 11 organ systems serves a specific body function, yet all systems work collaboratively to enable the human body to function as an independent organism. Although each organ system is equally important in maintaining a homeostasis environment for the human body, there are specific organ systems that are of significant importance in general diagnostic radiography. These organs systems include the respiratory system, digestive system, skeletal system, reproductive system, and urinary system. Other organ systems may be better visualized through advanced imaging modalities such as computed tomography, magnetic resonance imaging, nuclear medicine, and ultrasound. These systems include the cardiovascular system, nervous system, lymphatic system, and muscular system, and endocrine system. The integumentary system is a unique system in that it is located external to all other organ systems and can be visually assessed. Because of the functionality of each organ system, it is imperative for radiologic technologists to have a comprehensive understanding of the anatomic structures and physiological processes distinct to each system. For this reason, we will examine each system separately with emphasis on the systems routinely imaged in diagnostic radiography (digestive, respiratory, skeletal, cardiovascular, urinary, reproductive). The imaging profession calls for technologists not only to identify anatomic structures but also to identify normal and abnormal organ function. Pathological conditions can alter normal body function and even hinder visualization of anatomic areas of interest. Various patient conditions and imaging circumstances often require the technologist to apply critical thinking skills to image production techniques in order to capture optimal images for image interpretation by the radiologist. To detect basic anomalies, one must first have a thorough understanding of what is considered to be "normal" anatomic structure and function. The diagrams in this chapter depict standard anatomic structure and function for each organ system. However, it should be noted that there are times when anatomical structure may deviate from the standard and still be considered normal.

ORGAN SYSTEMS AND RELATED TERMS

organ systems – The human body is composed of 11 organ systems, each designed to perform specific functions while collectively working to create a homeostatic environment in which the human body can act as an independent organism. The 11 organs systems include the cardiovascular system, digestive system, endocrine system, integumentary system, lymphatic system, muscular system, nervous system, reproductive system, respiratory system, skeletal system, and urinary system.

■ **cardiovascular system** – The cardiovascular system consists of the heart, blood vessels, and blood. The cardiovascular system is a transport system to which oxygenated blood is pumped by the heart and carried throughout the body providing an array of nutrients essential for the body to sustain itself. Deoxygenated blood is circulated back to the lungs for gas exchange, whereas cellular waste is directed to the urinary system for excretion by the kidneys. The two main components that constitute the composition of blood are plasma and cellular elements *(see Table 14–1 and Figure 14–1).*

■ **digestive system** – The purpose of the digestive system is to break down food for the body to absorb nutrients and to eliminate any resulting waste product. The digestive tract or alimentary canal begins at the mouth, where food is chewed and broken down by enzymes of the salivary glands. Food is swallowed, passes through the pharynx to the esophagus, and proceeds to the stomach. Gastric juices of the stomach and juices produced by the accessory organs (liver, gallbladder, and pancreas) assist in a further breakdown of food (referred to as chyme), thus allowing the small intestine to absorb nutrients. Material that is indigestible proceeds to the large intestine, where water reabsorption occurs and fecal material is temporarily stored until defecation takes place at the anus. Common radiographic procedures of the upper digestive system include the esophagram or barium

TABLE 14–1   Blood Composition

BEST PRACTICE RULE	RATIONALE
Plasma (55% of blood volume)	Cellular elements (45% of blood volume)
▬ water	▬ erythrocytes (red blood cells)
▬ proteins	▬ leukocytes (white blood cells)
▬ nutrients	▬ thrombocytes (platelets)
▬ electrolytes	
▬ hormones	
▬ vitamins	
▬ enzymes	
▬ waste	

Source: Delmar/Cengage Learning.

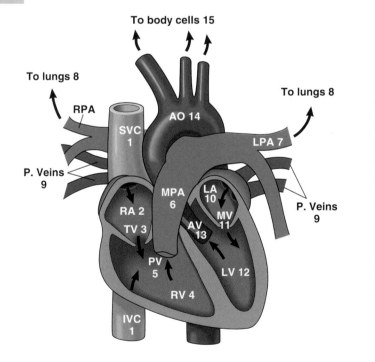

AO — Aorta
AV — Aortic valve
IVC — Inferior vena cava
LA — Left atrium
LPA — Left pulmonary artery
LV — Left ventricle
MPA — Main pulmonary artery
MV — Mitral valve
PV — Pulmonary valve
P.VEINS — Pulmonary veins
RA — Right atrium
RPA — Right pulmonary artery
RV — Right ventricle
SVC — Superior vena cava
TV — Tricuspid valve

1. Blood reaches heart through superior vena cava (SVC) and inferior vena cava (IVC)
2. To right atrium
3. To tricuspid valve
4. To right ventricle
5. To pulmonary valve (semilunar)
6. To main pulmonary artery
7. To left pulmonary artery and right pulmonary artery

8. To lungs—blood receives O_2
9. From lungs to pulmonary veins
10. To left atrium
11. To mitral (bicuspid) valve
12. To left ventricle
13. To aortic valve (semilunar veins)
14. To aorta (largest artery in the body)
15. Blood with oxygen then goes to all cells of the body

FIGURE 14–1. Physiology of the heart.

swallow and the upper gastrointestinal series (UGI). The esophagram involves imaging the pharynx and esophagus, whereas the UGI involves imaging the distal portion of the esophagus, the stomach, and the proximal portion of the small intestine, otherwise referred to as the duodenum. The most common radiographic procedures of the lower digestive system includes the small bowel series (SBS), often referred to as a small bowel follow-through, and the lower gastrointestinal series, commonly referred to as a barium enema (BE). The SBS involves imaging the entire small intestine, whereas the BE involves imaging the entire large intestine *(see Box 14-1, Table 14-2, and Figure 14-2 through Figure 14-6).*

BOX 14–1   Anatomy of the Pharynx and Esophagus

Pharynx

- nasopharynx – proximal pharynx
- oropharynx – mid pharynx
- laryngopharynx – distal pharynx

Esophagus

- proximal esophagus – approximate vertebral level of C5-C6
- mid esophagus – approximate vertebral level of T6
- distal esophagus – approximate vertebral level of T11

Source: Delmar/Cengage Learning.

TABLE 14–2   Anatomy of the Stomach, Small Intestine, and Large Intestine

proximal - → distal

STOMACH	SMALL INTESTINE	LARGE INTESTINE
Four main sections	Three main sections	Three main sections
▪ cardia	▪ duodenum (proximal)	▪ cecum (proximal)
▪ fundus	▪ jejunum	▪ colon
▪ body	▪ ileum (distal)	• ascending colon
▪ pylorus		• transverse colon
		• descending colon
		• sigmoid colon
		▪ rectum (distal)
		• anus

(Continued)

TABLE 14–2 **(Continued)**

proximal – → **distal**

STOMACH	SMALL INTESTINE	LARGE INTESTINE
Sphincters ■ lower esophageal sphincter ■ pyloric sphincter	Internal wall ■ plica ■ villi ■ lacteal	Sphincters ■ cecum ■ ileocecal valve ■ anus ■ internal anal sphincter ■ external anal sphincter
Curvatures ■ lesser curvature (medial) ■ greater curvature (lateral)	Three accessory organs (produce digestive secretions and have pathways to the small intestine via the duodenum) ■ liver ■ gallbladder ■ pancreas	Flexures ■ hepatic flexure (Rt) ■ splenic flexure (Lt)
Internal wall ■ rugae		External wall ■ haustra ■ taenia coli

Source: Delmar/Cengage Learning.

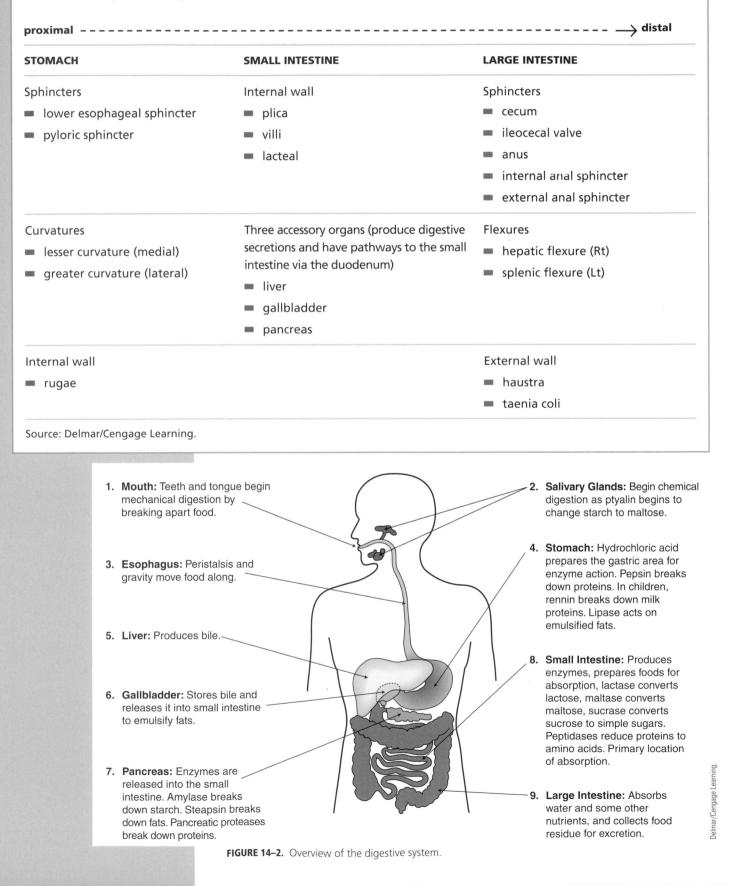

1. **Mouth:** Teeth and tongue begin mechanical digestion by breaking apart food.

2. **Salivary Glands:** Begin chemical digestion as ptyalin begins to change starch to maltose.

3. **Esophagus:** Peristalsis and gravity move food along.

4. **Stomach:** Hydrochloric acid prepares the gastric area for enzyme action. Pepsin breaks down proteins. In children, rennin breaks down milk proteins. Lipase acts on emulsified fats.

5. **Liver:** Produces bile.

6. **Gallbladder:** Stores bile and releases it into small intestine to emulsify fats.

7. **Pancreas:** Enzymes are released into the small intestine. Amylase breaks down starch. Steapsin breaks down fats. Pancreatic proteases break down proteins.

8. **Small Intestine:** Produces enzymes, prepares foods for absorption, lactase converts lactose, maltase converts maltose, sucrase converts sucrose to simple sugars. Peptidases reduce proteins to amino acids. Primary location of absorption.

9. **Large Intestine:** Absorbs water and some other nutrients, and collects food residue for excretion.

Delmar/Cengage Learning.

FIGURE 14–2. Overview of the digestive system.

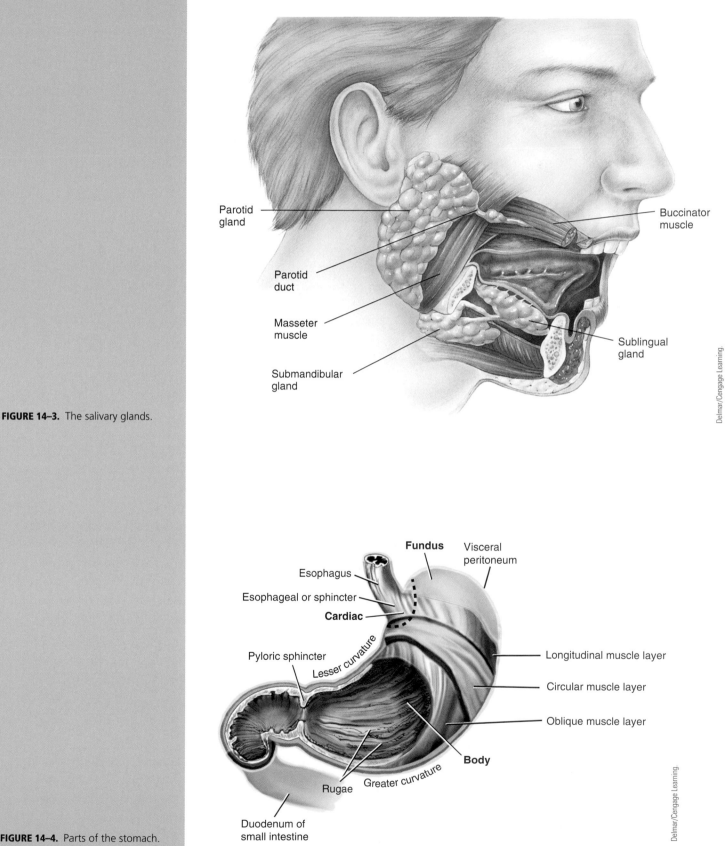

FIGURE 14–3. The salivary glands.

Parotid gland

Buccinator muscle

Parotid duct

Masseter muscle

Sublingual gland

Submandibular gland

Delmar/Cengage Learning.

Fundus
Visceral peritoneum

Esophagus

Esophageal or sphincter

Cardiac

Pyloric sphincter

Lesser curvature

Longitudinal muscle layer

Circular muscle layer

Oblique muscle layer

Body

Rugae

Greater curvature

Duodenum of small intestine

FIGURE 14–4. Parts of the stomach.

Delmar/Cengage Learning.

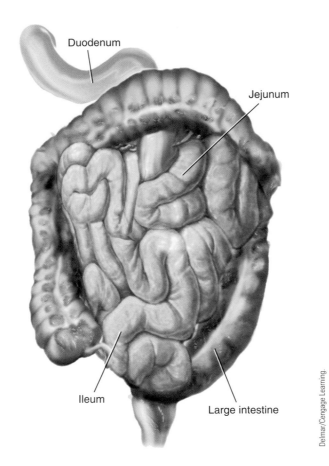

Duodenum

Jejunum

Ileum

Large intestine

Delmar/Cengage Learning.

FIGURE 14–5. The small intestine.

■ **digestive system accessory organs** – The digestive system has three main accessory organs: the liver, the gall bladder, and the pancreas. Each of these organs aids in the digestive process by producing or releasing digestive secretions into the small intestine through pathways or ducts that lead into an opening called the hepatopancreatic ampulla, located in the descending portion of the duodenum *(see Table 14–3, Figure 14–7, and Figure 14–8)*.

■ **endocrine system** – The endocrine system is an internal network of cellular communication through chemical secretions and hormones provided by various glands and organs. The endocrine system works collaboratively with the nervous system through a negative feedback system as a means of controlling the production and excretion of hormones *(see Table 14–4 and Figure 14–9)*.

■ **integumentary system** – The integumentary system consists of skin, nails, hair, sebaceous glands, and sweat glands. The skin is the largest organ of the body and serves as a protective layer against harmful pathogens. It also helps regulate body temperature, produce vitamin D, and provide a level of protection against the harmful effects of ultraviolet rays produced by the sun. The skin is composed of a superficial layer of epithelial cells known as the epidermis and a deeper layer of connective tissue referred to as the dermis *(see Box 14–2 and Figure 14–10)*.

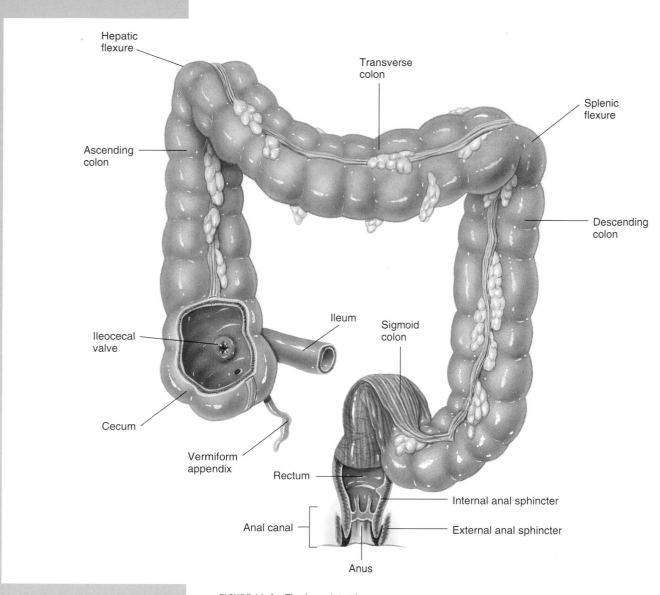

FIGURE 14–6. The large intestine.

Delmar/Cengage Learning.

TABLE 14–3 Anatomy of the Liver, Gallbladder, and Pancreas

ORGAN	FUNCTION
Liver	Serves more than 200 functions, including: • regulation of bile production • metabolic regulation • hematological regulation
Gallbladder	■ stores bile received from the liver ■ releases bile into the duodenum when foods high in fats are consumed
Pancreas	■ serves as both an endocrine gland and exocrine gland ■ produces digestive juices and releases them into the duodenum via the pancreatic duct

Source: Delmar/Cengage Learning.

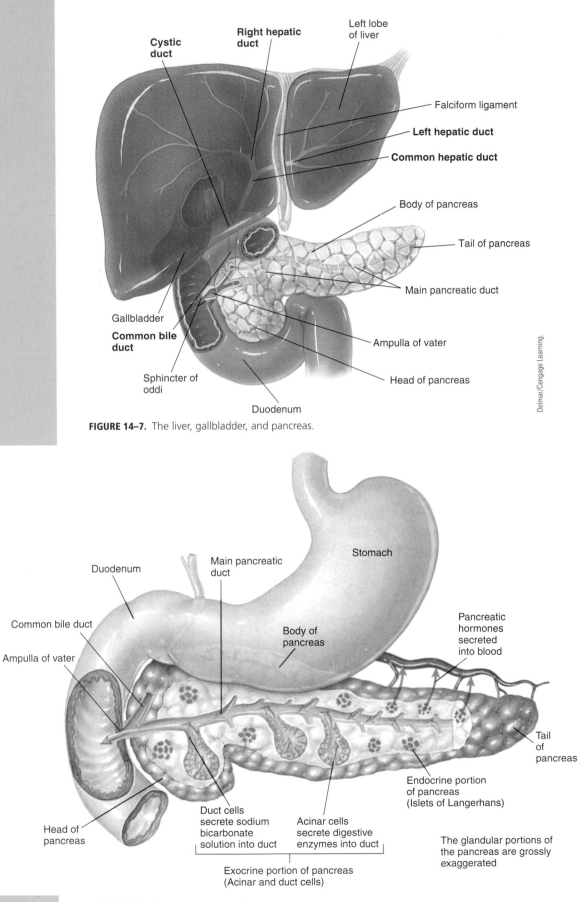

FIGURE 14–7. The liver, gallbladder, and pancreas.

Delmar/Cengage Learning.

FIGURE 14–8. The pancreas and duodenum.

Delmar/Cengage Learning.

TABLE 14–4   Organs and Glands of the Endocrine System

ORGAN/GLAND	HORMONE SECRETIONS
Hypothalamus (produces hormones)	Oxytocin
	Vasopressin: antidiuretic hormone (ADH)
Pituitary gland	
■ anterior lobe (produces hormones)	Thyroid-stimulating hormone (TSH)
	Adrenocorticotropic hormone (ACTH)
	Follicle-stimulating hormone (FSH)
	Luteinizing hormone (LH)
	Prolactin (PRL)
	Melanocyte-stimulating hormone (MSH)
	Growth hormone (GH)
■ posterior lobe (releases hormones)	Oxytocin
	Antidiuretic hormone (ADH)
Pineal gland	Melatonin
Parathyroid gland	Parathyroid hormone (PTH)
Thyroid gland	Triiodothyronine (T3), thyroxine (T4), and calcitonin (CT)
Thymus	Thymosins
Heart	Atrial natriuretic peptide
Adrenal glands	
■ cortex	Mineralocorticoids: aldosterone
	Glucocorticoids: cortisone, cortisol, androgens
■ medulla	Epinephrine (E)
	Norepinephrine (NE)
Kidneys	Erythropoietin (EPO)
	Calcitrol
	Renin
Pancreas	Glucagons
	Insulin
Male gonads	Testosterone
Female gonads	Estrogen
	Progesterone

Source: Delmar/Cengage Learning.

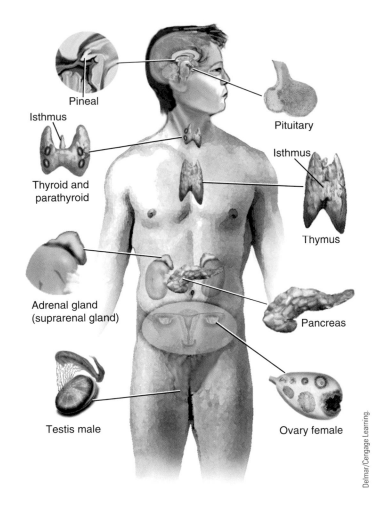

FIGURE 14–9. Locations of the endocrine glands.

Pineal

Isthmus

Pituitary

Isthmus

Thyroid and parathyroid

Thymus

Adrenal gland (suprarenal gland)

Pancreas

Testis male

Ovary female

Delmar/Cengage Learning.

BOX 14–2 Layers of the Skin

Epidermis (superficial layer) has five layers (listed from superficial to deep):

- stratum corneum
- stratum lucidum
- stratum granulosum
- stratum spinosum
- stratum germinativum

Dermis (deep layer) has two layers (listed from deep to deeper):

- papillary layer
- reticular layer

Source: Delmar/Cengage Learning.

- **lymphatic system** – The lymphatic system is the body's defense system. It protects the body against harmful pathogens and aids the body in building immunity to certain illnesses and diseases. Comprising the lymphatic system are the lymph vessels, lymph nodes, lymphoid tissues (tonsils), and lymphoid

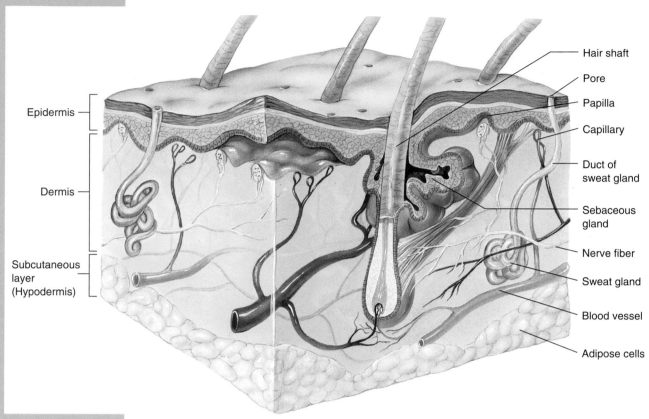

Epidermis

Dermis

Subcutaneous layer (Hypodermis)

Hair shaft

Pore

Papilla

Capillary

Duct of sweat gland

Sebaceous gland

Nerve fiber

Sweat gland

Blood vessel

Adipose cells

Delmar/Cengage Learning.

FIGURE 14–10. Cross-section of skin.

organs (spleen and thymus). Skeletal muscle contractions promote the circulation of lymphatic fluid (lymph) through the body *(see Figure 14–11)*.

■ **muscular system** – The muscular system is composed of approximately 650–700 skeletal muscles that collectively serve as a support structure for soft tissues, providing the body with shape and posture. Muscles also regulate the body's internal temperature, provide mobility to skeletal bones, and permit voluntary control over specific bodily functions such as urination and defecation. The body has three types of muscle tissue: cardiac muscle (located within the heart), smooth muscle (located within the internal lining of tubular structures and organs), and skeletal muscle (attached to skeletal bones; *see Table 14–5 and Figure 14–12 through Figure 14–16)*.

■ **nervous system** – The nervous system is composed of two main sections, the central nervous system and the peripheral nervous system, which work by sending and receiving sensory impulses. The central nervous system, or the body's control center, consists of the brain and spinal cord, by which nerve impulses are transmitted to and from the brain. The peripheral nervous system (PNS) includes 12 pairs of cranial nerves connected to the brain and 31 pairs of spinal nerves positioned along the vertebral column. The PNS also includes a subdivision known as the autonomic nervous system, which is designed to ensure involuntary actions to sustain life are carried out, including rhythmic heart beat, peristalsis, and respiration *(see Figure 14–17 through Figure 14–19)*.

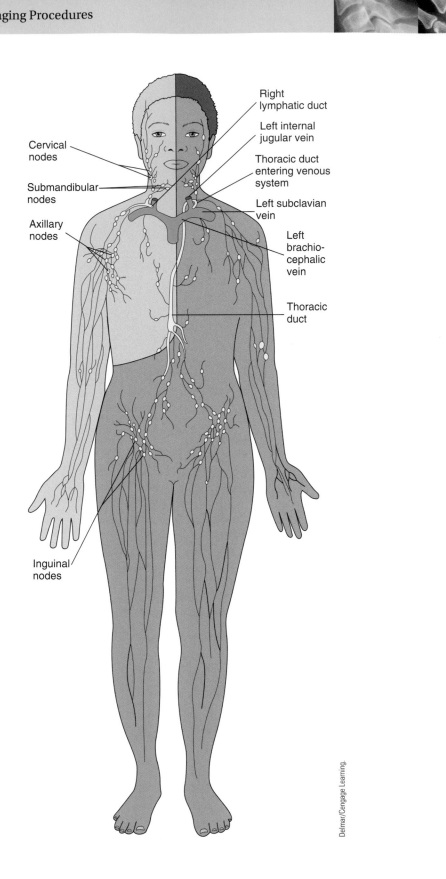

Right lymphatic duct

Left internal jugular vein

Thoracic duct entering venous system

Left subclavian vein

Left brachio-cephalic vein

Thoracic duct

Cervical nodes

Submandibular nodes

Axillary nodes

Inguinal nodes

FIGURE 14–11. Lymphatic system.

Delmar/Cengage Learning.

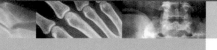

TABLE 14–5   Characteristics of Three Types of Muscle Tissue

CARDIAC	SMOOTH	SKELETAL
Intercalated discs	Spindle-shaped cell	Bundles of muscle cells
Single centrally located nuclei	Single centrally located nuclei	Multiple nuclei
Striations	No striations	Striations
Involuntary control	Involuntary control	Voluntary control
Location: heart	Location: visceral organs	Location: attached to skeletal bones

Source: Delmar/Cengage Learning.

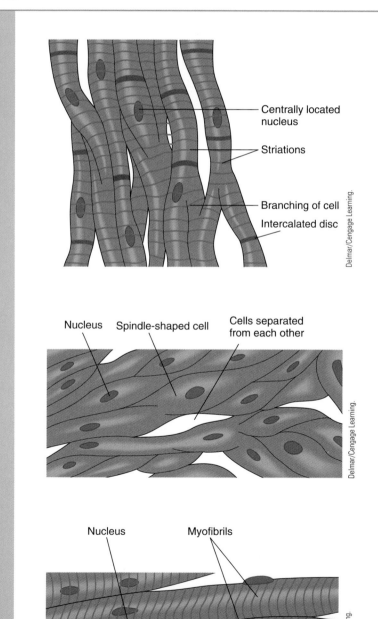

Centrally located nucleus

Striations

Branching of cell

Intercalated disc

Delmar/Cengage Learning.

FIGURE 14–12. Cardiac muscle cells.

Nucleus   Spindle-shaped cell   Cells separated from each other

Delmar/Cengage Learning.

FIGURE 14–13. Smooth muscle cells.

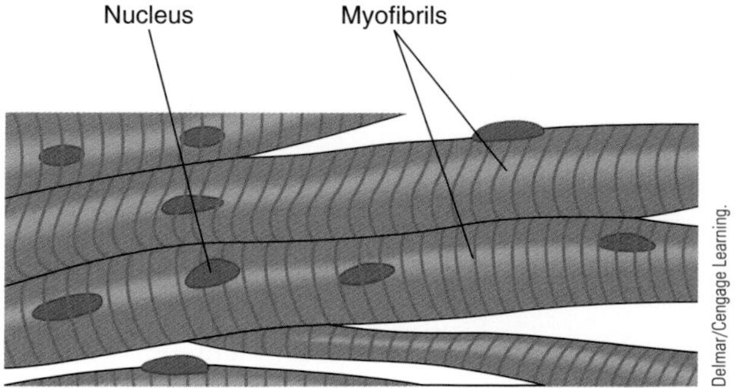

Nucleus   Myofibrils

Delmar/Cengage Learning.

FIGURE 14–14. Skeletal muscle cells.

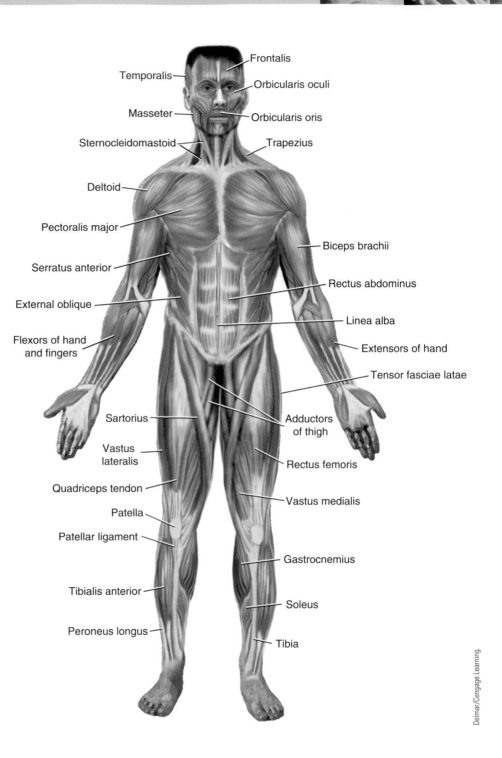

Frontalis
Temporalis
Orbicularis oculi
Masseter
Orbicularis oris
Sternocleidomastoid
Trapezius
Deltoid
Pectoralis major
Biceps brachii
Serratus anterior
Rectus abdominus
External oblique
Linea alba
Flexors of hand and fingers
Extensors of hand
Tensor fasciae latae
Sartorius
Adductors of thigh
Vastus lateralis
Rectus femoris
Quadriceps tendon
Vastus medialis
Patella
Patellar ligament
Gastrocnemius
Tibialis anterior
Soleus
Peroneus longus
Tibia

Delmar/Cengage Learning.

FIGURE 14–15. Principal skeletal muscles of the body (anterior view).

■ **reproductive system** – The reproductive system is designed for procreation. Human procreation requires the male reproductive organs (testes) to produce sperm and the female reproductive organs (ovaries) to produce ova. These two cells must unite in order for fertilization to occur. The result of fertilization is a zygote, which with continued growth will become an embryo and finally a fetus. A gestation period of nine months is considered normal fetal development time with birth estimated between 38 and 40 weeks (*see Table 14-6 and Figure 14-20 through Figure 14-22*).

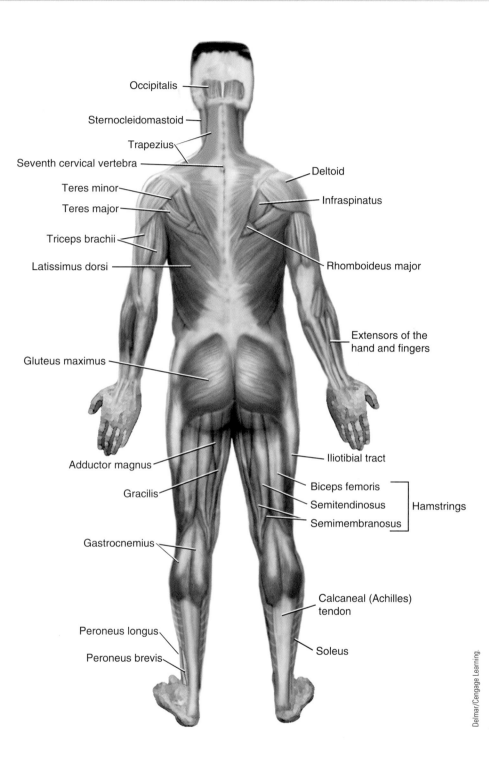

Occipitalis

Sternocleidomastoid

Trapezius

Seventh cervical vertebra

Teres minor

Teres major

Triceps brachii

Latissimus dorsi

Deltoid

Infraspinatus

Rhomboideus major

Extensors of the
hand and fingers

Gluteus maximus

Adductor magnus

Gracilis

Iliotibial tract

Biceps femoris

Semitendinosus

Semimembranosus

Hamstrings

Gastrocnemius

Calcaneal (Achilles)
tendon

Peroneus longus

Peroneus brevis

Soleus

Delmar/Cengage Learning.

FIGURE 14–16. Principal skeletal muscles of the body (posterior view).

■ **respiratory system** – The respiratory system permits the body to take air (oxygen) in through the respiratory tract to the lungs, where a gaseous exchange occurs between thin membranes of the alveoli and circulating blood cells (erthocytes). The oxygenated blood will travel throughout the body, sustaining organs and tissues, and the deoxygenated blood (carbon dioxide) will circulate back to the lungs to be expelled upon exhalation. Air

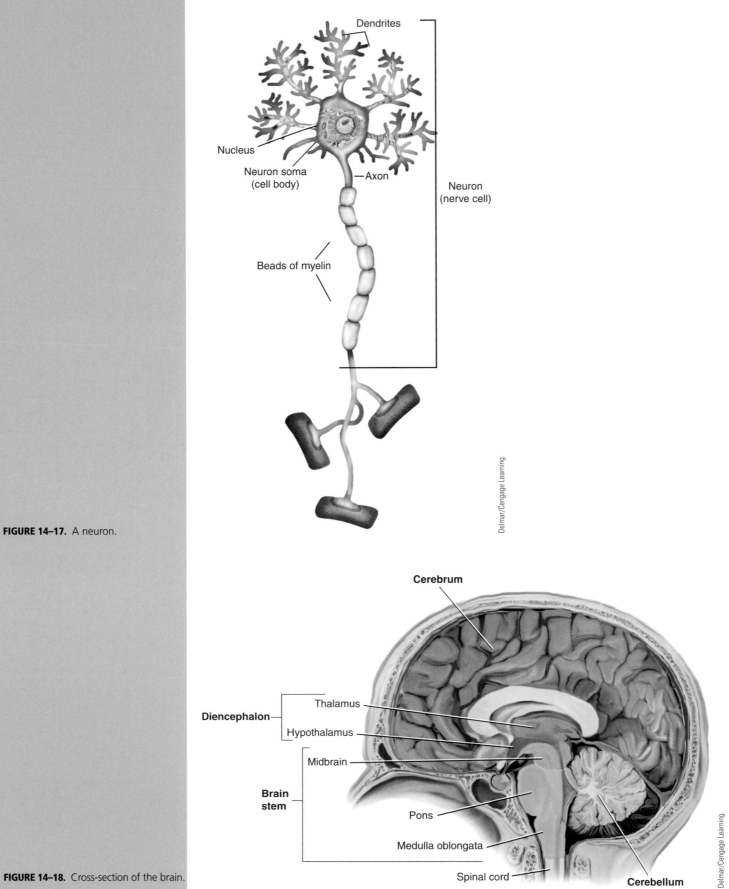

FIGURE 14–17. A neuron.

FIGURE 14–18. Cross-section of the brain.

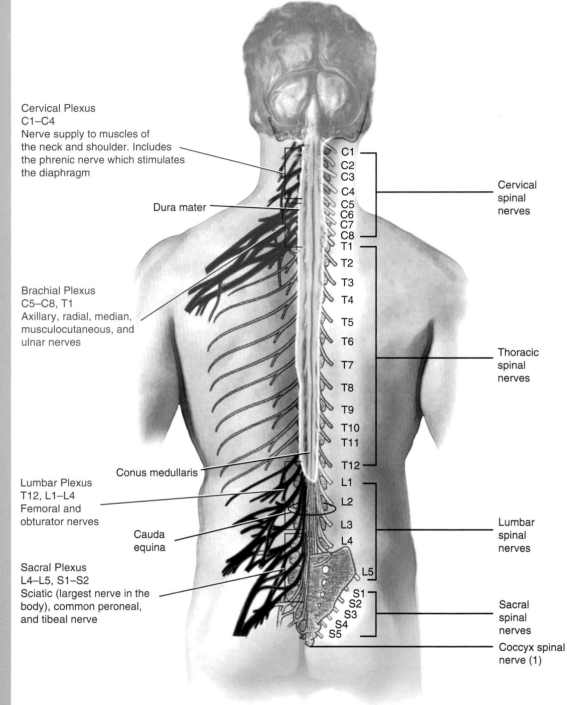

Cervical Plexus
C1–C4
Nerve supply to muscles of
the neck and shoulder. Includes
the phrenic nerve which stimulates
the diaphragm

Dura mater

Brachial Plexus
C5–C8, T1
Axillary, radial, median,
musculocutaneous, and
ulnar nerves

Conus medullaris

Lumbar Plexus
T12, L1–L4
Femoral and
obturator nerves

Cauda
equina

Sacral Plexus
L4–L5, S1–S2
Sciatic (largest nerve in the
body), common peroneal,
and tibeal nerve

Cervical
spinal
nerves

Thoracic
spinal
nerves

Lumbar
spinal
nerves

Sacral
spinal
nerves

Coccyx spinal
nerve (1)

C1
C2
C3
C4
C5
C6
C7
C8
T1
T2
T3
T4
T5
T6
T7
T8
T9
T10
T11
T12
L1
L2
L3
L4
L5
S1
S2
S3
S4
S5

Delmar/Cengage Learning.

FIGURE 14–19. Spinal nerve plexus and important nerves.

flow through the respiratory tract begins at the nasal cavity, passes through
the pharynx (nasopharynx, oropharynx, laryngopharynx) to the larynx (voice
box), to the trachea, through the right and left primary bronchi, secondary
bronchi, and tertiary bronchi to the bronchioles. Bronchioles branch into
smaller terminal bronchioles and finally into a lobule that consists of small
branching respiratory bronchioles that form alveolar sacs composed of
millions of alveoli *(see Table 14-7 and Figure 14-23 through Figure 14-25)*.

TABLE 14–6   Female and Male Reproductive Organs

FEMALE REPRODUCTIVE ORGANS	MALE REPRODUCTIVE ORGANS
Two ovaries	External genitalia ■ penis ■ scrotum
Two uterine tubes (fallopian tubes)	Two testes
Uterus	Epididymis
Vagina	Ductus deferens
External genitalia	Ejaculatory duct
Mammary glands	Urethra
Accessory glands	Accessory organs ■ seminal vesicles ■ prostate gland ■ bulbourethral glands

Source: Delmar/Cengage Learning.

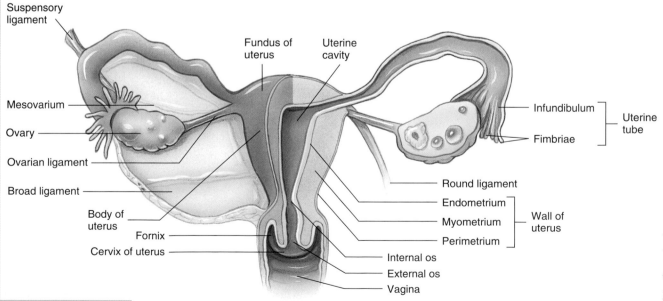

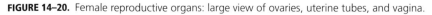

FIGURE 14–20. Female reproductive organs: large view of ovaries, uterine tubes, and vagina.

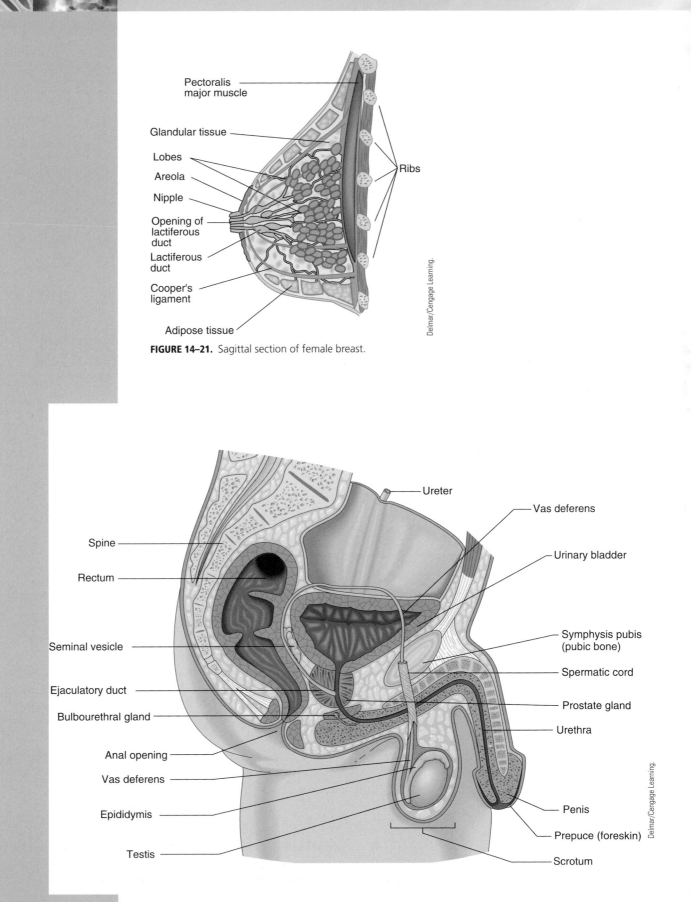

Pectoralis
major muscle

Glandular tissue

Lobes

Areola

Nipple

Opening of
lactiferous
duct

Lactiferous
duct

Cooper's
ligament

Adipose tissue

Ribs

Delmar/Cengage Learning.

FIGURE 14–21. Sagittal section of female breast.

Spine

Rectum

Seminal vesicle

Ejaculatory duct

Bulbourethral gland

Anal opening

Vas deferens

Epididymis

Testis

Ureter

Vas deferens

Urinary bladder

Symphysis pubis
(pubic bone)

Spermatic cord

Prostate gland

Urethra

Penis

Prepuce (foreskin)

Scrotum

Delmar/Cengage Learning.

FIGURE 14–22. Male reproductive organs.

TABLE 14–7   Four Main Sections of the Respiratory System

proximal --- ⟶ distal

LARYNX	TRACHEA	RIGHT AND LEFT BRONCHI	LUNGS
Three large cartilages ■ epiglottis ■ thyroid ■ cricoid Six smaller pairs cartilages ■ arytenoids ■ corniculate ■ cuneiform	Tubular structure ■ approximately 20 C-shaped Tracheal cartilages ■ approximately 1-inch diameter; 4–5 inches in length ■ anterior to esophagus ■ carina is the lowest tracheal cartilage (T5)*	Right primary bronchi vs left primary bronchi ■ wider than left primary bronchi ■ shorter than left primary bronchi ■ more vertical than left primary bronchi	Apex (superior) right lung ■ three lobes • superior • middle • inferior ■ two fissures left lung ■ two lobes • superior • inferior ■ one fissure • base (inferior)
False vocal cords True vocal cords	Proximal level of trachea - C6 (6th cervical vertebra) Distal level of trachea T5*	Division of primary bronchi begins at the carina (T5)	Pleura ■ visceral pleura ■ pleural cavity ■ parietal pleura

*T5 is the 5th thoracic vertebra.
Source: Delmar/Cengage Learning.

■ **skeletal system** – The skeletal system is composed of 206 bones, including the axial skeleton (80 bones) and the appendicular skeleton (126 bones). The skeletal system provides structural support for the body, protection of internal organs, production of erythrocytes and leukocytes, and bodily mobility *(see Table 14–8 and Figure 14–26 through Figure 14–28).*

■ **urinary system** – The urinary system is composed of two kidneys, two ureters, a bladder, and a urethra. The urinary system serves to regulate blood pH, produce urine (a concentration of metabolic waste), store urine, and eliminate urine. Urine production occurs at the kidneys via millions of nephrons located within the renal cortex of the kidneys. Urine then travels from the kidneys through long tubular structures referred to as the ureters to the urinary bladder. Urine is stored in the urinary bladder until the urge to urinate occurs, typically when urine volume reaches 200 mL *(see Table 14–9 and Figure 14–29 through Figure 14–31).*

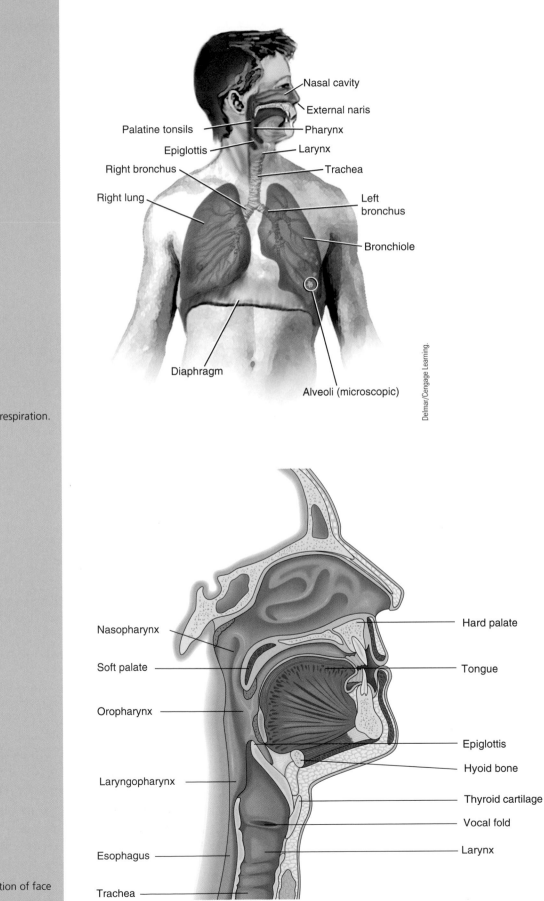

Nasal cavity
External naris
Pharynx
Palatine tonsils
Epiglottis
Larynx
Right bronchus
Trachea
Right lung
Left bronchus
Bronchiole

Diaphragm

Alveoli (microscopic)

Delmar/Cengage Learning.

FIGURE 14–23. Pathway of respiration.

Nasopharynx
Hard palate
Soft palate
Tongue
Oropharynx

Epiglottis
Hyoid bone
Laryngopharynx
Thyroid cartilage
Vocal fold
Esophagus
Larynx
Trachea

Delmar/Cengage Learning.

FIGURE 14–24. Sagittal section of face and neck.

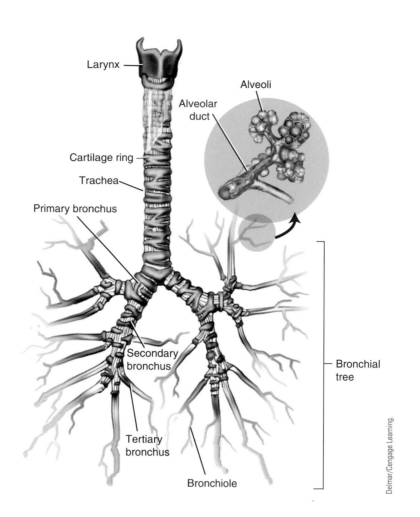

FIGURE 14–25. Larynx, trachea, and right and left bronchi.

Delmar/Cengage Learning.

TABLE 14–8 Skeletal System

AXIAL SKELETON (80 BONES)	APPENDICULAR SKELETON (126 BONES)
Auditory ossicles **(6 bones)**	Right and left upper extremities **(64 bones)**
Hyoid **(1 bone)**	■ 2 clavicle
Skull **(22 bones)**	■ 2 scapula
■ 8 cranial bones	■ 2 humerus
• 1 frontal bone	■ 2 radius
• 2 parietal bones	■ 2 ulna
• 2 temporal bones	■ 16 carpal bones (8 per wrist)
• 1 ethmoid	• proximal row
• 1 sphenoid	• scaphoid
• 1 occipital	• lunate
	• triquetrum
	• pisiform

(Continued)

TABLE 14-8   Skeletal System (Continued)

AXIAL SKELETON (80 BONES)	APPENDICULAR SKELETON (126 BONES)
■ 14 facial bones	• distal row
• 2 lacrimal bones	• trapezium
• 2 nasal bones	• trapezoid
• 2 inferior nasal conchae	• capitate
• 2 zygomatic bones	• hamate
• 1 vomer	■ 10 metacarpals (5 per hand)
• 2 palatine bones	■ 28 phalanges (14 per hand)
• 2 maxillary bones	
• 1 mandible	**Right and left lower extremities (62 bones)**
Thoracic cage (25 bones)	■ 2 coxal bone
■ 24 ribs	■ 2 femur
■ 1 sternum	■ 2 patella
	■ 2 tibia
Vertebral column (26 bones)	■ 2 fibula
■ 7 cervical vertebrae	■ 14 tarsals (7 per ankle)
• C-1 – atlas	• calcaneus
• C-2 – axis	• talus
■ 12 thoracic vertebrae	• navicular
■ 5 lumbar vertebrae	• cuboid
■ 1 sacrum	• lateral cuneiform
■ 1 coccyx	• intermediate cuneiform
	• medial cuneiform
	■ 10 metatarsals (5 per foot)
	■ 28 phalanges (14 per foot)

Source: Delmar/Cengage Learning.

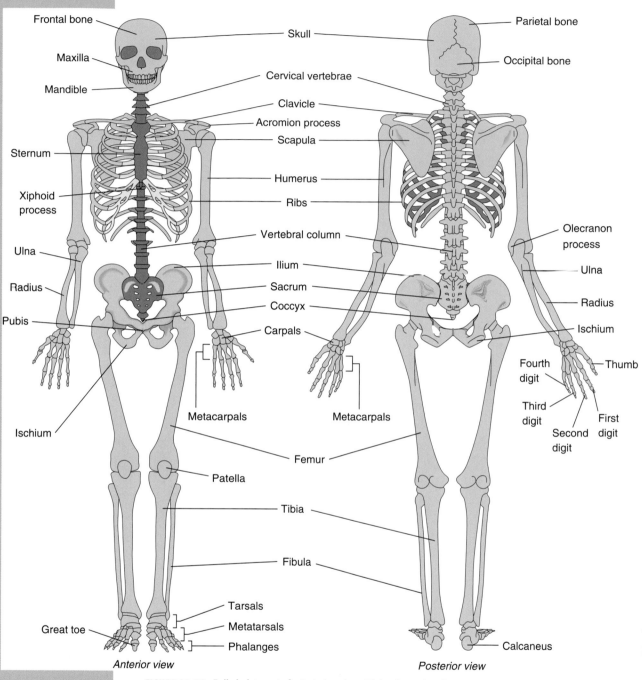

Frontal bone
Maxilla
Mandible
Sternum
Xiphoid process
Ulna
Radius
Pubis
Ischium
Great toe

Skull
Cervical vertebrae
Clavicle
Acromion process
Scapula
Humerus
Ribs
Vertebral column
Ilium
Sacrum
Coccyx
Carpals
Metacarpals
Femur
Patella
Tibia
Fibula
Tarsals
Metatarsals
Phalanges

Parietal bone
Occipital bone
Olecranon process
Ulna
Radius
Ischium
Thumb
Fourth digit
Third digit
First digit
Second digit
Metacarpals
Calcaneus

Anterior view

Posterior view

FIGURE 14–26. Full skeleton. *Left.* Anterior view. *Right.* Posterior view.

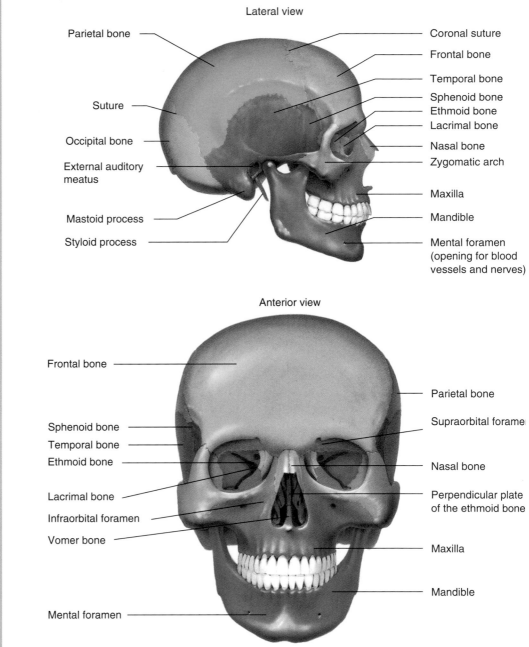

Lateral view

Parietal bone

Coronal suture

Frontal bone

Temporal bone

Sphenoid bone

Ethmoid bone

Lacrimal bone

Suture

Nasal bone

Occipital bone

Zygomatic arch

External auditory meatus

Maxilla

Mandible

Mastoid process

Styloid process

Mental foramen (opening for blood vessels and nerves)

Anterior view

Frontal bone

Parietal bone

Supraorbital foramen

Sphenoid bone

Temporal bone

Ethmoid bone

Nasal bone

Lacrimal bone

Perpendicular plate of the ethmoid bone

Infraorbital foramen

Vomer bone

Maxilla

Mandible

Mental foramen

FIGURE 14–27. Skull: lateral view *(top)* and anterior view *(bottom)*.

Delmar/Cengage Learning.

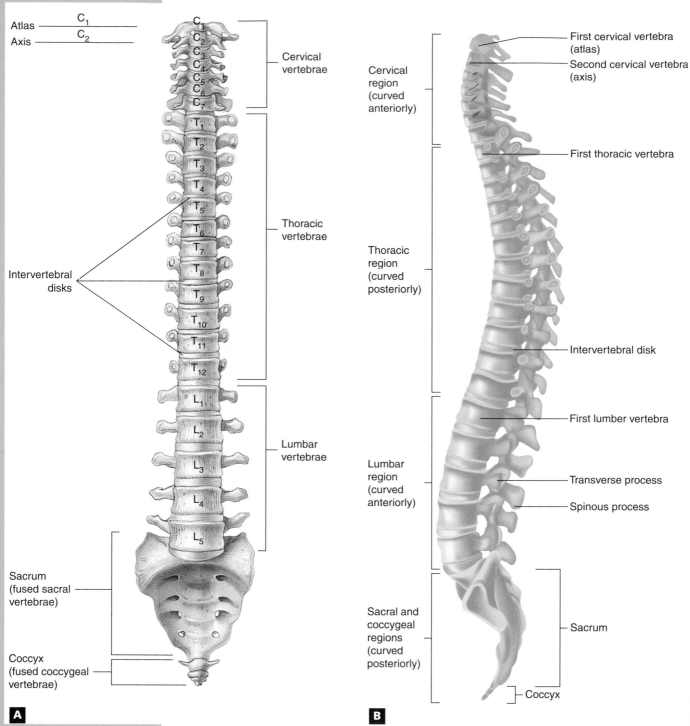

Atlas — C₁

Axis — C₂

Intervertebral disks

Sacrum (fused sacral vertebrae)

Coccyx (fused coccygeal vertebrae)

Cervical vertebrae

Thoracic vertebrae

Lumbar vertebrae

A

Cervical region (curved anteriorly)

Thoracic region (curved posteriorly)

Lumbar region (curved anteriorly)

Sacral and coccygeal regions (curved posteriorly)

First cervical vertebra (atlas)

Second cervical vertebra (axis)

First thoracic vertebra

Intervertebral disk

First lumber vertebra

Transverse process

Spinous process

Sacrum

Coccyx

B

Delmar/Cengage Learning.

FIGURE 14–28. *A.* Anterior view of the vertebral column. *B.* Lateral view of the vertebral column.

TABLE 14–9 **Anatomy of the Urinary System**

proximal - ⟶ **distal**

TWO KIDNEYS	TWO URETERS	BLADDER	URETHRA
Renal capsule (outside covering)	Proximally: enter kidney at the hilum	Trigone (triangular area between the two ureters and the urethra)	Female urine passageway extending from bladder to exterior of body (approximate length, 4–5 cm)
Renal cortex (outer portion) ▪ renal column ▪ nephrons (extend into both cortex and medulla)	Extend from kidney to bladder, with proximal portion bending slightly anterior and distal portion bending slightly posterior	Total volume capacity approximately 350–500 mL	Male urine passageway extending from bladder to exterior of body (approximate length, 18–20 cm)
Renal medulla (inner portion) ▪ renal pyramids ▪ nephrons (extend into both cortex and medulla)	Distally: enter the bladder lateral/posteriorly	Urethra extends from the bladder to the exterior of the body.	
Minor calyces Major calyces Renal pelvis (extends to ureter)			

The right kidney is positioned slightly lower in the posterior abdominal cavity than the left kidney because of the size and location of the liver.

The urinary system can function with only one kidney.

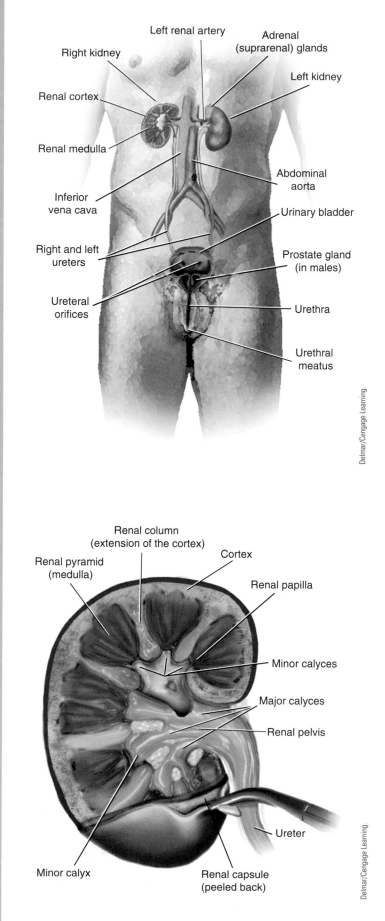

Left renal artery
Right kidney
Adrenal (suprarenal) glands
Left kidney
Renal cortex
Renal medulla
Abdominal aorta
Inferior vena cava
Urinary bladder
Right and left ureters
Prostate gland (in males)
Ureteral orifices
Urethra
Urethral meatus

Delmar/Cengage Learning.

FIGURE 14–29. Structures of the urinary system (kidneys, ureters, urethra, and bladder).

Renal column (extension of the cortex)
Cortex
Renal pyramid (medulla)
Renal papilla
Minor calyces
Major calyces
Renal pelvis
Minor calyx
Ureter
Renal capsule (peeled back)

Delmar/Cengage Learning.

FIGURE 14–30. Structures of the kidney.

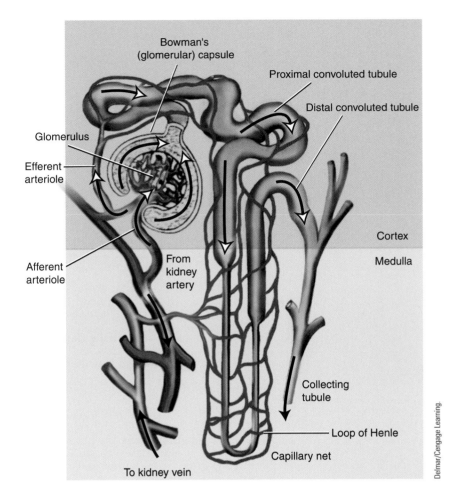

Delmar/Cengage Learning.

FIGURE 14–31. Structures of the nephron.

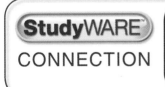

StudyWARE™ CONNECTION

After completing this chapter, review the Flashcards or play an interactive game on your StudyWARE™ CD-ROM that will help you learn the content in this chapter.

CONCEPT THINKING QUESTIONS

1. List two organ systems the pancreas is directly associated with.

2. Explain the purpose of the respiratory system.

3. Identify the two components that comprise the central nervous system (CNS).

4. How many bones make up the adult skeleton?

5. Identify the four main sections (proximal to distal) of the stomach.

6. What is the most proximal section of the small intestine?

7. What structure separates the small intestine from the large intestine?

8. What sections of the large intestine lie transverse in the body?

9. Explain the location of the kidneys within the body.

10. What bones make up the pelvis?

11. Explain the main function of the lymphatic system.

12. How many layers make up the epidermis of the integumentary system?

PRACTICE EXERCISES

1. List the four sections of the colon (proximal to distal).

2. Identify the eight carpal bones by proximal row (medial to lateral) and distal row (medial to lateral).

3. Identify the eight cranial bones of the skull.

4. Identify the 14 facial bones of the skull.

5. Which vertebral vertebrae have transverse foramina? Why?

6. Identify each structure (proximal to distal) of the alimentary canal.

7. How many lobes does the right lung have and what are the names of the lobes?

8. The pituitary gland belongs to what organ system?

9. Identify the three types of muscle tissue and explain where they may be found.

10. Provide an example of voluntary motion and identify organ systems in permit mobility.

11. Provide an example of involuntary motion and identify organ systems in which involuntary motion occurs.

12. Draw and label the components comprising a neuron.

MATCHING

Match each term to the appropriate description.

cardiac muscle tissue	appendicular	trachea
atlas	axis	tarsal bone
kidney	alveoli	PNS
5 rem	axial	carpal bone
T2	T5	smooth muscle tissue
heart	larynx	axon

Description	Term
1. 80 skeletal bones	_____
2. 12 pair of cranial nerves	_____

3. hamate _____

4. C-1 _____

5. nephron _____

6. neuron _____

7. carina _____

8. gas exchange _____

9. no striations _____

10. cuboid _____

11. mitral valve _____

12. thyroid cartilage _____

RETENTION OF MATERIAL

Retention requires practicing the use of previously learned material. Apply the knowledge you have regarding the 11 organ systems to answer the following questions.

1. Which organ system provides the body with an internal defense mechanism against harmful pathogens?

2. Explain where and how gas exchange (oxygen and carbon dioxide) occurs.

3. Identify similarities and differences between the cervical, thoracic, and lumbar vertebrae.

4. Which organ system produces cells through the process of meiosis?

5. Identify the steps of blood flow through the heart, beginning with the right atrium.

6. Which kidney sits slightly lower than the other? Explain why.

7. What cranial bone houses the pituitary gland?

8. What is the largest moveable facial bone? What is the largest immovable facial bone?

9. The epiglottis is part of what organ system, and what function does it serve?

10. Identify three organs that are able to send secretions directly into the duodenum.

11. How do haustra and the teniae coli work together to assist the colon in eliminating waste?

12. What are the smallest functional units of the kidney, and where are they located?

CHAPTER 15

Positioning Terms, Landmarks, and Lines

OBJECTIVES

Upon completion of this chapter, the reader will be able to:

- Distinguish between a projection and a position
- Differentiate between proximal and distal
- Discuss various positions the term *recumbent* encompasses
- Identify the three main body planes
- Discuss body quadrants and expected location of organs
- Discuss the relevance of positioning landmarks and lines
- Identify positioning lines associated with radiographic procedures involving skull and facial bones

CONCEPT THINKING

Positioning terms, bony landmarks, and positioning lines serve as a roadmap for the radiologic technologist to correctly position patients. Accurate positioning is critical in obtaining optimal images of anatomic areas of interest for image interpretation by a radiologist. Because of the body's three-dimensional shape and a small degree of inherent distortion caused by object-to-image distance and the diverging x-ray beam, a technologist must combine known imaging principles with learned technical skills to capture radiographic images that depict as true a representation as possible of the actual anatomic structures being imaged. Unwanted rotation or tilt of the body can hinder views of anatomical structures and be the cause for repeat radiographic images. A repeat exposure subjects the patient to 100% more radiation than necessary; although an occasional repeat image is inevitable, one should always be conscious of adhering to the *ALARA* principle and avoiding undo radiation exposure to a patient. The use of proper positioning landmarks and lines provides the technologist with a guideline for directing the central ray to the appropriate body part. However, the correlation of internal organs and structures to established positioning landmarks and lines is based on the anatomy of the "average" human being. Therefore, slight positioning adjustments may be necessary to accommodate body habitus and pathological conditions impacting the size, shape, or location of these anatomic organs and bony structures. One must also keep in mind that radiographic positioning terms are based upon anatomic structures as they are seen in "anatomical position" with the body erect, arms down by the side with palms facing forward, and feet slightly apart.

ABBREVIATIONS: RADIOGRAPHIC EXAMINATIONS

BE	barium enema
CXR	chest x-ray
IVP	intravenous pyelogram
IVU	intravenous urogram
KUB	kidneys, ureters, bladder
SBS	small bowel series
UGI	upper gastrointestinal

ABBREVIATIONS: PROJECTIONS AND POSITIONS

projection	projection refers to the path of the x-ray beam, where the central ray (CR) enters and exits
position	position refers to the placement of the body or body part in relation to the central ray (CR) and image receptor (IR)
AP	anterior posterior *(projection; see Figure 15–1)*
PA	posterior anterior *(projection; see Figure 15–1)*
LAO	left anterior oblique *(body position; see Figure 15–1)*
LPO	left posterior oblique *(body position; see Figure 15–1)*
RAO	right anterior oblique *(body position; see Figure 15–1)*
RPO	right posterior oblique *(body position; see Figure 15–1)*
SMV	submentovertex projection *(skull and mandible; see Figure 15–2)*
VSM	verticosubmental projection *(skull and mandible; see Figure 15–3)*
dorsoplantar	the central ray enters the dorsal surface of the foot and exits through the plantar part of the foot *(see Figure 15–4)*
plantodorsal	the central ray enters the plantar surface of the foot and exits through the dorsal part of the foot *(see Figure 15–5)*

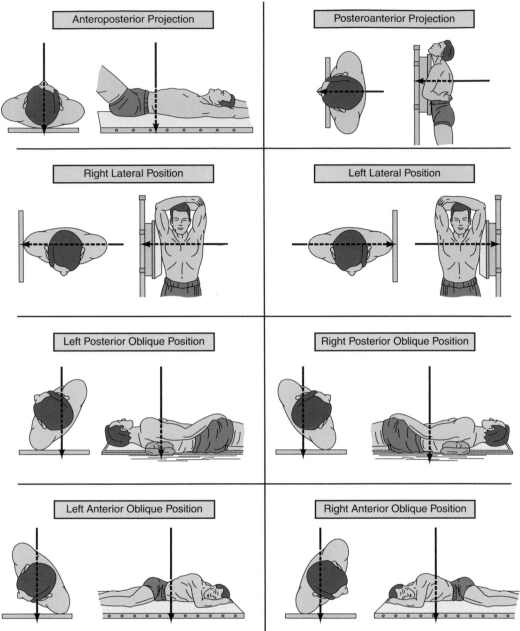

Anteroposterior Projection

Posteroanterior Projection

Right Lateral Position

Left Lateral Position

Left Posterior Oblique Position

Right Posterior Oblique Position

Left Anterior Oblique Position

Right Anterior Oblique Position

FIGURE 15–1. Standard terminology for positioning and projection.

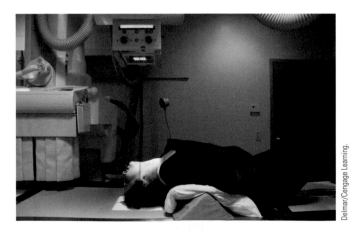

FIGURE 15–2. SMV projection.

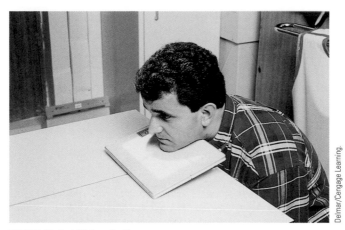

FIGURE 15–3. VSM projection.

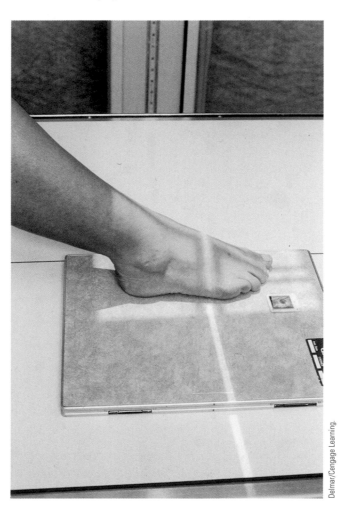

FIGURE 15–4. Dorsoplantar projection.

COMMON VOCABULARY/ POSITIONING TERMS

decubitus	recumbent position with a horizontal x-ray beam
erect	standing upright
Fowler's	recumbent position with body tilted so the head is at a level higher than the feet

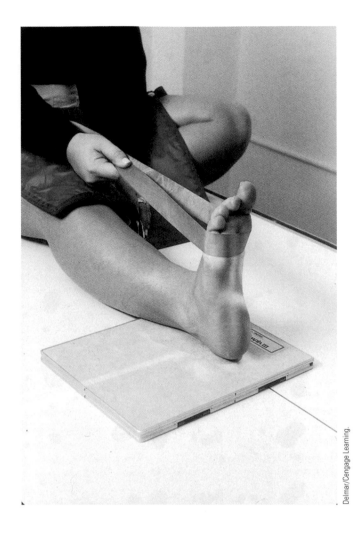

Delmar/Cengage Learning.

FIGURE 15–5. Plantodorsal projection.

lateral	lying or standing erect with side of the body closest to the image receptor *(see Figure 15–1)*
lithotomy	lying supine with knees flexed and abducted; both knees and ankles are held in position with resting supports
oblique	body or body part positioned so as to be neither parallel nor perpendicular to the image receptor *(see Figure 15–1)*
prone	lying face down with anterior part of body in contact with the surface of the x-ray table, examination table, bed, or stretcher
recumbent	lying down in any position (e.g., supine, prone, lateral)
Sim's	lying recumbent on left side with right leg flexed and placed over left flexed leg; left arm lies behind back
supine	lying face up with posterior part of body in contact with the surface of x-ray table, examination table, bed, or stretcher
trendelenburg	recumbent with body tilted so the head is at a level lower than the feet

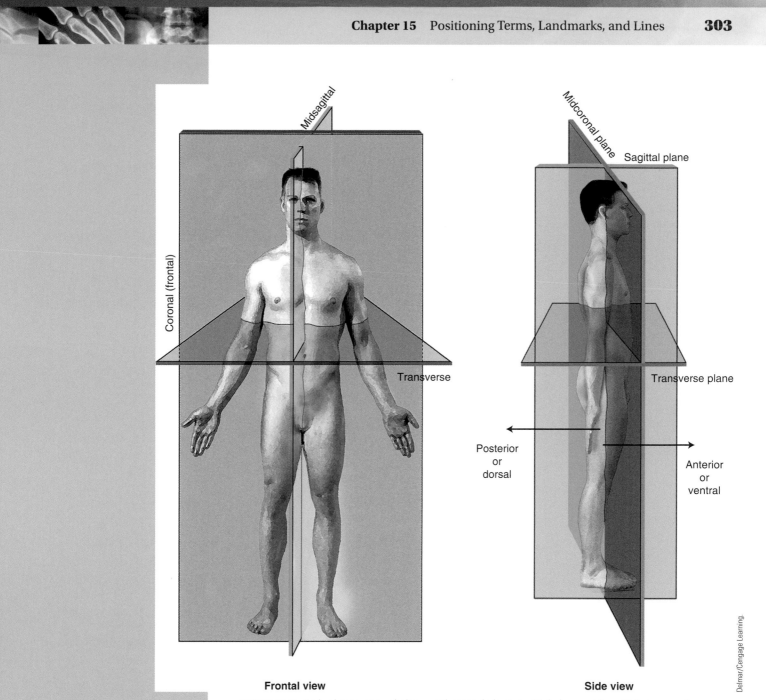

FIGURE 15–6. Body planes: coronal plane, mid-coronal plane, sagittal plane, mid-sagittal plane, and transverse plane.

body planes

- ■ **coronal plane** – The coronal plane *(or frontal plane)* runs longitudinally through the body, dividing the body into anterior and posterior sections *(see Figure 15-6)*.

- ■ **mid-coronal plane** – The mid-coronal plane runs longitudinally through the body, dividing the body into two equal sections of anterior and posterior *(see Figure 15-6)*.

- ■ **occlusal plane** – The parallel plane between the biting surface of the upper teeth and the mastoid process of the occipital bone.

- ■ **sagittal plane** – The sagittal plane divides the body into left and right sections running parallel to the long axis of the body and going through the body from anterior to posterior *(see Figure 15-6)*.

- **mid-sagittal plane** – The midsagittal plane *(or median plane)* runs parallel to the long axis of the body, directly down the center of the body anterior to posterior, dividing the body into two equal sections of left and right *(see Figure 15-6)*.

- **transverse plane** – The transverse plane *(or horizontal plane)* runs perpendicular to the long axis of the body, dividing the body into superior and inferior sections *(see Figure 15-6)*.

StudyWARE™ CONNECTION   To help visualize the location of each plane, view the Body Planes animation on your StudyWARE™ CD-ROM.

BODY QUADRANTS (ABDOMINOPELVIC)

LUQ   left upper quadrant – Organs found in this quadrant include fundus and body of stomach, spleen, left splenic flexure of the colon, tail of the pancreas, part of the small intestines (distal duodenum and jejunum), left suprarenal gland, and left kidney.

LLQ   left lower quadrant – Organs found in this quadrant include descending colon, sigmoid colon, and part of the small intestines (jejunum and ileum).

RUQ   right upper quadrant – Organs found in this quadrant include liver, gallbladder, pyloric antrum of the stomach, hepatic flexure of the colon, proximal part of the small intestines (duodenal bulb, duodenum, ileum), head of the pancreas, right suprarenal gland, and right kidney.

RLQ   right lower quadrant – Organs found in this quadrant include distal part of the small intestines (ileum and ileocecal valve), cecum and ascending colon, and appendix *(see Figure 15-7)*.

BODY REGIONS (ABDOMINOPELVIC)

right hypochondriac region (rhr)

epigastric region (er)

left hypochondriac region (lhr)

right lumbar region (rlr)

umbilical region (ur)

left lumbar region (llr)

right inguinal region (rir)

right hypogastric (pubic) region (rhgr)

left hypogastric (pubic) region (lhgr)

(see Figure 15-8)

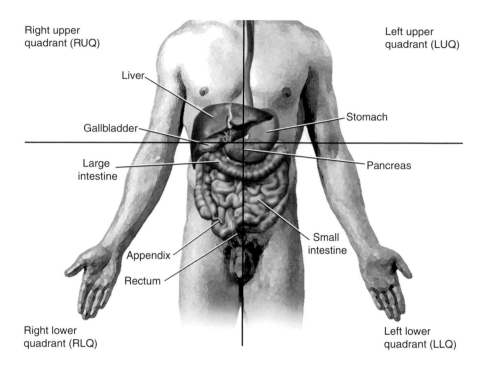

Right upper
quadrant (RUQ)

Left upper
quadrant (LUQ)

Liver

Gallbladder

Stomach

Large
intestine

Pancreas

Small
intestine

Appendix

Rectum

Right lower
quadrant (RLQ)

Left lower
quadrant (LLQ)

Delmar/Cengage Learning.

FIGURE 15–7. Abdominal quadrants.

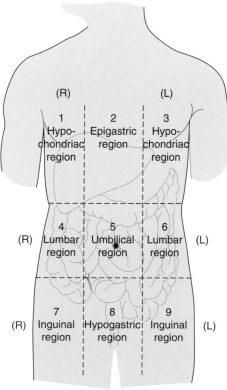

(R)   (L)

| 1 | 2 | 3 |
| Hypo-chondriac region | Epigastric region | Hypo-chondriac region |

(R)

| 4 | 5 | 6 |
| Lumbar region | Umbilical region | Lumbar region |

(L)

(R)

| 7 | 8 | 9 |
| Inguinal region | Hypogastric region | Inguinal region |

(L)

Delmar/Cengage Learning.

FIGURE 15–8. Nine abdominal regions.

DIRECTIONAL TERMS

anterior   front or ventral *(see Figure 15–9)*

abduction   to move a body limb away from the body; moving lateral *(see Figure 15–10)*

adduction   to move a body limb closer to the body; moving medial *(see Figure 15–10)*

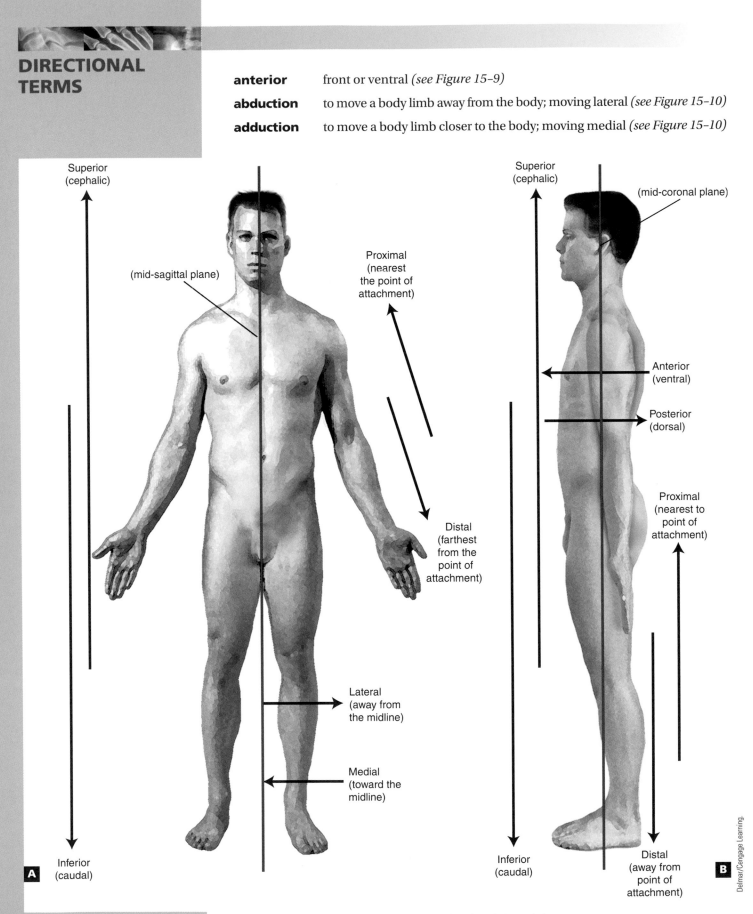

FIGURE 15–9. Directional terminology. *A.* Anterior view. *B.* Lateral view.

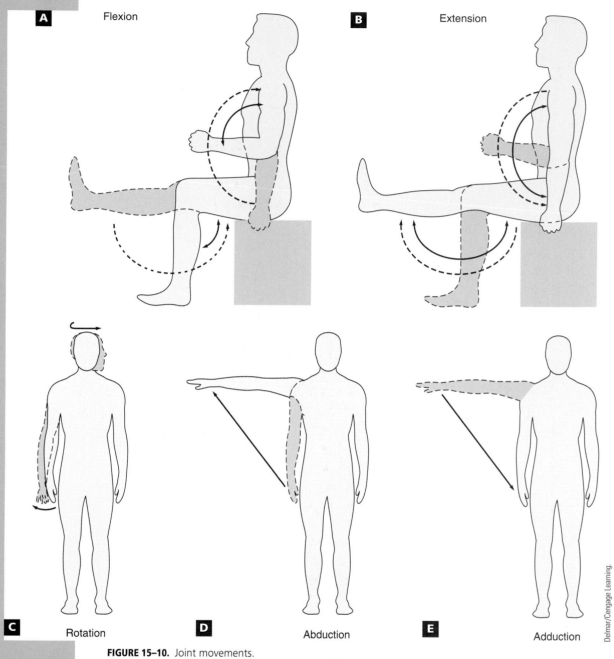

FIGURE 15–10. Joint movements.

cephalic	toward the head *(cephalad refers to x-ray tube angle directed toward the patient's head)*
caudal	toward the feet *(caudad refers to x-ray tube angle directed toward the patient's feet)*
deviation	to turn away from *(typically refers to movement of the wrist: radial deviation or ulnar deviation)*
distal	away from the source of attachment
extension	increasing the angle of a joint to increase distance between body parts *(see Figure 15–10)*
external rotation	*(see lateral rotation)*

eversion	lateral upward movement of the foot; outward stress movement (*see Figure 15–11*)
flexion	decreasing the angle of a joint to decrease distance between body parts plane (*see Figure 15–10*)
hyperextension	increasing the angle of a joint beyond normal extension (*see Figure 15–12*)

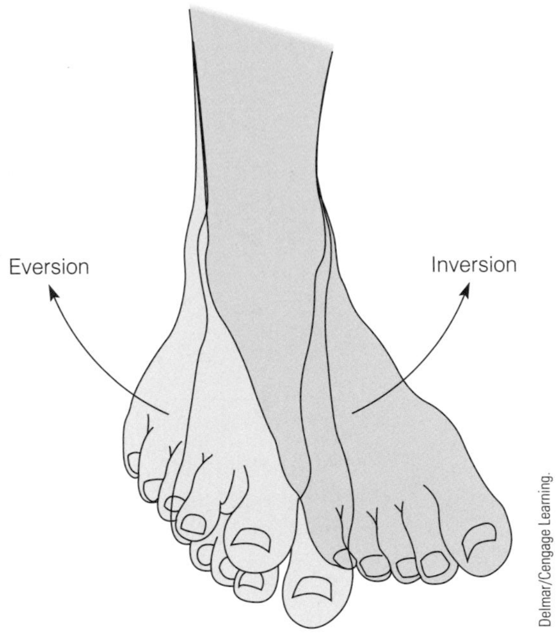

FIGURE 15–11. Right foot eversion and inversion.

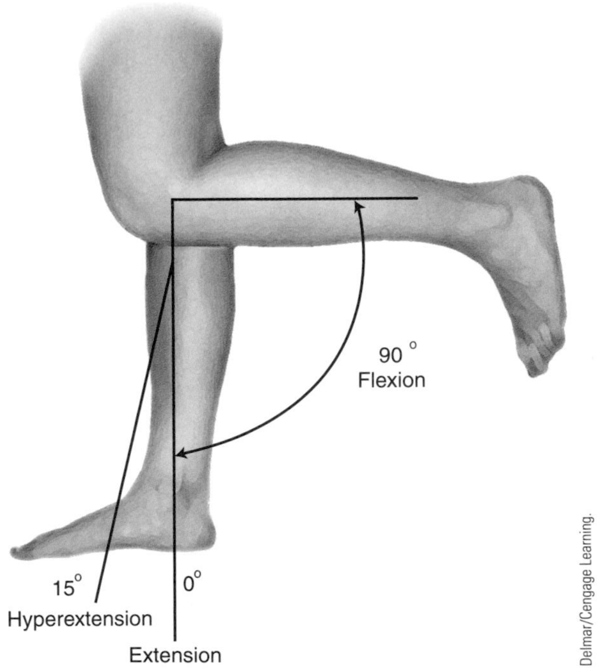

FIGURE 15–12. Hyperextension.

hyperflexion	decreasing the angle of a joint beyond normal flexion
inferior	below *(see Figure 15–9)*
internal rotation	*(see medial rotation)*
inversion	medial upward movement of the foot; inward stress movement *(see Figure 15–11)*
lateral	side of the body or body part furthest away from the median or midsagittal plane *(see Figure 15–9)*
medial	toward the median or mid-sagittal plane *(see Figure 15–9)*
neutral	body or body part in its relaxed state with no intentional movement
oblique	body is positioned to prohibit mid-sagittal plane from being perpendicular or parallel to the image receptor *(see Figure 15–13)*
palmar	palm of hand *(see Figure 15–14)*
posterior	back or dorsal *(see Figure 15–9)*
pronation	rotating the hand to show palm side down *(see Figure 15–15)*
proximal	closest to the source of attachment or closer to the mid-sagittal plane *(see Figure 15–9)*

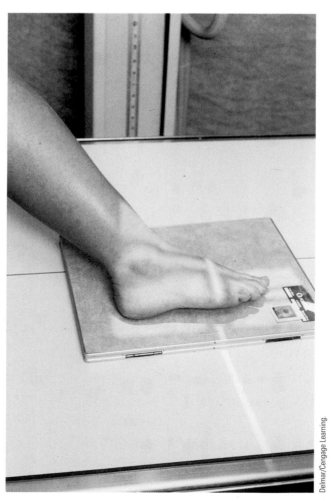

FIGURE 15–13. Oblique foot.

Delmar/Cengage Learning.

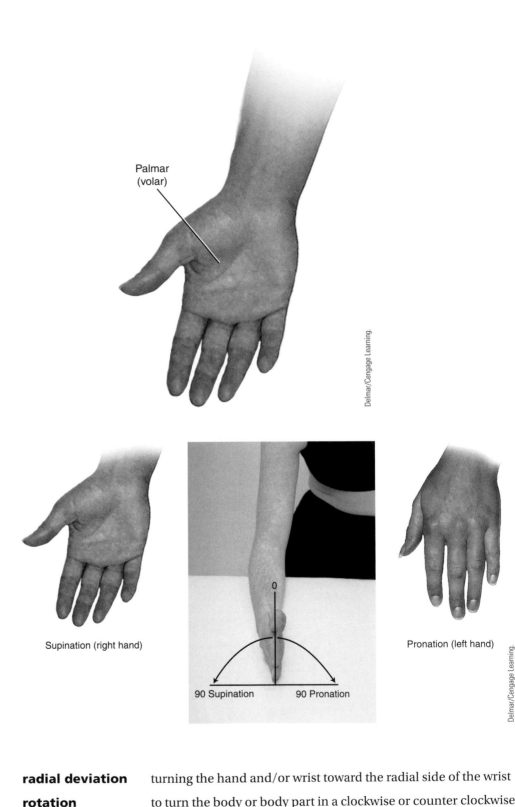

Palmar (volar)

Delmar/Cengage Learning.

FIGURE 15–14. Palmar.

Supination (right hand)

0

90 Supination   90 Pronation

Pronation (left hand)

Delmar/Cengage Learning.

FIGURE 15–15. Supination and pronation.

radial deviation	turning the hand and/or wrist toward the radial side of the wrist
rotation	to turn the body or body part in a clockwise or counter clockwise direction *(see Figure 15-10C)*
lateral rotation	external rotation; to turn the body part away from the medial plane so the anterior aspect is rotating outward *(see Figure 15-16)*
medial rotation	internal rotation; to turn the body part towards the medial plane so the anterior aspect is rotating inward *(see Figure 15-16)*

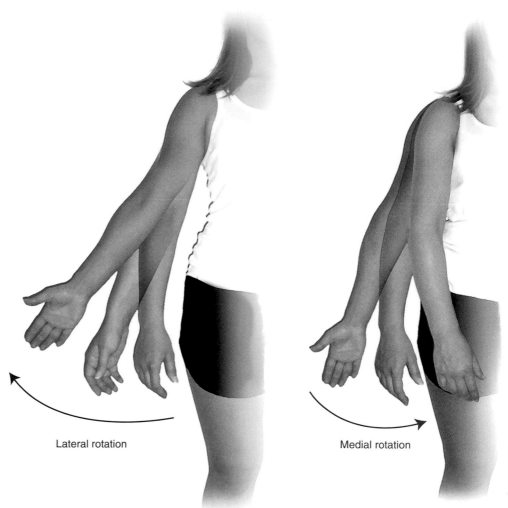

Lateral rotation

Medial rotation

Delmar/Cengage Learning.

FIGURE 15–16. Lateral and medial rotation.

supination	rotating the hand to show palm side up *(as seen in anatomical position)*
superior	above *(see Figure 15–9)*
tilt	mid-sagittal plane is not parallel to the image receptor
ulnar deviation	turning the hand and/or wrist toward the ulnar side of the wrist
ventral	front or anterior part of the body *(see Figure 15–9)*

DIRECTIONAL X-RAY TUBE TERMS

axial	angulation of the central ray *(see Figure 15–17)*
horizontal beam	path of the x-ray beam runs parallel to the floor and ceiling *(see Figure 15–18)*
parallel	refers to the relationship between a positioning line or body plane and the path of the x-ray beam, traveling in the same direction, never to intersect with each other *(see Figure 15–18)*

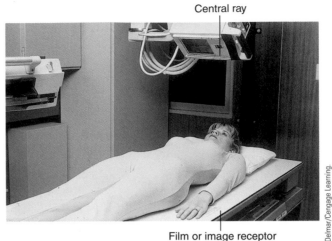

FIGURE 15–17. Axial projection (angled beam).

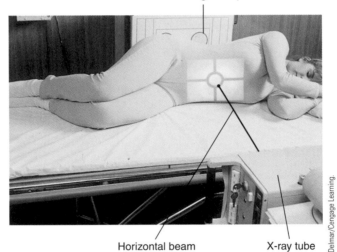

FIGURE 15–18. The horizontal beam runs parallel to the floor, ceilng, and sagittal body planes.

perpendicular	refers to the relationship between a positioning line or body plane and the path of the x-ray beam, traveling at right angles to each other; can intersect with one another (*see Figure 15–19*)
tangential	central ray is positioned to skim a body part as opposed to being centered to it (*see Figure 15–20*)

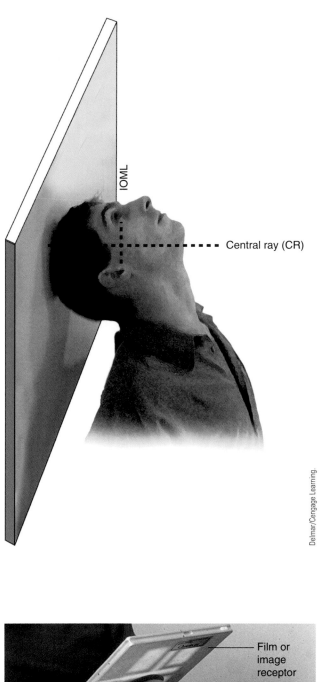

IOML

Central ray (CR)

Delmar/Cengage Learning.

FIGURE 15–19. The IOML positioning line is perpendicular to the central ray.

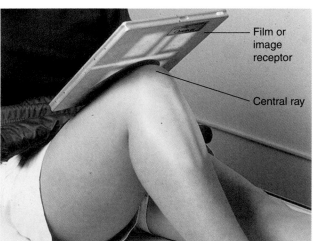

Film or image receptor

Central ray

Delmar/Cengage Learning.

FIGURE 15–20. Tangential position.

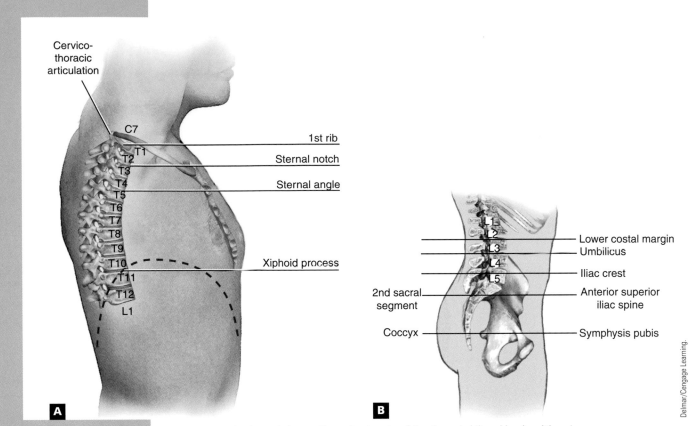

FIGURE 15–21. Lateral views of bony landmarks of the thoracic (*A*) and lumbar (*B*) regions.

Delmar/Cengage Learning.

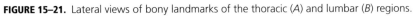

BONY LANDMARKS

See Figure 15–21.

ASIS	anterosuperior iliac spine is the anterior portion of the iliac spine located at the vertebral level of (sacral segments) S1–S2
greater trochanter	lateral prominence on the proximal part of the femur, located inferior to the head of the femur; lies at the level of the symphysis pubis
iliac crest	crest of the ilium; at a level between the 4th and 5th lumbar vertebrae
prominent rib	lowest costal rib margin lies at the vertebral level of L2–L3
symphysis pubis	a slightly movable joint at the junction of the inferior ramus of the innominate bones; lies at the level of mid-coccyx
vertebra prominens	spinous process of the 7th cervical vertebra
xiphoid process	tip of the sternum; at a level between the 9th and 10th thoracic vertebrae

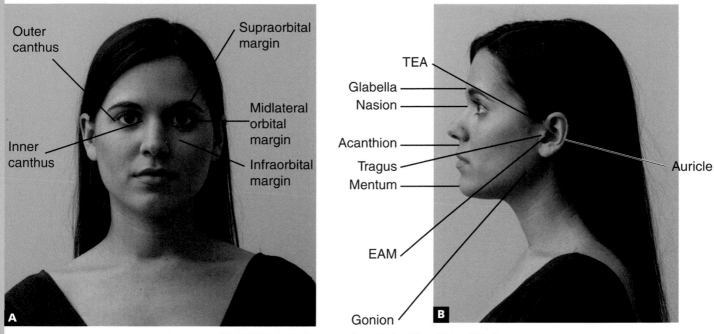

FIGURE 15–22. Skull topography: anterior (*A*) and lateral (*B*) views.

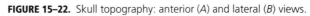

SKULL TOPOGRAPHY

See Figure 15–22.

EAM	external auditory meatus
IAM	internal auditory meatus
IOM	infraorbital margin
SOG	supraorbital groove
SOM	supraorbital margin
TEA	top of the ear attachment
acanthion	area just below the nasal septum and above the upper lip
auricle	large cartilaginous flap of ear
glabella	mid-sagittal point slightly above the eyebrows and superciliary ridges
gonion	angle of the posterior lateral portion of the mandible
inion	mid-sagittal prominence on the lower portion of the occipital bone
inner canthus	medial point of the orbit where the eyelids meet
mentum (mental point)	mid-sagittal point on the most anterior portion of the chin
nasion	mid-sagittal point just below the eyebrows and superciliary ridges; at the bridge of the nose
outer canthus	lateral point of the orbit where the eyelids meet

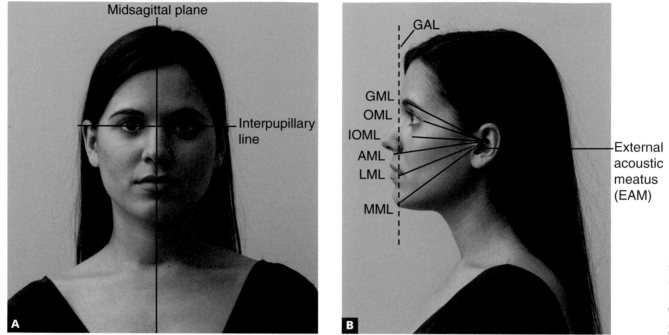

FIGURE 15–23. Skull positioning lines on anterior (*A*) and lateral (*B*) views.

superciliary ridge	bony arch above each eye where the eyebrows are located
tragus	small cartilaginous flap extending over the opening to the ear

SKULL POSITIONING LINES

See Figure 15–23.

AML	acanthiomeatal line; extends from the acathion to the EAM
GML	glabellomeatal line; extends from the glabella to the EAM
GAL	glabelloalveolar line; extends from the glabella to anterior portion of the alveolar process of the maxilla
IOML	infraorbitalmeatal line *(referred to as Reid's base line)*; extends from the inferior orbital margin to the EAM
IPL	interpupillary line; extends from one outer canthus to the other
LML	lipsmeatal line; extends from the junction of the lips to the EAM
MML	mentomeatal line; extends from the mental point to the EAM
MSP	midsagittal plane *(median plane)*; line that extends down the center of the body dividing the body into equal halves
OML	orbitalmeatal line *(referred to as canthomeatal line and radiographic baseline)*; line that extends from the outer canthus to the EAM

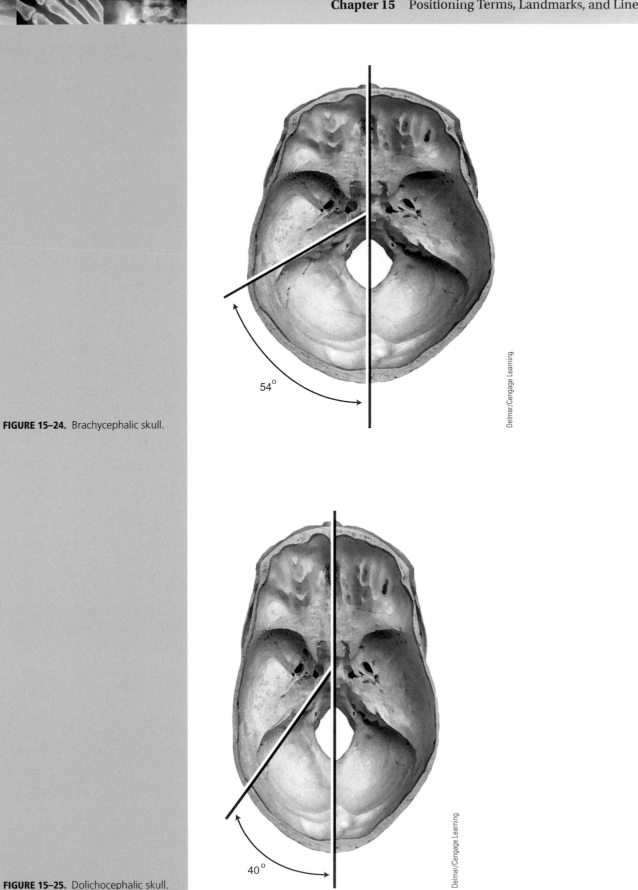

54°

Delmar/Cengage Learning.

FIGURE 15–24. Brachycephalic skull.

40°

Delmar/Cengage Learning.

FIGURE 15–25. Dolichocephalic skull.

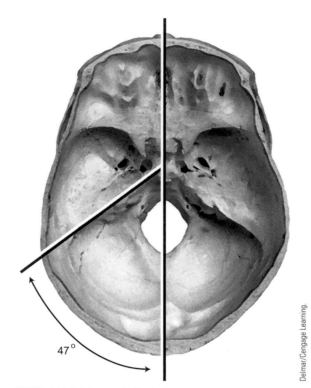

Delmar/Cengage Learning.

FIGURE 15–26. Mesocephalic skull.

SKULL MORPHOLOGY

brachycephalic   short, broad-shaped skull with petrous ridges angled more than 47° to the mid-sagittal plane *(see Figure 15–24)*

dolichocephalic   narrow, long-shaped skull with petrous ridges angled less than 47° to the mid-sagittal plane *(see Figure 15–25)*

mesocephalic   average-shaped skull with petrous ridges angled 47° to the mid-sagittal plane *(see Figure 15–26)*

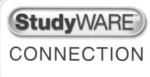 CONNECTION

After completing this chapter, play Concentration or another interactive game on your StudyWARE™ CD-ROM that will help you learn the content in this chapter.

CONCEPT THINKING QUESTIONS

1. List three organs that can be found in the left upper quadrant.

2. Which is the largest organ of the right upper quadrant and the largest organ of the left upper quadrant?

3. Which abdominal region is the majority of the transverse colon found?

4. With what vertebral level does the iliac crest correspond?

5. What part of the small intestine does the head of the pancreas make contact with?

6. Identify the abdominal quadrant and abdominal region to which the appendix is located.

7. What bony landmark could be palpated to locate the body of the stomach?

8. What projection describes the x-ray beam entering below the mandible and exiting at the top of the skull?

9. Which body plane divides the body into superior and inferior sections?

10. What is the name of the position in which the heart is placed closest to the image receptor and the body is rotated 45°?

11. What cranial positioning landmark is located at the mid-sagittal point slightly above the superciliary ridges?

12. What name is given to the angle of the mandible?

PRACTICE EXERCISES

1. List the three types of skull morphology and describe each by the angle of the petrous ridges to the mid-sagittal plane.

2. What skull positioning line is aligned with the mid-sagittal plane?

3. What bony landmark could be used to locate the level of the symphysis pubis?

4. Moving the hand to be in anatomic position requires what type of rotation?

5. Which vertebral vertebra is considered a bony landmark and why?

6. Identify the positioning line and body plane utilized for placing the skull in a true lateral position.

7. Explain why a horizontal beam is necessary when imaging the paranasal sinuses.

8. Identify the type of device that blurs grid lines during a radiographic exposure.

9. List the nine abdominopelvic regions in rows of three, beginning with the superior row, followed by the middle row, and lastly the inferior row.

10. A left lateral decubitus position with an anterior/posterior projection would be helpful in demonstrating what?

MATCHING

Match each term to the appropriate description.

posterior	**LML**	**ulnar deviation**
IOML	**pronation**	**L2-3**
L4-5	**OML**	**TEA**
diaphragm	**vertrebra prominens**	**plantar surface**
dorsal surface	**S1-2**	**supination**
MML	**posterior**	**inion**

Description   Term

1. level of the petrous ridges   _____

2. line from the outer canthus
   to the EAM   _____

3. C7   _____

4. mid-sagittal prominence on
   occipital bone   _____

5. prominent rib   _____

6. line extends from the mental
   point to the EAM   _____

7. to turn the hand or wrist
   toward the ulna   _____

8. at the level of the xyphoid
   process   _____

9. ASIS   _____

10. top of foot   _____

11. moving hand to show palm
    side up   _____

12. dorsal   _____

RETENTION OF MATERIAL

Retention requires practicing the use of previously learned material. Apply the knowledge you have regarding the 11 organ systems to answer the following questions.

1. The patient is lying on their right side and the beam is horizontal. What position is this?

2. With the patient lying supine, does the chin need to be tilted up or down in order to place the LML perpendicular to the IR?

3. Explain the location of the ASIS to the iliac crest?

4. Identify the seven bony landmarks and the vertebral level to which they correspond.

5. If the CR is perpendicular to the mid-sagittal plane and parallel to the interpulliary line, what position is the skull placed in?

6. The patient is prone with the mid-coronal plane parallel to the IR. Identify the projection.

7. Describe how the orbits will appear on the radiographic image when tilt occurs during a lateral projection of the facial bones.

8. Describe how the orbits will appear on the radiographic image when rotation occurs during a lateral projection of the facial bones.

9. Which is the preferred projection for imaging the paranasal sinuses and why?

10. The Reid's baseline is more commonly referred to as which skull positioning line?

11. The patient is lying supine with the feet placed higher than the head. Identify this position.

12. Identify the anatomic structures that are located in the RUQ of the abdominopelvic cavity.

Appendix A

asrt
American Society of Radiologic Technologists

Code of Ethics

1 The radiologic technologist conducts herself or himself in a professional manner, responds to patient needs and supports colleagues and associates in providing quality patient care.

2 The radiologic technologist acts to advance the principal objective of the profession to provide services to humanity with full respect for the dignity of mankind.

3 The radiologic technologist delivers patient care and service unrestricted by concerns of personal attributes or the nature of the disease or illness, and without discrimination on the basis of sex, race, creed, religion or socio-economic status.

4 The radiologic technologist practices technology founded upon theoretical knowledge and concepts, uses equipment and accessories consistent with the purpose for which they were designed and employs procedures and techniques appropriately.

5 The radiologic technologist assesses situations; exercises care, discretion and judgment; assumes responsibility for professional decisions; and acts in the best interest of the patient.

6 The radiologic technologist acts as an agent through observation and communication to obtain pertinent information for the physician to aid in the diagnosis and treatment of the patient and recognizes that interpretation and diagnosis are outside the scope of practice for the profession.

7 The radiologic technologist uses equipment and accessories, employs techniques and procedures, performs services in accordance with an accepted standard of practice and demonstrates expertise in minimizing radiation exposure to the patient, self and other members of the health care team.

8 The radiologic technologist practices ethical conduct appropriate to the profession and protects the patient's right to quality radiologic technology care.

9 The radiologic technologist respects confidences entrusted in the course of professional practice, respects the patient's right to privacy and reveals confidential information only as required by law or to protect the welfare of the individual or the community.

10 The radiologic technologist continually strives to improve knowledge and skills by participating in continuing education and professional activities, sharing knowledge with colleagues and investigating new aspects of professional practice.

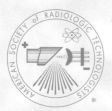

Appendix B

PROFESSIONAL ORGANIZATION	ADDRESS	WEBSITE
Radiology Associations		
Academy of Molecular Imaging	5839 Green Valley Circle, Suite 209 Los Angeles, CA 90230	http://www.ami-imaging.org
Academy of Radiology Research	1029 Vermont Ave NW, Suite 505 Washington, DC 20005	http://www.acadrad.org
American Association for Women Radiologists	4550 Post Oak Place, Suite 342 Houston, TX 77027	http://www.aawr.org
American Board of Nuclear Medicine	4555 Forest Park Boulevard, Suite 119 St. Louis, MO 63108	http://www.abnm.org
American Board of Radiology	5441 East Williams Boulevard, Suite 200 Tucson, AZ 85711	http://www.theabr.org
American College of Medical Physics	One Physics Ellipse College Park, MD 20740-3846	http://www.acmp.org
American College of Nuclear Medicine	1850 Samuel Morse Drive Reston, VA 20190	http://www.acnponline.org
American College of Radiology	1891 Preston White Drive Reston, VA 20191	http://www.acr.org
Association for Medical Imaging Managment	AHRA 490B Boston Post Rd, Suite 200 Sudbury, MA 01776	http://www.ahraonline.org
American Osteopathic College of Radiology	119 East Second Street Milan, MO 63556-1331	http://www.aocr.org
Association of Educators in Imaging and Radiological Sciences	P.O. Box 90204 Albuquerque, NM 87199-0204	http://www.aeirs.org
Association of Vascular and Interventional Radiographers	12100 Sunset Hills Road, Suite 130 Reston, VA 20190	http://www.avir.org

PROFESSIONAL ORGANIZATION	ADDRESS	WEBSITE
Radiology Societies		
American Radium Society	11300 W. Olympic Blvd, Suite 600 Los Angeles, CA 90064	http://www.americanradiumsociety.org
American Roentgen Ray Society	4421 Slatestone Court Leesburg, VA 20176-5109	http://www.arrs.org
American Society of Emergency Radiology	4550 Post Oak Place, Suite 342 Houston, TX 77027	http://www.erad.org
American Society of Head and Neck Radiology	2210 Midwest Road, Suite 207 Oak Brook, IL 60523-8205	http://www.ashnr.org
American Society of Radiologic Technologists	5000 Central Ave. SE Albuquerque, NM 87123-3909	http://www.asrt.org
Fleischner Society	1891 Preston White Drive Reston, VA 20191	http://www.fleischner.org
International Society of Radiology	7910 Woodmont Ave, Suite 400 Bethesda, MD 20814	http://www.isradiology.org
Radiological Society of North America	820 Jorie Blvd Oak Brook, IL 60523-2251	http://www.rsna.org
Society for Pediatric Radiology	1891 Preston White Drive Reston, VA 20191	http://www.pedrad.org
Society for the Advancement of Women's Imaging	P.O. Box 885 Schererville, IN 46375	http://www.sawi.org
Society of Breast Imaging	1891 Preston White Drive Reston, VA 20191	http://www.sbi-online.org
Society of Interventional Radiology	3975 Fair Ridge Drive, Suite 400 North Fairfax, VA 22033	http://www.sirweb.org
Society of Gastrointestinal Radiologists	International Meeting Managers, Inc. 4550 Post Oak Place, Suite 342 Houston, TX 77027	http://www.sgr.org
Society of Skeletal Radiology	1100 E. Woodfield Rd, Suite 520 Schaumburg, IL 60173	http://www.skeletalrad.org
Society of Uroradiology	International Meeting Managers, Inc. 4550 Post Oak Place, Suite 342 Houston, TX 77027	http://www.uroradiology.org

PROFESSIONAL ORGANIZATION	ADDRESS	WEBSITE
State Organizations		
Arizona Arizona State Society of Radiologic Technologists	ASSRT P.O. Box 40637 Tucson, AZ 85717-0637	http://www.assrt.com
Arkansas Arkansas Society of Radiologic Technologists	ArSRT P.O. Box 241492 Little Rock, AR 72223	http://www.arsrt.org
California California Society of Radiologic Technologists	CSRT 2196 Tanager Ct. Pleasanton, CA 945566	http://www.csrt.org
California Los Angeles Radiological Society	LARS P.O. Box 93125 Pasadena, CA 91109	http://www.larad.org
Colorado Colorado Society of Radiologic Technologists	No listing	http://www.csrt.net
Connecticut Connecticut Society of Radiologic Technologists	No listing	http://www.csrtinc.org
Florida Florida Radiological Society	FRS 620 West Sligh Avenue Tampa, FL 33634	http://www.flrad.org
Florida Florida Society of Radiologic Technologists	FSRT 6825 NW 15th Street Margate, FL 33063	http://www.fsrt.org
Georgia Georgia Society of Radiologic Technologists	GSRT, Corporate Office P.O. Box 767369 Roswell, GA 30076-7369	http://www.gsrt.org
Hawaii Hawaii Society of Radiologic Technologists	HSRT P.O. Box 23096 Honolulu, HI 96823-3096	

(continued)

PROFESSIONAL ORGANIZATION	ADDRESS	WEBSITE
State Organizations *(continued)*		
Idaho Idaho Society of Radiologic Technologists	No listing	http://www.isu.edu/isrt
Illinois Chicago Radiological Society	No listing	http://www.chi-rad-soc.org
Illinois Illinois State Society of Radiologic Technologists	ISSRT 1701 E. Empire St., Ste 360 Box 276 Bloomington, IL 61704	http://www.issrt.org
Indiana Indiana Society of Radiologic Technologists	No listing	http://www.isort.org
Iowa Iowa Society of Radiologic Technologists	No listing	http://www.isrt.org
Kansas Kansas Society of Radiologic Technologists	No listing	http://www.ksrad.org
Louisiana Louisiana Society of Radiologic Technologists	LSRT Executive Secretary, 520 Jackson Street Denham Springs, LA 70726	http://www.lsrt.net
Maryland Maryland Society of Radiologic Technologists	MSRT Executive Secretary P.O. Box 617 Fallston, MD 21047	http://www.msrtonline.org
Massachusetts Massachusetts Society of Radiologic Technologists	No listing	http://www.msrt-ma.org
Massachusetts Massachusetts Radiological Society	MRS 860 Winter Street Waltham Woods Corporate Center Waltham, MA 02451-1411	http://www.massrad.org
Michigan Michigan Society of Radiologic Technologists	No listing	http://www.msrt.org

PROFESSIONAL ORGANIZATION	ADDRESS	WEBSITE
Minnesota Minnesota Society of Radiologic Technologists	MnSRT 300 33rd Avenue South, Suite 101 Waite Park, MN 56387	http://www.mnsrt.com
Missouri Missouri Society of Radiologic Technologists	No listing	http://www.mosrt.org
Nebraska Nebraska Society of Radiologic Technologists	No listing	http://www.nsrt.net
New Jersey Radiological Society of New Jersey	RSNJ 26 Eastmans Road Parsippany, NJ 07054	http://www.rsnj.org
New Mexico New Mexico Society of Radiologic Technologists	NMSRT 47 Yucca Lane Placitas, NM 87043	http://www.nmsrt.org
New York New York State Society of Radiologic Sciences, Inc.	No listing	http://www.nyssrs.org
New York New York State Society of Radiologic Technologists	No listing	http://www.nyssrs.og
New York The Association of Educators In Radiologic Technology of the State of New York, Inc.	No listing	http://www.aertsny.org
North Carolina North Carolina Society of Radiologic Technologists	NCSRT, Central Office P.O. Box 38 Jamestown, NC 27282	http://www.ncsrt.org
Ohio Ohio Society of Radiologic Technologists	No listing	http://www.osrt.org
Oklahoma Oklahoma Society of Radiologic Technologists	OSRT P.O. Box 3434 Edmond, OK 73083-3434	http://www.osrt.net

(continued)

PROFESSIONAL ORGANIZATION	ADDRESS	WEBSITE
State Organizations (continued)		
Oregon Oregon Society of Radiologic Technologists	OSRT P.O. Box 7863 Salem, OR 97303	http://www.oregonsrt.org
South Carolina South Carolina Society of Radiologic Technologists	SCSRT P.O. Box 25568 Greenville, SC 29601	http://www.scsrt.org
South Dakota South Dakota Society of Radiologic Technologists	No listing	http://www.sdsrt.org
Texas Texas Society of Radiologic Technologists	TSRT Executive Office 806 Woodlawn Kilgore, TX 75662	http://tsrtorg.tripod.com
Virginia Virginia Society of Radiologic Technologists	No listing	http://www.vsrt.org
Washington Washington Society of Radiologic Technologists	No listing	http://www.wsrt.com
Wisconsin Wisconsin Society of Radiologic Technologists	No listing	http://www.wsrt.net
Wyoming Wyoming Society of Radiologic Technologists	WSRT P.O. Box 82 Torrington, WY 82240	http://www.wsrt.org

Note: Not all states provide a website listing and/or mailing address.

National and International Organizations

Australia The Royal Australian and New Zealand College of Radiologists	Level 9 51 Druitt Street Sydney NSW 2000 Australia	http://www.ranzcr.edu.au

PROFESSIONAL ORGANIZATION	ADDRESS	WEBSITE
Austria		
European Society of Radiology	ESR Office Neutorgasse 9 1010 Vienna, Austria	http://www.myesr.org
Canada		
British Columbia Radiological Society	30-1210 Summit Drive, Ste. 128 Kamloops, BC V2C 6M1	http://www.bcrs.bc.ca
Canadian Association of Radiologists	377 Dalhousie Street, Suite 310 Ottawa, Ontario K1N 9N8	http://www.car.ca
Germany		
International Commission on Non-Ionizing Radiation Protection	ICNIRP, c/o BfS Ingolstaedter Landstr. 1 85764, Oberschleissheim, Germany	http://www.icnirp.de
South Africa		
The Society of Radiographers of South Africa	P.O. Box 6014 Roggebaai 8012, South Africa	http://www.sorsa.org.za
United Kingdom		
British Institute of Radiology	Membership 36 Portland Place London W1B 1AT	http://www.bir.org.uk
Society and College of Radiographers	207 Providence Square, Mill Street London SE1 2EW	http://www.sor.org
Society of Radiologists in Training	Consultant Radiologist Christie Hospital, NHS Trust Withington, Manchester M20 4BX	http://www.thesrt.org.uk
United States		
International Commission on Radiation Units and Measurements	7910 Woodmont Avenue, Suite 400 Bethesda, MD 20841-3095	http://www.icru.org
The National Association for Proton Therapy	1301 Highland Drive Silver Spring, MD 20910	http://www.proton-therapy.org
Professional Organization by Imaging Modality		
Magnetic resonance imaging International Society for Magnetic Resonance in Medicine	2030 Addison Street, 7th Floor Berkeley, CA 94704 USA	http://www.ismrm.org

(continued)

PROFESSIONAL ORGANIZATION	ADDRESS	WEBSITE
Professional Organization by Imaging Modality *(continued)*		
Nuclear medicine		
Society of Nuclear Medicine	1850 Samuel Morse Drive Reston, VA 20190	http://www.snm.org
Radiology		
American Society of Neuroradiology	ASNR 2210 Midwest Road, Suite 207 Oak Brook, IL 60523	http://www.asnr.org
American Society for Therapeutic Radiation and Oncology	ASTRO 8280 Willow Oaks Corporate Dr. Suite 500 Fairfax, VA 22031	http://www.astro.org
North American Society for Cardiac Imaging	NASC 1891 Preston White Drive Reston, VA 20191	http://www.nasci.org
Society for Computer Applications in Radiology	9440 Golf Vista Plaza, Suite 330 Leesburg, VA 20176-8264	
Sonography		
American Registry of Diagnostic Medical Sonographers	51 Monroe Street, Plaza East One Rockville, MD 20850-2400	http://www.ardms.org

Appendix C

ASRT SCOPE OF PRACTICE (PRACTICE STANDARDS FOR MEDICAL IMAGING AND RADIATION THERAPY)

Radiography Scope of Practice

The scope of practice of radiography includes:

1. Performing diagnostic radiographic procedures.

2. Corroborating the patient's clinical history with procedure, ensuring information is documented and available for use by a licensed independent practitioner.

3. Maintaining confidentiality of the patient's protected health information in accordance with the Health Insurance Portability and Accountability Act.

4. Preparing the patient for procedures, providing instructions to obtain desired results, gaining cooperation, and minimizing anxiety.

5. Selecting and operating imaging equipment and/or associated accessories to successfully perform procedures.

6. Positioning the patient to best demonstrate the anatomic area of interest, respecting the patient's ability and comfort.

7. Immobilizing the patient as required for appropriate examination.

8. Determining radiographic technique exposure factors.

9. Applying principles of radiation protection to minimize exposure to the patient, self, and others.

10. Evaluating radiographs or images for technical quality, ensuring proper identification is recorded.

11. Assuming responsibility for the provision of physical and psychological needs of the patient during procedures.

12. Performing venipunctures where state statute(s) and/or institutional policy permits.

13. Preparing, identifying, and/or administering contrast media and/or medications as prescribed by a licensed independent practitioner, where state statute(s) and/or institutional policy permits.

14. Verifying informed consent for, and assisting a licensed independent practitioner with, interventional procedures.

15. Assisting a licensed independent practitioner with fluoroscopic and specialized interventional radiography procedures.

16. Performing noninterpretive fluoroscopic procedures as appropriate and consistent with applicable state statutes.

17. Initiating basic life support action when necessary.

18. Providing patient education.

19. Providing input for equipment purchase and supply decisions.

20. Providing practical instruction for students and/or other health care professionals.

21. Participating in the department's quality assessment and improvement plan.

22. Maintaining control of inventory and purchase of supplies for the assigned area.

23. Observing universal precautions.

24. Performing peripherally inserted central catheter placement where state statute(s) and/or institutional policy permits.

25. Applying the principles of patient safety during all aspects of radiographic procedures, including assisting and transporting patients.

26. Administering medications at the physician's request according to policy.

27. Starting and maintaining intravenous (IV) access per orders when applicable.

Comprehensive Practice

Radiographic procedures are performed on any or all body organs, systems, or structures. Individuals demonstrate competency to meet state licensure, permit, or certification requirements defined by law for radiography or they maintain appropriate credentials.

Appendix D

2010 AMERICAN HEART ASSOCIATION GUIDELINES FOR CPR AND EMERGENCY CARDIOVASCULAR CARE: LAY RESCUER ADULT CARDIOPULMONARY RESUSCITATION (CPR)

1. Attempt to wake the victim by gently tapping or shaking the shoulder and loudly asking whether he or she is okay.

2. If victim is unresponsive, call 911 or local emergency medical system (EMS).

3. If victim is not breathing or is gasping for breath, follow the C-A-B sequence* for CPR with a compression-ventilation ratio of 30:2.

C: Initiate Chest Compressions

1. The rescuer should place heel of one hand on the center (middle) of the victim's chest (which is the lower half of the sternum) and the heel of the other hand on the top of the first so that the hands are overlapped and parallel (*see Figure D-1*).

2. To provide effective chest compressions, push hard and push fast. It is reasonable for laypersons and health care providers to compress the adult chest at a rate of at least 100 compressions per minute with a compression depth of at least 2 inches/5 cm. Rescuers should allow complete recoil of the chest after each compression to allow the heart to fill completely before the next compression (AHA 2010; *see Figure D-2*).

3. Rescuers should attempt to minimize the frequency and duration of interruptions in compressions to maximize the number of compressions delivered per minute. A compression-ventilation ratio of 30:2 is recommended (AHA 2010).

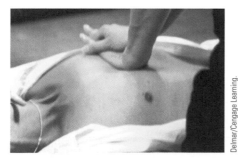

FIGURE D–1. Proper hand position.

Delmar/Cengage Learning.

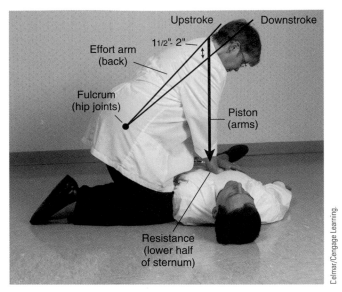

FIGURE D–2. Proper position of rescuer.

A: Establish Airway

1. Open airway by using the *head-tilt/chin-lift* method. This is accomplished by placing one hand on the victim's forehead and applying a steady backward pressure to tilt the head back while placing the fingers of the other hand below the jaw at the location of the chin and lifting the chin (*see Figure D–3*).

   - **In the event of a suspected head or neck injury**, the head-tilt/chin lift is modified and the jaw thrust is used without head extension. To perform the *jaw thrust*, place hands at the angles of the victim's lower jaw and lift, displacing the mandible forward (*see Figure D–4*).

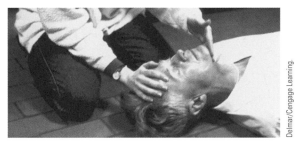

FIGURE D–3. Open airway by using *the head-tilt/chin-lift* method.

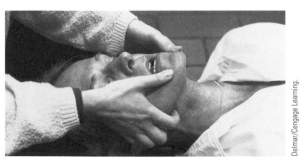

FIGURE D–4. In the event of a suspected head or neck injury, *jaw thrust* is used without head extension.

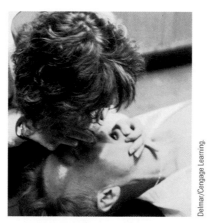

FIGURE D–5. Occlude the victim's nostrils.

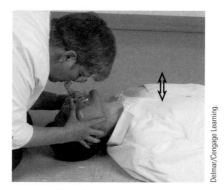

FIGURE D–6. Deliver two rescue breaths.

B: Delivery Rescue Breaths

1. Occlude the victim's nostrils with the thumb and index finger of the hand on the forehead that is tilting the head back (*see Figure D-5*).

2. Place mouth over the victim's mouth and form a seal to prevent air leakage during rescue breaths.

3. Deliver two rescue breaths sufficient to produce a visible rise in the victim's chest (*see Figure D-6*).

4. Continue CPR with a 30:2 compression-ventilation ratio until emergency responders arrive.

* Source: 2010 AHA Guidelines for CPR and ECC.

Appendix E

381.026 FLORIDA PATIENT'S BILL OF RIGHTS AND RESPONSIBILITIES

(1) SHORT TITLE. This section may be cited as the "Florida Patient's Bill of Rights and Responsibilities."

(2) DEFINITIONS. As used in this section and s. 381.0261, the term:

(a) "Department" means the Department of Health.

(b) "Health care facility" means a facility licensed under chapter 395.

(c) "Health care provider" means a physician licensed under chapter 458, an osteopathic physician licensed under chapter 459, or a podiatric physician licensed under chapter 461.

(d) "Responsible provider" means a health care provider who is primarily responsible for patient care in a health care facility or provider's office.

(3) PURPOSE. It is the purpose of this section to promote the interests and well-being of the patients of health care providers and health care facilities and to promote better communication between the patient and the health care provider. It is the intent of the Legislature that health care providers understand their responsibility to give their patients a general understanding of the procedures to be performed on them and to provide information pertaining to their health care so that they may make decisions in an informed manner after considering the information relating to their condition, the available treatment alternatives, and substantial risks and hazards inherent in the treatments. It is the intent of the Legislature that patients have a general understanding of their responsibilities toward health care providers and health care facilities. It is the intent of the Legislature that the provision of such information to a patient eliminates potential misunderstandings between patients and health care providers. It is a public policy of the state that the interests of patients be recognized in a patient's bill of rights and responsibilities and that a health care facility or health care provider may not require a patient to waive his or her rights as a condition of treatment. This section shall not be used for any purpose in any civil or administrative action and neither expands nor limits any rights or remedies provided under any other law.

(4) RIGHTS OF PATIENTS. Each health care facility or provider shall observe the following standards:

(a) *Individual dignity.*

   1. The individual dignity of a patient must be respected at all times and upon all occasions.

2. Every patient who is provided health care services retains certain rights to privacy, which must be respected without regard to the patient's economic status or source of payment for his or her care. The patient's rights to privacy must be respected to the extent consistent with providing adequate medical care to the patient and with the efficient administration of the health care facility or provider's office. However, this subparagraph does not preclude necessary and discreet discussion of a patient's case or examination by appropriate medical personnel.

3. A patient has the right to a prompt and reasonable response to a question or request. A health care facility shall respond in a reasonable manner to the request of a patient's health care provider for medical services to the patient. The health care facility shall also respond in a reasonable manner to the patient's request for other services customarily rendered by the health care facility to the extent such services do not require the approval of the patient's health care provider or are not inconsistent with the patient's treatment.

4. A patient in a health care facility has the right to retain and use personal clothing or possessions as space permits, unless for him or her to do so would infringe upon the right of another patient or is medically or programmatically contraindicated for documented medical, safety, or programmatic reasons.

(b) *Information.*

1. A patient has the right to know the name, function, and qualifications of each health care provider who is providing medical services to the patient. A patient may request such information from his or her responsible provider or the health care facility in which he or she is receiving medical services.

2. A patient in a health care facility has the right to know what patient support services are available in the facility.

3. A patient has the right to be given by his or her health care provider information concerning diagnosis, planned course of treatment, alternatives, risks, and prognosis, unless it is medically inadvisable or impossible to give this information to the patient, in which case the information must be given to the patient's guardian or a person designated as the patient's representative. A patient has the right to refuse this information.

4. A patient has the right to refuse any treatment based on information required by this paragraph, except as otherwise provided by law. The responsible provider shall document any such refusal.

5. A patient in a health care facility has the right to know what facility rules and regulations apply to patient conduct.

6. A patient has the right to express grievances to a health care provider, a health care facility, or the appropriate state licensing agency regarding alleged violations of patients' rights. A patient has the right to know the health care provider's or health care facility's procedures for expressing a grievance.

7. A patient in a health care facility who does not speak English has the right to be provided an interpreter when receiving medical services if

the facility has a person readily available who can interpret on behalf of the patient.

(c) *Financial information and disclosure.*

1.   A patient has the right to be given, upon request, by the responsible provider, his or her designee, or a representative of the health care facility full information and necessary counseling on the availability of known financial resources for the patient's health care.

2.   A health care provider or a health care facility shall, upon request, disclose to each patient who is eligible for Medicare, in advance of treatment, whether the health care provider or the health care facility in which the patient is receiving medical services accepts assignment under Medicare reimbursement as payment in full for medical services and treatment rendered in the health care provider's office or health care facility.

3.   A health care provider or a health care facility shall, upon request, furnish a patient, prior to provision of medical services, a reasonable estimate of charges for such services. Such reasonable estimate shall not preclude the health care provider or health care facility from exceeding the estimate or making additional charges based on changes in the patient's condition or treatment needs.

4.   A patient has the right to receive a copy of an itemized bill upon request. A patient has a right to be given an explanation of charges upon request.

(d) *Access to health care.*

1.   A patient has the right to impartial access to medical treatment or accommodations, regardless of race, national origin, religion, handicap, or source of payment.

2.   A patient has the right to treatment for any emergency medical condition that will deteriorate from failure to provide such treatment.

3.   A patient has the right to access any mode of treatment that is, in his or her own judgment and the judgment of his or her health care practitioner, in the best interests of the patient, including complementary or alternative health care treatments, in accordance with the provisions of s. 456.41.

(e) *Experimental research.* In addition to the provisions of s. 766.103, a patient has the right to know if medical treatment is for purposes of experimental research and to consent prior to participation in such experimental research. For any patient, regardless of ability to pay or source of payment for his or her care, participation must be a voluntary matter, and a patient has the right to refuse to participate. The patient's consent or refusal must be documented in the patient's care record.

(f) *Patient's knowledge of rights and responsibilities.* In receiving health care, patients have the right to know what their rights and responsibilities are.

(5) RESPONSIBILITIES OF PATIENTS.   Each patient of a health care provider or health care facility shall respect the health care provider's and health care facility's right to expect behavior on the part of patients which, considering the nature of their illness, is reasonable and responsible. Each patient shall observe the responsibilities described in the following summary.

(6) SUMMARY OF RIGHTS AND RESPONSIBILITIES.   Any health care provider who treats a patient in an office or any health care facility licensed under chapter 395 that provides emergency services and care or outpatient services and care to a patient, or admits and treats a patient, shall adopt and make available to the patient, in writing, a statement of the rights and responsibilities of patients, including the following:

SUMMARY OF THE FLORIDA PATIENT'S BILL OF RIGHTS AND RESPONSIBILITIES

Florida law requires that your health care provider or health care facility recognize your rights while you are receiving medical care and that you respect the health care provider's or health care facility's right to expect certain behavior on the part of patients. You may request a copy of the full text of this law from your health care provider or health care facility. A summary of your rights and responsibilities follows:

- A patient has the right to be treated with courtesy and respect, with appreciation of his or her individual dignity, and with protection of his or her need for privacy.
- A patient has the right to a prompt and reasonable response to questions and requests.
- A patient has the right to know who is providing medical services and who is responsible for his or her care.
- A patient has the right to know what patient support services are available, including whether an interpreter is available if he or she does not speak English.
- A patient has the right to know what rules and regulations apply to his or her conduct.
- A patient has the right to be given by the health care provider information concerning diagnosis, planned course of treatment, alternatives, risks, and prognosis.
- A patient has the right to refuse any treatment, except as otherwise provided by law.
- A patient has the right to be given, upon request, full information and necessary counseling on the availability of known financial resources for his or her care.
- A patient who is eligible for Medicare has the right to know, upon request and in advance of treatment, whether the health care provider or health care facility accepts the Medicare assignment rate.
- A patient has the right to receive, upon request, prior to treatment, a reasonable estimate of charges for medical care.
- A patient has the right to receive a copy of a reasonably clear and understandable itemized bill and, upon request, to have the charges explained.
- A patient has the right to impartial access to medical treatment or accommodations, regardless of race, national origin, religion, handicap, or source of payment.
- A patient has the right to treatment for any emergency medical condition that will deteriorate from failure to provide treatment.
- A patient has the right to know if medical treatment is for purposes of experimental research and to give his or her consent or refusal to participate in such experimental research.

- A patient has the right to express grievances regarding any violation of his or her rights, as stated in Florida law, through the grievance procedure of the health care provider or health care facility which served him or her and to the appropriate state licensing agency.
- A patient is responsible for providing to the health care provider, to the best of his or her knowledge, accurate and complete information about present complaints, past illnesses, hospitalizations, medications, and other matters relating to his or her health.
- A patient is responsible for reporting unexpected changes in his or her condition to the health care provider.
- A patient is responsible for reporting to the health care provider whether he or she comprehends a contemplated course of action and what is expected of him or her.
- A patient is responsible for following the treatment plan recommended by the health care provider.
- A patient is responsible for keeping appointments and, when he or she is unable to do so for any reason, for notifying the health care provider or health care facility.
- A patient is responsible for his or her actions if he or she refuses treatment or does not follow the health care provider's instructions.
- A patient is responsible for assuring that the financial obligations of his or her health care are fulfilled as promptly as possible.
- A patient is responsible for following health care facility rules and regulations affecting patient care and conduct.

History. s. 1, ch. 91-127; s. 65, ch. 92-289; s. 656, ch. 95-148; s. 21, ch. 98-89; s. 178, ch. 98-166; s. 64, ch. 99-397; s. 7, ch. 2001-2053; s. 2, ch. 2001-2116.

Appendix F

INFORMED CONSENT

PATIENT'S CONSENT STATEMENT FOR RADIOGRAPHIC PROCEDURE

I, _____, understand that my doctor, _____
 _____(physician performing procedure)

has ordered a _____ which requires the injection or introduction of
 _____(type of procedure)

_____ into my body for diagnostic purposes.
 _____(contrast medium)

I have answered the following questions as far as I know them to be true according to my personal
knowledge.

Are you allergic to any types of: medication ☐   food ☐   shellfish ☐   other ☐

If so, what? _____

_____

Have you ever had any of the following? (Check all that apply)

    ☐ Asthma   ☐ Diabetes   ☐ Neurological Problems

    ☐ Cardiac (Heart) Disease   ☐ Renal (Kidney) Disease   ☐ Do not know

If you have had this radiographic procedure before or any similar type procedure that included an
injection, did you have any problems after the injection?

_____

_____

After reading and discussing this form, and having my questions answered satisfactorily by the physician performing the procedure, I voluntarily consent to the injection of contrast medium for the
following procedure: _____

_____   Date: _____
 (Signature of Patient)

Witness: _____

Patient is unable to consent because: _____

_____

_____   Date: _____
 (Signature of legal guardian or
 closest available relative)

Witness: _____   Witness: _____

_____

Note. This is a sample only. Consent forms are designed for specific use and must be checked with
legal counsel before use. Consent forms should be obtained by the performing physician or other
qualified persons trained in managing such procedures.

Delmar/Cengage Learning.

Appendix G

STEPS FOR CONTRAST ADMINISTRATION (VENIPUNCTURE)

1. Technologist verifies the correct patient for the procedure by checking the patient's identification bracelet (information included: patient's name, medical record number, date of birth, name of medical facility, and date of admittance; other information may be included depending on the medical facility).

2. Technologist introduces him or herself to the patient and explains the procedure and potential side effects of the contrast agent.

3. Technologist performs a patient screening to determine possible risk factors.

4. Technologist answers patient questions and obtains a signed informed consent form from the patient, permitting the medical facility to perform the procedure.

5. Technologist checks for appropriate contrast agent (content, expiration date, route of administration).

   A. First check when taking the contrast agent from the storage shelf

   B. Second check when drawing the contrast agent into the syringe for bolus injection

   C. Third check before administering contrast agent to the patient

6. Draw contrast agent into syringe for bolus injection.

7. Wash hands.

8. Apply tourniquet approximately 3 inches above the injection site.

9. Ask the patient to close his or her hand. The patient must not be allowed to pump the hand. Place the patient's arm in a downward position if possible.

10. Select a vein, noting the location and direction of the vein *(see Figure G-1A)*. Clean the injection site in a circular motion, beginning inward and moving outward with 70% isopropyl alcohol swab *(see Figure G-1B)*.

11. Put on gloves while alcohol is drying. Do not touch the venipuncture site.

12. Draw the patient's skin taut with your thumb. The thumb should be 1–2 inches below the puncture site *(see Figure G-1C)*.

13. With the bevel up, align the needle with the vein and perform venipuncture, depressing the plunger with even pressure to administer contrast agent.

14. Ask patient to open the hand.

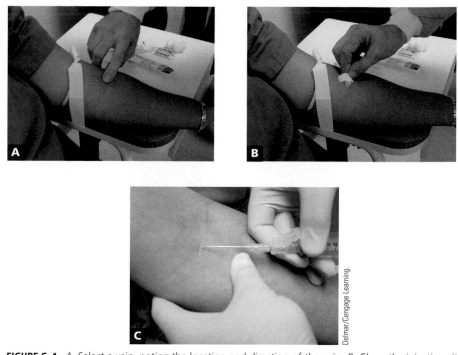

FIGURE G–1. *A.* Select a vein, noting the location and direction of the vein. *B.* Clean the injection site in a circular motion, beginning inward and moving outward with 70% isopropyl alcohol swab. *C.* Draw the patient's skin taut with your thumb. The thumb should be 1–2 inches below the puncture site.

15. Release tourniquet.

16. Lightly place gauze square or cotton ball above the venipuncture site while removing the needle from the arm. Slide gauze square or cotton ball onto the injection site once needle is removed.

17. Dispose of syringe and needle in a sharps container. Dispose of device intact.

18. Apply pressure to the injection site for 3–5 minutes. The patient may assist if able.

Appendix H

KMR Medical Centre

INCIDENT REPORT FORM
(Incidents involving employees, students, visitors)

This is a confidential report and should not be made a part of an employee's personnel record. It is completed
to allow us to obtain advice from legal counsel and for the protection of the medical centre/university regarding potential liability.

************ **PLEASE PRINT LEGIBLY**************

INFORMATION ABOUT THE PERSON INVOLVED IN THE INCIDENT	
Full Name:	Social Sec. #:
Home Address:	Gender: M F
Circle: Employee (Full-time, part-time, perm., temp.) Student Visitor	
Date of Birth: Home phone: Campus Phone:	
Campus address:	
Job Title: Supervisor:	

INFORMATION ABOUT THE INCIDENT
Date of Incident: Time: Police notified: Yes   No   Case #:
Location of Incident:
Describe what happened, how it happened, factors leading to the event, substances or objects involved. **Be as specific as possible** (attach seperate sheet if necessary):
Were there any witnesses to the incident? Yes   No If yes, attach seperate sheet with names, addresses and phone numbers, or campus depts and phone.
Was the individual injured? If so, describe the injury (laceration, spain, etc.), the part of body injured, and any other information known about the resulting injury(s):
Was incident reported to immediate supervisor? Yes   No   Work/clinical time
Was medical treatment provided?   Yes   No   Refused If so, where (circle) :   Emerg. Rm.   The Workplace   Walk-in Clinic   Other:
Will the employee/student miss time from work/clinical time as a result of this incident?   Yes   No   Unknown

REPORTER INFORMATION
Print Name if Reporter:
Reporter Signature: Title:
Date Report Completed:

EMPLOYEE REPORTS - Send to HR or School   **VISITOR/STUDENT to Risk Management**

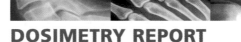

Appendix I

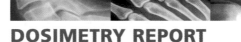

DOSIMETRY REPORT

LANDAUER®

Landauer, Inc. 2 Science Road Glenwood, Illinois 60425-1586
Telephone: (708) 755-7000 Facsimile: (708) 755-7016
www.landauerinc.com

luxel®

SAMPLE ORGANIZATION
RADIATION SAFETY OFFICER
1000 HIGH TECH AVENUE
GLENWOOD, IL 60425

RADIATION DOSIMETRY REPORT

ACCOUNT NO.	SERIES CODE	ANALYTICAL WORK ORDER	REPORT DATE	DOSIMETER RECEIVED	REPORT TIME IN WORK DAYS	PAGE NO.
103702	RAD	9920800151	06/11/04	06/07/04	4	1

PARTICIPANT NUMBER	NAME			DOSIMETER	USE	RADIATION QUALITY	DOSE EQUIVALENT (MREM) FOR PERIODS SHOWN BELOW			QUARTERLY ACCUMULATED DOSE EQUIVALENT (MREM)			YEAR TO DATE DOSE EQUIVALENT (MREM)			LIFETIME DOSE EQUIVALENT (MREM)			RECORDS FOR YEAR	INCEPTION DATE (MM/YY)
	ID NUMBER	BIRTH DATE	SEX				DEEP DDE	EYE LDE	SHALLOW SDE	DEEP DDE	EYE LDE	SHALLOW SDE	DEEP DDE	EYE LDE	SHALLOW SDE	DEEP DDE	EYE LDE	SHALLOW SDE		
FOR MONITORING PERIOD:							05/01/04 - 05/31/04			QTR 2			2004							
0000H	CONTROL			Ja	CNTRL		M	M	M										5	07/97
	CONTROL			Pa	CNTRL		M	M	M											07/97
	CONTROL			U	CNTRL				M											07/97
00191	ADDISON, JOHN			Ja	WHBODY	PN	90	90	90	90	90	90	100	100	100	200	200	200	5	07/97
	336235619	08/31/1968	M			P	60	60	60	60	60	60	70	70	70	170	170	170		
						NF	30	30	30	30	30	30	30	30	30	30	30	30		
00192	JORGENSON, MIKE			Pa	WHBODY		M	M	M	M	M	M	M	M	M	M	M	M	5	07/97
	471740095	10/04/1968	M	U	RFINGR				M			M			70			100		07/97
00193	THOMAS, LEE			Pa	WHBODY		ABSENT			M	M	M	M	M	M	M	M	M	5	07/97
	384846378	11/22/1964	M	U	RFINGR		ABSENT					M			M			M		07/97
00196	WALKER, JANE			Pa	WHBODY		3	3	3	12	11	11	12	11	11	22	21	21	5	11/97
	587336640	06/09/1960	F																	
00197	EDWARD, CHRIS			Pa	WHBODY		M	M	M	M	M	M	M	M	M	M	M	M	5	01/98
	489635774	02/14/1966	M																	
00198	ZERR, ROBERT			Pa	WHBODY		40	40	40	160	160	160	200	200	200	240	240	240	5	07/98
	982446591	07/15/1945	M		NOTE		CALCULATED													
00199	ADAMS, JANE			Pa	WHBODY		M	M	M	M	M	M	9	10	12	9	10	12	5	07/98
	335148621	08/25/1951	F																	
00200	MEYER, STEVE			Pa	COLLAR	PL	105	105	105										5	08/98
	416395887	03/21/1947	M	Pa	WAIST		M	M	M											08/98
					ASSIGN		4	105	105	6	162	165	11	327	334	51	1247	1284		
					NOTE		ASSIGNED DOSE BASED ON EDE 1 CALCULATION													
				U	RFINGR				140			400			690			2180		08/98
00202	HARRIS, KATHY			Pa	WHBODY		M	M	M	M	M	M	M	M	M	M	M	M	4	02/99
	352235619	06/15/1972	F	U	RFINGR				M			M			30			30		02/99

M: MINIMAL REPORTING SERVICE OF 1 MREM
ELECTRONIC MEDIA TO FOLLOW THIS REPORT

QUALITY CONTROL RELEASE: VS

20 - PR 6774 - RPT130 - N1   - 02013

NVLAP®
NVLAP LAB CODE 100518-0**

Answer Key

CHAPTER 1
IMAGING MODALITIES AND PROFESSIONAL ORGANIZATIONS

Concept Thinking Questions

1. Accreditation is important because it validates the education delivered to recipients and meets the highest possible standards of the profession. This is important to the institution, the program, educators of the institution or programs, as well as currently enrolled students, future enrolled students, and employers hiring graduates of the program.

2. Accreditation is a voluntary process.

3. Joint Review Committee on Education in Radiologic Technology (JRCERT)

4. The Joint Commission (TJC) formerly known as the Joint Commission on Accreditation of Healthcare Organizations (JCAHO)

5. The American Registry of Radiologic Technologists is a national organization that provides certification (in various disciplines of radiologic technology) through examination and annual registration of certification to individuals who maintain compliance with ARRT standards. The American Society of Radiologic Technologists is a worldwide professional organization offering membership to registered technologists. Membership types are listed on the ASRT website (http://www.asrt.org).

6. The ARRT requires individuals seeking certification as a radiologic technologist to have completed all educational requirements (both didactic and clinical) from an ARRT-approved educational program and to have followed the ARRT Standards of Ethics.

7. ARRT certification is initial certification granted to an individual who has successfully met ARRT requirements and received a passing score on the credentialing examination, whereas ARRT registration refers to the annual renewal of certification.

8. To ensure certified technologists or radiologist assistants are abreast of new technologies and technical skills that may be required of the imaging profession.

9.
   - magnetic resonance imaging
   - nuclear medicine
   - radiation therapy
   - radiography
   - sonography

10. nuclear medicine

Practice Exercises

1. Radiologic technology is an umbrella term that encompasses various imaging disciplines within the radiologic profession, including radiography, nuclear medicine, radiation therapy, sonography, magnetic resonance imaging, computed tomography, quality management, bone densitometry, cardiac-interventional radiography, vascular-interventional radiography, vascular sonography, breast sonography, and radiologist assistant.

2. The role of the radiologic technologist is to obtain static and dynamic images of the human body for interpretation by a radiologist. A registered radiologic assistant (R.R.A.) has acquired additional formal education beyond the scope of a radiologic technologist to be able to perform more complex radiographic procedures under the supervision of a radiologist.

3. Joint Review Committee on Education in Radiologic Technology (JRCERT)

4. Joint Commission on Accreditation of Healthcare Organizations

5. American Registry of Radiologic Technologists (ARRT)

6. The American Society of Radiologic Technologists (ASRT) is known to be the largest professional worldwide organization for registered technologists. The ASRT provides registered technologists with a broad scope of knowledge

reflecting current technological advancements within the imaging profession, along with providing an array of continuing education activities. The organization promotes the profession's Code of Ethics and the importance of delivering consistently high-quality patient care. The ASRT supports and encourages technologists to pursue life-long learning and professional advancement within the imaging profession.

7. Accreditation standards provide compliance guidelines and assessment evaluation criterion for institutions or educational programs to measure the quality of education or patient care being delivered to the public. For an institution or educational program to be awarded an accreditation status, proof of compliance must be demonstrated.

8.

- Middle States Association of Colleges and Schools (Middle States Commission on Higher Education)
- New England Association of Schools and Colleges (Commission on Institutions of Higher Education)
- North Central Association of Colleges and Schools (The Higher Learning Commission)
- Northwest Commission on Colleges and Universities
- Southern Association of Colleges and Schools (Commission on Colleges)
- Western Association of Schools and Colleges (Accrediting Commission for Community and Junior Colleges; Accrediting Commission for Senior Colleges and Universities)

9. Sonography

10.

- A. R.T.(MR)(ARRT) – Registered Technologist in MRI; by the American Registry of Radiologic Technologists
- B. R.T.(R)(ARRT) – Registered Technologist in Radiography; by the American Registry of Radiologic Technologists
- C. R.T.(T)(ARRT) – Registered Technologist in Radiation Therapy; by the American Registry of Radiologic Technologists
- D. R.R.A.(ARRT) – Registered Radiologic Assistant; by the American Registry of Radiologic Technologists

Matching

1. biennium

2. TJC

3. ARRT

4. fractionated

5. Tesla

6. accreditation

7. radioisotopes

8. transducer

9. Category A credit

10. BMD

11. quality management

12. R.T.

Retention of Material

1.

- A. Accreditation is a voluntary process an institution of higher education or a specialized program chooses to undergo in order to demonstrate compliance with an accrediting agency's standards.
- B. Certification is granted by the ARRT to an eligible candidate who has successfully met the ARRT requirements and received a passing score on the credentialing examination.
- C. The term *registration* as it pertains to the radiologic profession is a national database listing of ARRT registered technologists who hold current ARRT certification and remain in compliance with ARRT credentialing requirements.

2.

- A. Method requiring the use of ionizing radiation and image receptors (i.e., film, photostimulable phosphor plates [PSP] with computed radiography [CR], solid-state detector plates with digital radiography [DR], and an image intensifier with fluoroscopy to demonstrate anatomical structures within the human body).
- B. Imaging method requiring the use of ionizing radiation and an array of detectors to image structures in thin slices. Data are collected and digitally manipulated to view images in various body planes on a computer monitor; three-dimensional images can be produced.
- C. Imaging method that uses a magnetic field strength of generally <2.0 tesla and the manipulation of radiofrequency (RF) interactions with hydrogen nuclei of the body. Images are viewed on a computer monitor.

D. Imaging method that requires the patient to receive radiopharmaceuticals targeted to specific areas within the body. The gamma scintillation camera detects radioactivity of targeted areas to depict the presence or nonpresence of disease. Images can be viewed via film or computer monitor.

E. Imaging method that uses high-frequency sound waves (1–17 MHz) via a transducer (probe) containing one or multiple specialized crystals. Sound waves are reflected back from the body's internal structures to the transducer, where they are transformed into an electrical signal and sent to the scanning unit to be processed into a digital image for viewing on a TV monitor. Multidimensional images can be produced. Sonography has therapeutic application with frequencies in the kilohertz (kHz) range.

3. This radiation safety mnemonic *(as low as reasonably achievable)* serves as a reminder to technologists to always use the lowest amount of radiation necessary when producing optimal images.

4. A radiologist interprets images depicting anatomical structures within the body that have been obtained through various imaging modalities. This information is then used in the diagnosis or treatment of patients.

5. A primary pathway is considered the foundation pathway to certification in which a base knowledge in a specific imaging discipline has been achieved and the eligible candidate is prepared to take the national certification examination. The postprimary pathway requires initial certification in a supporting discipline along with additional education and proof of competent technical skills (mandated by the ARRT) in the discipline for which the candidate seeks advanced certification.

6. The ARRT provides a primary and postprimary pathway to certification to ensure the safety of patients by not allowing individuals to skip steps in the educational process or skill competency requirements necessary for delivering appropriate patient care.

7. MRI and sonography

8. Certification by the ARRT is a voluntary process an eligible candidate can pursue.

9. bone densitometry

10. The patient can call the medical facility and ask whether the technologists they employ are ARRT-certified, or the patient can ask to see the technologist's credentials before the technologist performs the procedure. Although the ARRT website has a directory of registered technologists, some technologists choose to not have their credentialing information listed. The ARRT can confirm whether a technologist is certified if the proper name of the technologist is provided.

CHAPTER 2
ABBREVIATIONS AND WORD PARTS

Concept Thinking Questions

1. asthenic

2. dys and algia

3.

    A. $\bar{c}$

    B. $\bar{s}$

    C. $\bar{a}$

Practice Exercises

1. leukocytes

2. cyanosis

3. dysuria

4. bradycardia

5. apnea

6. appendectomy

7. nephroma

8. pneumothorax

9. polydipsia

10. tachypnea

Matching

1. hypersthenic

2. sthenic

3. asthenic

4. hyposthenic

Retention of Material

1. endo

2. ecto

3. super

4. infra

5. inter

6. osis

7. oma

8. itis

9. otomy

10. ectomy

CHAPTER 3
MEDICAL AND LEGAL TERMS

Concept Thinking Questions

1. A tort is a civil wrongdoing resulting in injury or harm to an individual (patient) or to his or her property because of a lack of care by the caregiver. Torts can be classified into two main categories, *intentional misconduct* and *unintentional misconduct*, often referred to as negligence.

2.

   intentional misconduct – Intentional misconduct is an action taken by an individual with the purpose or intent to cause harm to another (e.g., assault, battery, defamation, false imprisonment).

   unintentional misconduct – Unintentional misconduct is an action taken by an individual with no intent to cause harm to another (e.g., negligence).

3.

   blood pressure rate – Blood pressure rate is a measurement of the force of blood against the walls of the arteries as the heart pumps blood through the circulatory system.

   temperature – Normal body temperature is considered the temperature at which homeostasis exists between heat produced within the body and heat exerted by the body.

   respiration rate – Respiration rate is a measurement of the body's ability to move air (oxygen) into the lungs and move carbon dioxide out of the lungs.

   pulse rate – Pulse rate or heart rate is a measurement of the hearts ability to beat or pump blood through the circulatory system.

4.

   objective data – Objective data are factual data.
   - Observing the patient: coughing, spitting up blood, fainting, vomiting

   subjective data – Subjective data are based on emotions and feelings.
   - Patient statement of "feeling sick," "feeling tired," or "feeling out of sorts"

5.

   assault – Assault is a legal term meaning to threaten someone or to imply harm may occur.

   battery – Battery is a legal term meaning to bring physical harm to an individual or to make unwanted physical contact with another individual.

6. Under federal HIPAA law (*Health Insurance Portability Act*), a patient's identifying health care information or medical record is protected and secured from public access.

7. A **felony** is a crime that is considered serious in nature and may or may not involve a violent act. There are various classifications of felonies with degrees of punitive actions, including incarceration. A **misdemeanor** is a crime considered less serious than a felony and results in a lesser degree of punitive action. Often misdemeanor offenses result in a fine imposed by the court.

8.

   blood pressure rate – A blood pressure rate of less than 120 mmHg systolic and less than 80 mmHg diastolic is considered the normal blood pressure range for the average healthy adult.

   temperature – An oral body temperature reading of 97.8°–99.1°F is considered within the normal body temperature range for the average healthy adult, with 98.6°F being the average.

   respiration rate – A respiration rate of 12–18 breaths per minute is considered within the normal respiration range for the average healthy adult.

   pulse rate – A pulse rate of 60–80 beats per minute (bpm) is considered within the normal pulse range for the average healthy adult.

9.

> **morals/morality** – Morality refers to what we have been taught to be right and wrong. To have morals or morality is to be able to recognize right from wrong and then choose to do the right thing not because you have to, but because it is the right thing to do.
>
> **values** – Values are a set of beliefs an individual or organization deems important to achieving success.
>
> **ethics, ethical** – Ethics and ethical behavior refer to adapting our moral belief (knowing right from wrong) to make appropriate professional decisions/judgments expected within the scope of practice for a given profession.

10. An advanced health care directive (AHCD) is a legal document declaring the wishes of an individual regarding their own health care and/or treatment in the event that they are unable to convey their choices and/or decisions for their well being.

Practice Exercises

1.

> **onset** – Onset is marking the first moment the pain, injury, or illness manifested and detailing possible circumstances or events that might have lead up to it.
>
> **localization** – Localization is the process of establishing the exact point of pain, injury, or illness.
>
> **chronology** – Chronology is a determined timeframe that spans the onset of pain, injury, or illness to the present time of the imaging procedure in terms of *duration*, *frequency*, and *symptoms*.
>
> **quality** – Quality is a description by the patient as to how the pain feels (e.g., hot, itchy, burning, stabbing, sharp, dull, pressure, radiating, throbbing, wavelike, constant ache). The radiologic technologist would indicate apparent symptoms if present (e.g., coughing, sweating, bleeding, spitting, vomiting, diarrhea, lesions, dizziness) as acute (sudden onset) or chronic (during a long period of time).
>
> **severity** – Severity refers to the degree of pain or illness the patient is experiencing. Oftentimes a rating scale can be used to determine the "severity" of pain. For example, one might ask the patient on a scale of 1–10, with 10 being the most severe pain, "What rating number would you equate to the level of pain you are experiencing?"
>
> **associated manifestations** – Associated manifestations apply to any other accompanying complaints the patient

may have. This information is important in determining whether a relationship exists between the accompanying complaints and the patient's chief complaint.

> **aggravating and alleviating factors** – Aggravating factors are factors that have a negative impact on the pain, injury or illness, causing an increase in symptoms or severity. Alleviating factors are factors that have a positive impact on the pain, injury or illness, causing a decrease in symptoms or severity.

2.

> **plaintiff's case** – The technologist left me alone in the x-ray room on the x-ray table and I had to go to the bathroom. I called out, but no one came to assist me.
>
> **defendant's case** – I instructed the patient to not move from the table and that I would retrieve her walker to help assist her to the bathroom. The walker was adjacent to the x-ray room; it only took a minute or two to retrieve the walker. The patient was combative and fell as I attempted to help her down from the x-ray table.

3. The systolic reading is a recording of the blood flow force as the ventricles of the heart contract, whereas the diastolic reading is a recording of the blood flow force while the ventricles of the heart are at rest.

4. breathing fast; excitable

5. The technologist performs an imaging procedure on a patient as per physician orders. The procedure performed was the wrong procedure. Although the technologist performed the incorrect procedure, the technologist followed the medical requisition. The medical facility would take responsibility for the wrongful action.

6.

> **veracity** – A technologist asks the mother of a child how the child obtained injury to the eye. The mother explains the child was hit in the face with a baseball during a practice session at school. The technologist can see the mother is sincere and truthful about the explanation.
>
> **malice** – A schoolmate intentionally inflicts physical pain on another schoolmate at the bus stop each day.

7. minimum expectations of professional conduct and ethical behavior specific to the radiologic imaging profession

8. A pedestrian stops to help an accident victim who was struck by a car. Despite the pedestrian's best effort to assist the injured person, the person dies. The family sues the pedestrian for administering CPR incorrectly.

The pedestrian volunteered in good faith to help the injured person and therefore may introduce the Good Samaritan Law as a means of defense.

9.

  A. Establish a good base of support.
  B. Be aware of the body's center of gravity; position the center of gravity over the base of support when lifting a heavy object.
  C. Keep chest up and slightly forward with waist extended.
  D. Hold head erect with chin in to avoid curvature of neck.
  E. Bend knees slightly when lifting an object.
  F. Keep buttocks tucked in and abdomen up and in.
  G. Inform patient of a move or a lift before initiating the action.
  H. Align the patient's body prior to lifting, moving, or transferring.

10. invasive procedures

Matching

1. ADA Amendments Act

2. deception

3. warning

4. 70 bpm

5. open

6. 102°F

7. mmHg

8. negligence

9. compliance

10. intentional misconduct

11. medical record

12. female patient scheduling

Retention of Material

1. Obtaining a "good patient history" is essential to establishing a foundation upon which to provide appropriate patient care.

2. A mission statement is a statement declaring an organizations focus or purpose. A company mission statement is designed to provide its employees with an overall goal that all work is aimed toward in an effort to maintain or achieve the vision for the company's existence.

3. to recognize when a patient's health may be in danger

4. a patient unable to speak or move, a comatose patient, a severely ill patient, a pediatric patient, a geriatric patient

5. to have a documented record of the incident/accident that occurred in case it becomes a legal matter

6. Velcro straps, sandbags, and the pig-o-stat are considered simple immobilization methods. Special restraints that are considered more sophisticated and require a physician's order include but are not limited to wrist and ankle restraints, vest restraints, mitts, and full bed rails.

7.

  diagnosis – Diagnosis refers to the recognition of an illness, disorder, or disease by a physician.
  prognosis – Prognosis refers to an expected outcome as it relates to an illness, disorder, or disease diagnosed by a physician. A therapeutic plan may be discussed in the prognosis of an illness, disorder, or disease.

8. assault, battery, and false imprisonment

9. negligence

10.

  - duty
  - breach of duty
  - causation
  - damage

11. IVU was performed on the wrong patient; patient ID was not checked.

12. Incorrect contrast media (ionic vs nonionic) was administered to the patient. The technologist prepared ionic contrast media rather than nonionic for injection; however, the radiologist was the person who administered the contrast media to the patient. Patient experienced a severe allergic reaction.

CHAPTER 4
INFECTION CONTROL

Concept Thinking Questions

1. Standard precautions are infection control guidelines for health care workers to assist in reducing the spread of pathogens within health care settings.

2. A pathogen is a microorganism capable of producing a disease; a nonpathogen is a microorganism not capable of producing a disease.

3. bacteria, virus, fungi, protozoan parasites

4. Bacteria have no nuclei and are classified according to their shape.

   Fungi are not considered a plant or animal, and they can be helpful or deadly to the body.

   Viruses need a host to survive; they alter cellular function by depositing their own genetic information into a cell.

   Protozoan parasites are one-celled organisms classified by their method of movement.

5. Direct contact or indirect contact

6. The CDC (Centers for Disease Control and Prevention)

7. fungi

8. Toxins are poisonous substances that can be lethal to the body.

9. Friction reduces the spread of microorganisms.

10. A "superbug" is resistant to antibiotics.

Practice Exercises

1. *Refer to Figure 4–2.*

2.
   - susceptible host – human
   - pathogenic organism – bacteria
   - means of transmission – direct contact
   - reservoir of infection – bodily fluid within the host

3. Kill bacteria within the host or eliminate direct contact with host.

4.
   - Remove jewelry (e.g., rings, bracelets, watches).
   - Wet hands under warm running water (do not touch the faucet again).
   - Use antibacterial soap and rub together to create friction for at least 15 seconds.
   - Wash palms of hands, between fingers, under the fingernails, tips of the fingers, and the back of hands.
   - Rinse hands thoroughly and dry with a towel or paper towel.
   - Turn off faucet with the use of the towel or paper towel to avoid contamination to the hands.

5.
   - **numbered stroke method** – This method involves counting a predetermined number of brush strokes using a nailbrush for each finger, anterior hand (palm side), posterior hand (knuckle side), and lower arm beginning slightly above the elbow.
   - **timed scrub method** – The timed scrub method is very similar to the numbered stroke method except that, instead of counting brush strokes, the surgical scrub is performed for a predetermined amount of time as dictated by facility protocol.

6.
   - **medical asepsis** – Medical asepsis is an infection control practice utilized to reduce the presence of microorganisms.
   - **surgical asepsis** – Surgical asepsis is an infection control practice utilized to eliminate the presence of microorganisms (i.e., surgical procedures).

7.
   - spheric-shaped
   - comma-shaped
   - rod-shaped
   - spiral-shaped

8. Conditions that promote a continuum of the cycle of infection.

9. It is a method for testing air leakage gaps around the face where the particulate respirator (N95) should fit securely.

10. A virion is a virus particle that invades a cell and alters it by depositing its own genetic information in the form of DNA or RNA.

11. When having direct or indirect contact with a patient

12. A patient with a compromised immune system, patients with open wounds (burn victims), and patients who are vulnerable to illness should be placed in protective isolation.

Matching

1. organism

2. kills bacteria

3. disinfectant

4. MSDS

5. direct contact

6. N95

7. idiopathic

8. HAI

9. vector

10. sterile

11. fomite

12. pathogens

Retention of Material

1. Use a skin prep kit to reduce the chance for infection to enter the body at the puncture or incision site.

2. myleography, angiography, lumbar puncture

3. virus

4. bacteria

5. The MSDS contains information on how best to handle workplace chemicals or substances regarding storage, temperature, ventilation, skin contact, spills, or other occurrences that could pose potential health risks.

6. Gloves, goggles, face mask, face shield, gown, hair cap and particular respirators. Disposable gloves are considered a "standard precaution" and should be used when health care workers have direct or indirect contact with patients. Other PPEs are used in accordance to the patient's condition, fluid contact, and type of patient interaction (sterile technique).

7. contact (direct and/or indirect contact), airborne, and droplet

8. contact – scabies; airborne – tuberculosis; droplet – common cold

9. Humans, animals, vectors, and fomites

10. bile, blood, blood plasma, chyme, interstitial fluid, lymph, pleural fluid, saliva, sebum, sputum, sweat, tears, and gender-specific fluids such as female vaginal secretions, breast milk (produced after childbirth), and male semen

CHAPTER 5
PHARMACOLOGY AND CONTRAST MEDIA

Concept Thinking Questions

1.
- right patient
- right drug
- right amount
- right route
- right time

2.

ionic contrast – Ionic contrast contains a complex molecular arrangement of iodine and other compounds resulting in a contrast agent with high osmolality. Although ionic contrast is more cost-efficient than nonionic contrast media, the likelihood of an adverse reactions is greater.

nonionic contrast – Nonionic contrast agents are two to three times more expensive than ionic contrast agents, and, although they still contain an iodine compound, the molecular arrangement produces a low-osmolality contrast agent with fewer adverse reactions.

3. An IV push is a bolus intravenous injection of a solution given rapidly at one time.

4. urticaria, itching

5. shock, respiratory arrest

6. plunger, barrel, and tip

7. oral route, parenteral route, sublingual route, and topical route

8. An ampule is a sealed container that holds a single dose of medication. A vial is a sealed container holding more than one dose of medication.

9. Solutions of low viscosity flow easily with little required force or pressure, whereas solutions of high viscosity are slow to flow and require increased force or pressure.

10. A tourniquet is often used for venipuncture procedures to dilate the veins, making them more pronounced; this helps to access the vein easily when performing intravenous injections.

Practice Exercises

1. *Refer to Box 5–1.*

2.

   - Have you ever had a contrast procedure before? If so, did you experience an adverse reaction?
   - Do you have allergies? If so, what types of things are you allergic to?
   - Are you allergic to shellfish?
   - What kind of medications are you currently taking?
   - Do you currently take allergy medication or receive allergy shots?

3. An informed consent is a document provided by a health care facility to a patient in which the procedure or treatment being considered is explained and any associated risks are disclosed. Invasive procedures require an informed consent be signed by the patient (or legal guardian in the case of a minor) for the procedure or treatment to legally be performed.

4. *Refer to Appendix G.*

5. A positive contrast agent or radio-opaque contrast agent has a higher atomic number than the tissue to which it will be introduced. Positive contrast agents will appear light (white) on a radiographic image. Examples of positive contrast agents include barium sulfide ($BaSO_4$) and iodinated (water-soluble and fat-soluble) contrast agents. A negative contrast agent or radiolucent contrast agent has a lower atomic number than the tissue to which it will be introduced. Negative contrast agents will appear dark on a radiographic image. Examples of negative contrast agents include air, oxygen (O_2), carbon dioxide (CO_2), and nitrous oxide.

6. An intravenous injection is an injection of a solution directly into a vein.

   An intrathecal injection is an injection of a solution directly into the subarachnoid space of the spinal canal.

7. Drugs can be classified by their chemical name, generic name, and the trade name.

8. The greater the atomic number of tissue, the greater the absorption of radiation.

9. Tissue density and radiographic density have an indirect relationship. As tissue density increases, radiographic density (overall blackness on a radiographic film) decreases.

10. Nitroglycerin is a common nitrate vasodilator prescribed to patients with angina pectoris (chest pain caused by a narrowing of the coronary arteries) to lessen the workload on the heart and allow oxygenated blood to flow with ease to the heart.

11. A vasodilator dilates blood vessels to increase blood flow, and a vasoconstrictor constricts blood vessels decreasing blood flow.

12. Ionic contrast contains a complex molecular arrangement of iodine and other compounds resulting in a contrast agent with high osmolality. High osmolality refers to a solution that contains a high concentration of solute particles and a low concentration of solvent molecules. Nonionic contrast agents still contain an iodine compound; however, the molecular arrangement produces a low-osmolality contrast agent with less adverse reactions. Low osmolality refers to a solution, which contains a low concentration of solute particles and a high concentration of solvent molecules.

Matching

1. air-entrainment nebulizer

2. sublingual

3. Levin tube

4. barium

5. Groshong

6. nitroglycerin

7. air

8. Harris tube

9. epinephrine

10. sacred seven

11. viscosity

12. radio-opaque

Retention of Material

1. Invasive procedures require an informed consent be signed by the patient (or legal guardian in the case of a minor) for the procedure or treatment to legally be performed.

2.

   - **intramuscular injection** – injection into the muscle at a 90° angle.

- **intrathecal injection** – injection into the subarachnoid space of the spinal canal. For cervical puncture, C1–C2; for lumbar puncture, L3–L4.
- **intravenous injection** – injection into the vein at a 15°–20° angle.
- **subcutaneous injection** – injection below the skin at a 45° angle.

3. For adults, the nasal cannula, transtracheal catheter, oxygen mask, air entertainment mask, or an air-entertainment nebulizer can be used. Enclosure delivery systems are generally used for pediatric patients and include the oxygen tent (for children) and the oxyhood (for infants).

4. The technologist should immediately remove the injection needle and apply light pressure and warm compresses to the puncture site.

5. Radiolucent materials appear dark on a radiographic image, and radio-opaque materials appear light on a radiographic image.

6. Double contrast studies (positive and negative contrast agents used together) of the digestive tract are very useful in demonstrating the mucosal lining of the esophagus, stomach, small intestine, and large intestine.

7. Osmolarity affects the osmosis process in which water molecules will move across a semipermeable membrane from an area of low solute particle concentration to an area of high solute particle concentration in order to create balance.

8. Cantor tube, Harris tube, and the double lumen Miller-Abbott tube

9. Dobbhoff feeding tube, the single lumen Levin tube, and the double lumen Salem-Sump tube

10. presurgical patients, suspected perforation (organ, intestines), suspected large bowel obstruction

11. The greater the atomic number of tissue and or contrast agents, the more radiation absorption occurs. The result of radiation absorption on the radiographic image is areas with little or no radiographic density/image receptor exposure (appearing light).

12.

   A. The PICC line is a small catheter inserted into a vein located within the anterior part of the elbow and advanced into the superior vena cava for short-term use in drug administration/therapy and blood drawings.

   B. The Groshong catheter has a single or double lumen and is inserted under the skin of the chest wall and tunneled to a specific vein (usually the subclavian vein), where it is advanced into the superior vena cava for long-term use in drug administration and blood drawings.

   C. The Swan-Ganz catheter may have one lumen or several lumens. This catheter contains a small electrode at the distal end along with a balloon tip to secure the catheter's position (balloon inflation). Once the tip is advanced from the subclavian vein, internal vein, external vein, or femoral vein into the right atrium of the heart, cardiac function/pressures can be monitored.

   D. The infusion port (*Port-a-Cath*) or venous access port is an infusion port implanted under the skin of the upper arm or chest designed for long-term use in drug administration, blood transfusions, and/or blood drawings from the superior vena cava. Other names of venous access ports include the *Infusa-Port* and *Mediport*.

CHAPTER 6
PHYSICS TERMINOLOGY

Concept Thinking Questions

1. Wave-particle duality describes the dual characteristics of an x-ray photon. X-ray photons travel through space in a wave-like manner and have the ability to ionize matter. Therefore, they resemble both a wave (by their motion through space) and a particle (by their impact on atoms).

2. in the patient

3. Because of the various energy values produced, characteristic energy values are limited.

4. at the anode

5. Velocity remains constant at the speed of light, 186,000 miles per second.

6. indirect

7. direct

8. source, force, and a target

9. If a stable atom loses an electron, the atom would be considered unstable and would have a *positive* charge.

10. Isotopes are considered to be atoms that have the same number of *protons* but a different number of *neutrons*.

Practice Exercises

1. 127 indicates the atomic mass number (total number of protons and neutrons in the atom).

2. 53 indicates the atomic number (number of protons in the atom).

3. $2 \times n\,(3)^2 = 2 \times 9 = 18$. The maximum number of electrons that could occupy the M shell is 18.

4. The element $^{184}_{74}\text{W}$ is a stable atom; therefore, the atom should contain 74 electrons.

5. The A# is the atomic mass number (total number of protons and neutrons in the atom). The Z# is the atomic number (total number of protons in the atom).

6. $^{132}_{56}\text{Ba}$

7. A positive ion has more protons than it does electrons, which is the reason for its positive charge.

8. protons and neutrons

9. K shell, because it is positioned closest to the nucleus

10. P shell, because it is positioned furthest way from the nucleus

Matching

1. heat

2. neutron

3. work

4. A#

5. alpha particles

6. hertz

7. Z#

8. scatter

9. binding energy

10. electron

11. kinetic energy

12. wavelength

Retention of Material

1. *Refer to Figure 6–22.* A high-energy sinusoidal wave looks like a high-energy Bremsstrahlung x-ray photon (many peaks and valleys). See below.

2. *Refer to Figure 6–22.* A low-energy sinusoidal wave . *See below.*

3. *Refer to Figure 6–5.*

4.

   A. coherent scattering
   B. Compton scattering
   C. pair production
   D. photodisintegration
   E. photoelectric absorption

5.

   1. are a type of electromagnetic radiation
   2. are invisible
   3. are highly penetrating
   4. are polyenergetic (consisting of various energies)
   5. are capable of ionizing matter
   6. travel at the speed of light (186,000 miles per second or, as listed in the British SI system, 3×10^8 m/s [*meters per second*] or 3×10^{10} cm/s [*centimeters per second*] in a vacuum)
   7. travel in straight diverging lines
   8. cannot be focused by a lens
   9. cause fluorescence (emit light) of certain types of phosphor crystals
   10. affect photographic film
   11. cause biological changes
   12. have no mass
   13. have no electrical charge
   14. produce secondary radiation

CHAPTER 7
CIRCUITRY

Concept Thinking Questions

1. control console, high-voltage section, and x-ray tube

2.

   • move a conductor through a magnetic field
   • move a magnetic field past a conductor
   • vary the strength of a magnetic field while keeping the conductor stationary

3. Self-induction involves one coil wrapped around an iron core (referred to as an *electromagnet*). When

alternating current passes though the primary coil, a magnetic field will be produced. It is the continuous variation of the magnetic field (caused by AC) that will induce an opposing voltage. Mutual induction involves two coils, a *primary coil* wrapped around an iron core (referred to as an *electromagnet*) and a *secondary coil* placed in close proximity to the primary coil. When alternating current passes through the primary coil (electromagnet), a magnetic field will be produced. If a variation in alternating current occurs as it passes through the primary coil (electromagnet) a variation in the strength of the induced magnetic field will also occur. It is the continuous variation of the magnetic field that will cause alternating current to be induced in the secondary coil.

4. A conductor permits electrons to flow easily; aluminum and copper.

5. An insulator hinders the flow of electrons; rubber, dielectric oil.

6.

- an autotransformer
- a high-tension transformer (HTT), also referred to as a step-up transformer
- a filament transformer, also referred to as a step-down transformer

7. indirect

8. An autotransformer serves to supply a range of voltage (approximately 100–400 V) to the high-tension transformer (HTT). The autotransformer is also designed to assist the line voltage compensator, should the incoming line of voltage deviate from the 220-V requirement necessary to operate the unit.

9. The HTT or step-up transformer is a variable transformer that operates through the principles of mutual induction to convert voltage to kilovoltage. The filament transformer can also be referred to as a step-down transformer. The filament or step-down transformer is a variable transformer that operates through the principles of mutual induction to convert mA to amperage.

10. self-induction, autotransformer; mutual induction, HTT and the FT.

11. Resistance is an opposing force that hinders the flow of electric current. The five main variables that greatly impact the amount of resistance present within an electrical circuit are conducting material, diameter of conductor, length of conductor, straight-line conductor, and temperature of conductor.

12. There is a direct relationship between voltage and number of coil windings on a HTT; more windings on the secondary side of the HTT create an increase in voltage. There is an indirect relationship between voltage and number of coils on a FT; less windings on the secondary side of the FT create a decrease in voltage.

Practice Exercises

1. *Refer to Figure 7–11.*

Circuit Component:	Component Purpose:
1. Main power switch	On and off power to x-ray unit
2. Line monitor	Indicate incoming voltage level
3. Line compensator	Alter line supply to autotransformer
4. Autotransformer	Supplies a range of voltage from 100-400 V
5. Major kVp selector	Adjust voltage sent to HTT* (increments 10 kVp)
6. Minor kVp selector	Adjust voltage sent to HTT (increments 2 kVp)
7. Prereading kVp meter	Indicates anticipated kVp
8. Exposure timer circuit	Initiate, time and terminates exposure
9. mA selector	Adjust current sent to FT* (filament transformer)

*Note: *HTT, high voltage transformer or step-up transformer. *FT, filament transformer or step-down transformer.*

2. *Refer to Figure 7–11*

1. HTT* (High tension transformer)	Increases voltage to kilovoltage and decreases amperage
2. Four-diode rectification circuit	Converts AC to DC
3. mA meter	Indicates mA in Secondary HTT Circuit
4. Focal spot selector	Select filament to be heated
5. FT* (filament transformer)	Increases amperage and decreases voltage

3. *Refer to Figure 7–11*

1. X-ray tube
   anode (+) electrode
   cathode (−) electrode

   Produces radiation (Bremsstrahlung and characteristic radiation)

2. Induction motor
   Rotor
   Electromagnetic stators

   Operates by mutual induction to cause the rotating anode to spin and dissipate heat

4. *Refer to Figure 7–8.*

5.

$$V = I \times R$$
$$I = V/R$$
$$R = V/I$$
$$I \times R = (6 \times 2) = 12 \, V$$

6. $R = V/I$; $R = 110/3 = 36.6$ ohms or 37 Ω

7. Transformer law for voltage demonstrates a direct relationship between the number of turns or transformer windings and the voltage created through mutual induction. This is represented mathematically as: **Np/Ns = Vp/Vs**.

Transformer law for current demonstrates an indirect relationship between the number of turns or transformer windings and the voltage created through mutual induction. This is represented mathematically as: **Np/Ns = Is/Ip**.

8. $N_p(1)/N_s(1000) = V_p(220)/V_s(?) = 220,000$ volts or 220 kV

9. $N_p(10)/N_s(1) = I_s(?)/I_p(300) = 3000$ mA or 3 A

10. Current must be alternating (AC current).

Matching

1. (A) or (mA)

2. autotransformer

3. rheostat

4. ohm

5. inverter circuit

6. three-phase, 12-pulse

7. EMF

8. diode

9. motor

10. 100% voltage ripple

11. step-down transformer

12. hysteresis loss

Retention of Material

1.

- **ionization chamber** – The ionization chamber is considered the most common AEC imaging system used today. The parallel-plate ion chamber operates by collecting ion pairs; when a predetermined amount has been detected, the exposure timer will terminate the exposure. The ionization chamber is located between the patient and the image receptor.

- **photomultiplier tube** – The photomultiplier tube is considered to be outdated and not common in modern imaging equipment. The photomultiplier tube operates by the use of a fluorescent screen, which gives off light when struck by radiation. When a predetermined amount of light (via radiation) has been detected, the exposure timer will terminate the exposure. The photomultiplier tube is located behind the image receptor.

2. Diagnostic x-ray units need a potential difference of approximately 25–150 kVp to accelerate electrons across the x-ray tube.

3.

- **helix** – A helix is a spiral coil of wire.
- **solenoid** – A solenoid is a helix (spiral coil of wire) serving as a conductor for current flow.
- **choke coil** – A choke coil is a type of variable resistor that employs a fluctuating magnetic field (created by the forward and backward movement of an iron core within a solenoid) to create variations of resistance within an electrical circuit.

4. When an electrical circuit is wired in *series*, the current across the circuit will always be the same as the current across any *component* of the circuit. Current flow in a series circuit travels in one continuous line along a conductor. When an electrical circuit is wired in *parallel*, the voltage across the circuit will always be the same as the voltage across *any component* of the circuit.

Current flow in a parallel circuit does not travel in one continuous line along a conductor, rather it has bridges or connections that permit current to flow along various pathways within the circuit.

5. Fleming's right-hand rule is often referred to as the right-hand generator rule or right-hand dynamo rule. This hand technique mnemonic is very helpful in understanding electromagnetic relationships that arise when using a *generator*. The right hand is positioned with the thumb pointing in the same direction in which the conductor or armature is moving, the index finger points in the direction of the induced magnetic lines of flux, and the third finger points in the direction of conventional current flow. To ensure proper positioning of the fingers, all three fingers should be held at a right angle to each other.

6. *Refer to Figure 7-9.* Voltage ripple can be described as a loss of voltage during the rectification process.

7. Power loss = $I^{(2)} R$. Employ a circuit that uses high voltage and low amperage to decrease the amount of power loss.

8. 150 volts *(apply the transformer law formula for voltage)*: $N_p(1)/N_s(500) = V_p(?)/V_s(75) = 0.15$ kVp or 150 V

9. 0.4 A = 400 mA *(apply the transformer law formula for current)*:

   $N_p(15)/N_s(1) = I_s(6)/I_p(?) = 0.4$ A, or 400 mA

10. 120 kVp and 100 mA *(apply the transformer law formulas for voltage and current)*: $N_p(1)/N_s(500) = V_p(240)/V_s(?) = 120,000$ volts or 120 kV; $N_p(1)/N_s(500) = I_s(?)/I_p(50) = 0.1$ A or 100 mA

11. 15 mAs

   $$\frac{mAs_1(30)}{mAs_2(?)} = \frac{PCF_1(1)}{PCF_2(0.5)} = 30 \times 0.5 = 15/1 = 15 \text{ mAs}$$

   mAs_1 = original mAs

   mAs_2 = new mAs

   PCF_1 = original rectified unit

   PCF_2 = new rectified unit

RECTIFIED UNIT	PHASE CONVERSION FACTOR (PCF)
full-wave rectification	1
three-phase, 6-pulse rectification	0.67
three-phase, 12-pulse rectification	0.5

12. Increase the mAs from 8 to 12 (mAs is indicated in whole numbers) to maintain original density/image receptor exposure of the image produced via the three phase-6 pulse x-ray unit.

   $$\frac{mAs_1(8)}{mAs_2(?)} = \frac{PCF_1(0.67)}{PCF_2(1)} = 8 \times 1 = 8/0.67 = 11.9 \text{ mAs}$$

CHAPTER 8
X-RAY TUBE

Concept Thinking Questions

1. The vacuum tube enhances x-ray production by keeping air molecules out of the path of the accelerated electrons.

2. The focusing cup has a negative charge to repel the electrons produced at the filament.

3. The beveled edge allows for the line-focus principle in which the effective focal spot remains smaller than the actual focal spot size.

4. 11° or 12°

5. direct relationship

6. The lesser the degree of anode angle, the greater the ability of the anode to dissipate heat.

7. A smaller effective focal spot will result.

8. X-ray tube anodes are designed with an angled beveled edge in which the focal track resides. Line focus principle states that if the angle of the anode is less than 45°, the effective focal spot size will always be smaller than the actual focal spot size, thus creating better image resolution and a greater surface area for heat dissipation.

9. The anode heel effect is a variation of radiation intensity (approximately 45% difference) along the longitudinal axis of the image from anode end to cathode end. This variation is caused by the reabsorption of x-ray photons at the heel of the anode as photons are isotropically emitted. Although this variation of radiation intensity occurs during every x-ray exposure, it becomes more noticeable with the use of a small focal spot, a large image receptor size, a steep anode angle, and a short source-to-image distance (SID).

10. mAs

Practice Exercises

1. *Refer to Figure 8–11.*

    A. Bearings – provides steady and consistent rotation of the anode

    B. Tungsten anode – positive electrode that attracts electrons and serves as the "target" for x-ray production

    C. Envelope – houses the anode and cathode and provides a vacuum for more efficient x-ray production

    D. Filament – part of the cathode assembly that produces thermionic emission

    E. Electromagnetic stators – part of the induction motor (outside the envelop) that serves to rotate the tungsten anode

    F. Anode rotor – part of the induction motor (within the envelop) that serves to rotate tungsten anode

    G. Molybdenum anode neck and base – permits greater heat dissipation of the rotating tungsten anode

2.

    A. Large filament

    B. Small filament

    C. Actual focal spot

    D. Effective focal spot; changing from a large focal spot to a small focal spot results in an increase in recorded detail, decrease in penumbra, more noticeable anode heel effect, and an increase in heat loading capacity.

3. rotor and stators

4.

    A. Unsafe (above the 200 mA line)

    B. Unsafe (above the 200 mA line)

    C. Safe (below the 125 mA line)

5.

    A. kVp (85) × mA (300) × time (0.4) × 1 = 10,200 kHU

    B. kVp (110) × mA (200) × time (0.2) × 1.35 = 5,940 kHU

    C. kVp (95) × mA (400) × time (0.4) × 1.45 = 22,040 kHU

6.

    A. 15 min − 1.5 min = 13.5 minutes

    B. 6 min − 1 min = 5 minutes

    C. One exposure produces 17,280 kHU; the maximum amount of exposures that could be taken without exceeding 350 kHU is 20.

7. A space charge is the accumulation of electrons around the cathode filament and is caused by thermionic emission. A space charge can also be referred to as a *thermionic cloud*. The negative (−) force created by a space charge makes it difficult for additional electrons (possessing a negative [−] charge) to be boiled off the filament; this phenomenon is known as a space charge effect.

8. The fulcrum is the imaginary pivot point at which the x-ray tube and the image receptor cross paths as they move longitudinally to the x-ray table from opposite directions.

9. Bremsstrahlung interactions at the anode target cause the primary x-ray beam to be heterogeneous.

10. Vaporization occurs when the cathode filament and anode target receive a tremendous amount of heat, causing some of the tungsten atoms to transform from a solid to a gas.

Matching

1. kilovoltage

2. focusing cup

3. stators

4. tungsten

5. aluminum

6. heat

7. Coolidge tube

8. polyenergetic

9. anode

10. focal track

11. milliampere

12. conduction

Retention of Material

1. a source, a force, and a target

2. dual-focus x-ray tube

3. approximately 3–6 amperes

4. X-ray tube components, glass envelope, dielectric oil, and collimator assembly contribute to inherent filtration. The glass envelope (window port) is the largest contributor to inherent filtration.

5. X-ray tube anodes are designed with an angled beveled edge in which the focal track resides. Line focus principle states that if the angle of the anode is less than 45°, the effective focal spot size will always be smaller than the actual focal spot size, thus creating better image resolution and a greater surface area for heat dissipation. If the target angle exceeds 45°, no longer would the effective focal spot be smaller than the actual focal spot size. This would result in poor resolution and a decrease in the rotating anode's ability to dissipate heat.

6. Place the anode side of the x-ray tube toward the thinner part of the body and the cathode side toward the thicker part of the body.

7. rotor and electromagnetic stators

8.
- Single-phase; full-wave rectification: kVp × mA × time × 1 (multiplier factor) = kHU
- three-phase, 6-pulse unit: kVp × mA × time × 1.35 (multiplier factor) = kHU
- three-phase, 12-pulse unit: kVp × mA × time × 1.41 (multiplier factor) = kHU
- High-frequency unit: kVp × mA × time × 1.45 (multiplier factor) = kHU
- Fluoroscopic unit: kVp × mA × time × (multiplier factor for generator) × 60 = kHU

9. high anode speed rotation, tungsten target material (with rhenium-alloy added to the focal track and graphite and molybdenum added behind the tungsten), an anode diameter of approximately 5–12 cm with a small target angle

10. The tungsten vaporized gas adheres to the inside of the vacuum x-ray tube and exhibits the same characteristics of filtration in that low-energy photons are absorbed, causing a decrease of x-ray photons exiting the window port.

11. Decrease the actual focal spot size, or decrease the target angle.

12. The x-ray tube and the image receptor move in opposite directions simultaneously along the longitudinal axis of the x-ray table during the x-ray exposure. It is the degree of tomographic angle that determines the thickness of the body section or body plane. The larger the tomographic angle (greater movement of the tube and image receptor), the thinner the slice of anatomical area or object plane.

CHAPTER 9
FLUOROSCOPY

Concept Thinking Questions

1. The ABC system maintains a consistent level of image brightness by increasing mA or kVp.

2. When magnifying a fluoroscopic image, the diameter of the input phosphor size is reduced, causing the focal spot to shift away from the anode.

3. FOV decreases.

4. It produces a high dose of radiation to the patient.

5. CCD (charge-coupled device) or the TV camera tube (vidicon or Plumbicon)

6. 25,000 volts, or 25 kVp

7. Fluoroscopy produces a greater degree of noise because of the many processes that take place in converting incident x-rays to a visual image for monitor display. The fluoroscopic chain of events involved for image production is not a direct process, whereas conventional film/screen imaging involves few processes and is considered a much more direct mode of image production.

8. No. The image intensifier is moved out of the way, allowing the remnant x-rays (x-rays exiting the patient) to reach the image receptor cassette.

9. Spatial resolution increases when using the middle area of the input phosphor as opposed to the periphery.

10. Contrast resolution increases because more x-ray photons are needed to maintain the brightness level when shifting to a smaller input phosphor diameter.

Practice Exercises

1. *Refer to Figure 9–7.* A. Output fluorescent screen; B. Anode; C. Glass envelope; D. Electrostatic lens; E. Electron stream; F. Photocathode and input fluorescent screen.

2.
- **glass envelope** – The glass envelop creates a vacuum tube for efficient flow of electrons from photocathode to output phosphor.
- **input phosphor** – The input phosphor converts incident x-ray photons into light photons.
- **photocathode** – The photocathode converts light photons into electrons (photoemission).

- **electrostatic focusing lens** – The electrostatic focusing lens directs the stream of electrons from the photocathode to the output phosphor.
- **anode** – The anode attracts the electrons with a positive electrical charge.
- **output phosphor** – The output phosphor converts electrons into an increased number of light photons.

3. Identify the material or element associated with each of the following image intensifier components.

   A. input phosphor – cesium iodide (CsI)
   B. photocathode – cesium and antimony compounds
   C. output phosphor – zinc cadmium sulfide

4.
   - cine or spot-film camera
   - video monitor
   - image intensifier tube
   - bucky slot cover (bucky diaphragm for overhead film)
   - protective curtain
   - fluoroscopic x-ray tube under table
   - cassette-loaded spot-film
   - tilt x-ray table

5. Minification gain refers to a comparison between the input phosphor diameter and the output phosphor diameter of the image intensifier tube. MG is mathematically depicted as:

$$\text{Minification gain} = \frac{(\text{diameter of input phosphor})^2}{(\text{diameter of output phosphor})^2}$$

6. Flux gain refers to the increased number of light photons from the image intensifier output phosphor in comparison to the number of x-ray photons striking the image intensifier input phosphor. FG is mathematically depicted as:

$$\text{Flux gain} = \frac{\text{\# of output light photons}}{\text{\# of input x-ray photons}}$$

7. Total brightness gain refers to the increased amount of light or brightness of an image by the use of an image intensifier tube. It is the product of *minification gain* and *flux gain*. BG is mathematically depicted as:

   Brightness gain = minification gain × flux gain

8. Photoemission refers to the ability of the photocathode to emit electrons when struck by incident *light photons*. This process is very similar to the x-ray tube filament cathode emitting electrons (thermionic emission) when current in the range of 3–6 amperes is applied.

This amount of current causes the tungsten filament to become very hot and emit electrons.

9. The spot-film camera or photospot camera permits a rapid secession of static images in either 70-mm or 105-mm film format. When viewed at high speeds, the static images resemble a dynamic study. This type of image format would be appropriate for evaluating structures that rapidly perform a function.

10. When implementing the magnification mode, the FOV decreases and the structures appear larger as the focal spot shifts further away from the anode.

11. Total brightness gain is 6240, calculated by using the following formulas:

$$\text{Minification gain} = \frac{(\text{diameter of input phosphor})^2}{(\text{diameter of output phosphor})^2}$$

$$\frac{25^2}{2^2} = \frac{625}{4} = 156.3$$

flux gain × minification gain = brightness gain
(40)   ×   (156)   =   6240

12. The image size is 2.5 times larger (25/10 = 2.5).

Matching

1. zinc cadmium sulfide
2. anode
3. cones
4. photocathode
5. electrostatic focusing lens
6. dual-field tube
7. ABC
8. mL
9. resolution
10. CsI (cesium iodide)
11. brightness gain
12. vidicon

Retention of Material

1. Kilovoltage applied to the image intensifier tube serves to accelerate the electrons toward the anode.

2. between 0.5 and 5.0 mA

3. As the fluoro scope operator moves the carriage (image intensifier) over the patient to visualize different anatomic structures, the ABC automatically adjusts the kVp and/or mA to maintain the level of brightness, compensating for the differences in tissue density.

4. millilamberts (mL) or Lamberts (L)

5. The typical range of illumination levels for fluoroscopic images is between 100 mL and 1000 mL.

6. Fluoroscopic images are viewed in daylight; therefore, the cones of the eye are responsible for phototopic vision.

7. *Refer to Figure 9-7*, Image intensifier tube.

8. Dynamic studies (real-time motion) demonstrate structure and function and can depict normal and abnormal function. Static studies demonstrate structure but not function.

9. Resolution increases when FOV decreases, resulting in a magnified view of structures. This is caused by the centralized area of the input phosphor being used as opposed to the entire diameter of the input phosphor being used. Vignetting will come into play as you involve more of the input phosphor diameter, which results in a loss of spatial resolution.

10. Contrast resolution decreases when FOV increases. This is caused by a decrease in the number of x-ray photons present for a visible image to be created when decreasing the FOV. (More x-ray photons are needed to create a visible image when FOV decreases.)

11. Brightness levels increase (brightness gain) due to minification gain and flux gain.

12. The image on the 105-mm film size would have better resolution than the image on the 70-mm film due to a larger format and more x-ray photons.

CHAPTER 10
IMAGE PRODUCTION

Concept Thinking Questions

1. direct

2. indirect

3. Umbra is the best-recorded detail on the image; penumbra is loss of recorded detail around periphery of image.

4. A grid should be used when a body part measures more than 10 cm and when using more than 60 kVp.

5. collimation, compression, low kVp

6. The air-gap technique is the use of a 4- to 6-inch OID in place of a grid to reduce scatter from reaching the image receptor. An air-gap technique will increase image contrast.

7. kVp is the controlling factor for radiographic contrast.

8. mAs is the controlling factor for radiographic density and image receptor exposure.

9. Recorded detail refers to the structural detail captured on the recording medium. Visibility of detail refers to how well you can see the structural detail on the recording medium. VD can be hindered by scatter, fog, or overexposure.

10. Use the 15% rule when a change in contrast is desired without changing image density.

11. The characteristic curve is a graph depicting specific density readings obtained from the film of gradient densities. These density readings depict three important aspects of a radiographic film: sensitivity to x-ray exposure (referred to as film speed), inherent contrast, and exposure latitude. The graph is designed to demonstrate density readings on the vertical axis in correlation to the log relative exposure noted on the horizontal axis. When density readings are obtained (via a densitometer), plotted, and connected, an "s"-shaped curve (characteristic curve) becomes apparent and can be used for characteristic comparisons of more than one film type.

12. Both systems are film-less; however, CR uses PSP plates and a CR laser scan reader to capture the image to convert to an electrical signal for computer enhancement processing, whereas DR uses detector arrays to capture the image to convert to an electrical signal for computer enhancement processing.

13. Elongation caused by angling the x-ray tube. Foreshortening occurs when a perpendicular beam is used but the body part is not parallel to the IR. Spatial distortion is inherent on a radiographic image because of the three-dimensional relationship between the patient's body parts (as well as the thickness of the patient) and the divergence of the x-ray beam.

14. focal spot size, SID, OID.

15. Window level refers to adjusting the brightness level of the image. Window width refers to adjusting the scale of contrast of the image.

Practice Exercises

1. 100 mA × 4 s = 400 mAs; 200 mA × 2 s = 400 mAs; 400 mA × 1 s = 400 mAs; 800 mA × 0.5 s = 400 mAs

2. *Refer to Figure 10–2.*
- **toe** – The toe area indicates underexposure.
  - **base plus fog** – The base plus fog density is considered an inherent density on a radiographic film that can be measured and recorded once it has undergone film processing. The base plus fog density is attributed to the way in which radiographic film is manufactured, the blue tint of the radiographic film, and the chemical processing the film undergoes in the transformation of latent image to manifest image.
- **threshold** – The threshold area on the curve is located between the toe and average gradient, where the useful density range begins.
- **average gradient/straight line portion** – The average gradient or straight line portion of the curve represents the useful densities of the film. The useful range of optical densities typically lies between 0.25 and 2.5.
- **shoulder** – The shoulder portion of the curve represents overexposure. Shoulder range of densities lie between 2.5 and 4.0.
- **D-max** – The D-max portion of the curve represents the highest degree of measurable density on a radiographic film. D-max is close to or at an optical density of 4.0.

3. *Refer to Figure 10–12.* A focused grid would be preferred over a non-focused grid because the lines of the grid match the lines of the diverging x-ray beam, therefore reducing grid cutoff on the lateral margins of the image.

4. unwanted absorption of primary radiation

5.
- off-centered grid
- off-focus (incorrect focal distance)
- off-level grid
- upside down grid
- central ray angled perpendicular to the grid lines

6. *Refer to Figure 10–4.*

7.
- double mAs
- double mA
- double time
- increase kVp by 15%

8. The anode heel effect is a variation in density across a radiographic image from the anode side to the cathode side due to photon absorption occurring at the heel of the anode. The anode side would have less density than the cathode side. This can be used to an advantage by placing the thinner part of the body toward the anode and the thicker body part toward the cathode (e.g., AP femur projection with the head of the femur positioned toward the cathode end of the x-ray tube and the distal portion of the femur, where the knee is located, is positioned toward the anode).

9. A densitometer is a device that measures radiographic density on a film, whereas a sensitometer is a device that uses light (not x-ray photons) to put radiographic density on a film.

10. To increase contrast from the original technique of 75 kVp at 20 mAs, you must lower the kVp by 15% and double the mAs. The new technique would be 64 kVp at 40 mAs. 15% of 75 kVp = 11.3; subtract 11.3 from the 75 kVp for a sum of 63.7. Round this number to the nearest whole number at 64 kVp. To maintain the original density, a doubling of mAs is required to compensate for the decrease in density that resulted from lowering the kVp.

11. The units are mAs and distance; this math problem requires one to use the density maintenance formula:

$$\frac{mAs_1}{mAs_2} = \frac{D_1^{(2)}}{D_2^{(2)}}$$

$$\frac{mAs_1(12)}{mAs_2(?)} = \frac{D_1(40)^{(2)}}{D_2(72)^{(2)}} = \frac{(1600)}{(5184)}$$

Cross multiply 12 × 5184 = 62,208 ÷ 1600 = 38.8. The answer is 39 mAs.

12. The low grid ratio is expected to produce an image with less contrast and more density than the image produced with the higher grid ratio.

Matching

1. lp/mm

2. quantum mottle

3. scatter

4. penumbra

5. crossover

6. sodium sulfite

7. geometric properties

8. gadolinium

9. target angle <45°

10. blue tint

11. penetrability

12. small effective focal spot

13. mAs

14. matrix

Retention of Material

1. The inverse square law states that the radiation intensity will change by a factor of 4 as SID is doubled or halved. Mathematical formula depicting this concept is:

$$\frac{I_1}{I_2} = \frac{D_2^{(2)}}{D_1^{(2)}}$$

I_1 = original x-ray beam intensity
I_2 = new x-ray beam intensity (after a change in distance)
$D_1^{(2)}$ = original SID squared
$D_2^{(2)}$ = new SID squared

2. The direct square law or exposure maintenance law is the same as the density maintenance formula. The exposure maintenance formula is a mathematical equation used to calculate for the amount of mAs required to maintain radiographic density (for film) or image receptor exposure (for CR/DR images) after a change in SID has occurred. The mathematical formula depicting this concept is:

$$\frac{mAs_1}{mAs_2} = \frac{D_1^{(2)}}{D_2^{(2)}}$$

mAs_1 = original mAs
mAs_2 = new mAs (to maintain density/image receptor exposure after a change in SID has occurred)
$D_1^{(2)}$ = original SID (squared)
$D_2^{(2)}$ = new SID (squared)

3. The relationship between the actual focal spot size and the effective focal spot is a direct relationship. An increase in the actual FSS will result in an increase in the effective FSS.

4. It doesn't affect the quantity of photons produced; however, it does affect the quantity of photons that reach the patient and the IR.

5. Tube angulation increases the SID, causing a decrease in radiographic density. This is why the technologist must lower the SID to maintain the 40-inch SID and maintain radiographic density whenever the x-ray tube is angled. The rule of thumb is to decrease the SID 1 inch for every 5 degrees of tube angle.

6. A large actual focal spot size along with a small anode target degree provides for a small effective focal spot and a greater area for heat dissipation. For maximum heat dissipation, a large focal spot and a small target angle are best.

7.

- **film components** – base, adhesive layer (joins emulsion to the base), emulsion layer, and a protective coating (can be referred to as a supercoat)
- **intensifying screen components** – base (with light reflective surface) and active layer (active layer contains phosphors that emit light when struck by x-ray photons)

8. Methods to reduce scatter from reaching the IR:

- decrease body part thickness
- increase collimation
- decrease kVp
- use a grid or an air-gap technique
- increase grid ratio
- use lead strip absorbers

9. Increasing collimation (or reducing the collimated field size) results in a decrease in radiographic density and an increase in radiographic contrast.

10. The OID can never be reduced to zero because of the three-dimensionality of the body and the construct of the image receptor.

11.

$$\frac{\text{image size}}{\text{object size}} = \text{magnification factor (MF)}$$

$$\frac{3.5}{3.0} = 1.16 \text{ or } 1.2 \text{ MF}$$

12.

Penumbra = FSS × OID/SOD

FSS (1.2) × OID (2) = 2.4/38 (SOD) = 0.06 mm

SID of 40 inches minus the 2-inch OID will provide a SOD of 38 inches.

Penumbra = 0.06 mm

CHAPTER 11
IMAGING PRINCIPLES AND MATHEMATICAL EQUATIONS

Concept Thinking Questions

1. direct

2. direct

3. direct

4. indirect

5. 15% rule

6. mR and centimeters, inches, or feet (distance)

7. Radiation intensity changes by a factor of 4 as SID is doubled or halved.

8. Squaring the distances takes into account the radiation area that is changing by length (top and bottom) and width (side to side) as the SID is adjusted.

9. kVp and density share a direct relationship; it takes a 15% change in kVp to double or halve the radiographic density of an image.

10. The inverse square law states that a doubling or halving of SID will cause a change in the x-ray beam intensity by a factor of 4. For example, radiation intensity at an 80-inch SID using the technical factors of 75 kVp at 20 mAs yields an exposure rate (intensity) of 25 mR; when the SID is cut in half to a 40-inch SID, the x-ray beam's intensity or exposure rate will increase by a factor of 4, to 100 mR. Using the same scenario and applying the direct square law, we can determine the new mAs required to maintain density after the SID has changed from 80 to 40 inches without the use of a calculator simply by applying the concept. If radiation intensity (which determines radiographic density) has increased by a factor of 4 (from 25 mR to 100 mR), then to maintain density a decrease in mAs by a factor of 4 would be necessary. The new mAs at the 40-inch SID would need to be 5 mAs to maintain the density of the radiographic image that was taken at 75 kVp at 20 mAs at an 80-inch SID.

11. Applying the use of a grid will cause a decrease in radiographic density. Using the multiplier factor that correlates to the grid ratio of the grid used will tell the technologist how much more mAs is necessary to maintain radiographic density when going from no grid to a grid.

12. A grid multiplier of 4 tells the technologist they are using a grid with a grid ratio of 8:1 and will need 4 times the mAs required without the use of a grid.

13. Velocity is determined by the following formula v = distance (*d*) / time (*t*). However, because the velocity of electromagnetic radiation is constant at 186,000 miles per second, the formula depicts velocity as the speed of light, represented by the lower case (*c*) and the two changing variables of frequency (*f*) and wavelength (λ):

velocity (*c*) = frequency (*f*) × wavelength (λ)

14. The larger unit is the gray; 100 rads = 1 gray.

15. If the tube is moved from a perpendicular beam to an angled beam of 30°, the SID will have increased. If no compensation has been made to adjust the SID or technical factors, then the image will result in less overall density.

Practice Exercises

1.

100 mA at 1.5 s = 150 mAs
200 mA at 0.75 s = 150 mAs
600 mA at 0.33 s = 150 mAs

2. The number of transformer turns and current are inversely related. The number of transformer turns and voltage are directly related.

3. The curie (Ci) is the traditional unit to measure radioactivity.

4. The traditional unit for measuring radiation absorbed dose is the rad. The SI unit for measuring radiation absorbed dose is the gray.

5. 1000 mrads = 1 rad; 100 rads = 1 gray

6. To show a decrease in contrast, the technique would be 81 kVp at 7.5 mAs. To show an increase in contrast, the technique would be 60 kVp at 30 mAs. Both techniques maintain original density.

7.

75 kVp at 200 mA, 0.05 s

75 kVp at 100 mA, 0.1 s

86 kVp at 100 mA, 0.05 s

8. 400 RSV is four times more efficient in converting x-ray photon energy to light energy than the 100 RSV; therefore, the mAs would need to decrease by a factor of 4 to maintain the original density. New mAs required with the 400 RSV is 3 mAs.

$$\frac{mAs_1 (12)}{mAs_2 (?)} = \frac{RSV_2 (400)}{RSV_1 (100)}$$

Cross-multiply $12 \times 100 = 1200/400 = 3$ mAs.

3 mAs is required to maintain density when going from a RSV of 100 to a RSV of 400, with all other factors remaining constant.

9.

$$\frac{mAs_1 (15)}{mAs_2 (?)} = \frac{GMF_1 (1)}{GMF_2 (4)}$$

Cross-multiply $15 \times 4 = 60 /1 = 60$ mAs.

60 mAs is required to maintain density when going from no grid to a 8:1 grid, with all other factors remaining constant.

10.

$$\frac{mAs_1 (10)}{mAs_2 (?)} = \frac{PCF_1 (1)}{PCF_2 (0.5)}$$

Cross-multiply $10 \times 0.5 = 5/1 = 5$ mAs.

5 mAs is required to maintain density when going from a single-phase, fully rectified unit to a three-phase, 12-pulse unit, with all other factors remaining constant.

11.

$$\frac{\text{image size} (?)}{\text{object size} (6)} = \frac{\text{SID} (40)}{\text{SOD} (36)}$$

Cross-multiply $6 \times 40 = 240/36 = 6.66$ inches.

The image size of the hand would measure 6.7 inches.

12.

$$GR = h/d$$

h (3)/interspace distance (0.6) = 5:1 grid ratio

Matching

1. f × d

2. mR

3. PCF 0.67

4. inverse square law

5. 8 electrons

6. $2n^2$

7. W/t

8. Ohm's law

9. OID

10. 12:1 grid

11. mrad

12. 1000 V

Retention of Material

1. The units involved in the inverse square law are mR and distance (typically centemeters, inches, or feet). There is an inverse relationship between the intensity of the beam and the SID.

2. The units involved in the direct square law are mAs (and any portion of mAs) and distance (typically centemeters, inches, or feet). There is a direct relationship between a change in SID and the amount of mAs required to maintain radiographic density/image receptor exposure.

3. Ohm's law states that within a given circuit there is voltage (V), current (I), and resistance (R), and that the voltage within the circuit (total voltage or voltage at various points within the circuit) will always be equal to the amount of current flowing through the circuit times the amount of resistance present. Mathematically, Ohm's law can be depicted in any one of three ways:

$$V = I \times R$$
$$I = V/R$$
$$R = V/I$$

V = voltage

I = intensity of current

R = resistance to current flow

4. The beam intensity or exposure rate decreases.

5. Solve for the new mAs by using the density maintenance formula:

$$\frac{mAs_1\,(25)}{mAs_2\,(?)} = \frac{D_1(40)^{(2)}}{D_2(72)^{(2)}} = \frac{(1600)}{(5184)}$$

Cross-multiply $25 \times 5184 = 129{,}600/1600 = 81$ mAs.

81 mAs is required to maintain density when going from a 40-inch SID to a 70-inch SID, with all other factors remaining constant.

6. A factor of 4; you would need four times more mAs than the original mAs of 40. Therefore, 160 mAs would be required to maintain density when changing from a 40-inch SID to an 80-inch SID with all other factors remaining constant.

7. Increasing kVp would lower image contrast and increase the scale of contrast.

8. The voltage on the secondary side of a step-up transformer will be greater (kilovoltage) than the voltage on the primary side.

9. $N_1/N_2 = V_1/V_2$ or $N_P/N_S = V_P/V_S$

10. Voltage and current have an inverse relationship. Voltage increases to kilovoltage and current decreases from amperage to milliamperage.

11. To determine digital pixel size (measured in millimeters) divide the FOV (in mm) by the matrix size (50 cm = 500 mm):

$$\text{Pixel size} = \frac{\text{FOV}\,(500)}{\text{matrix size}\,(2500)}$$

$500/2500 = 0.2$ mm pixel size

12. Percent of magnification is determined by:

$$\frac{\text{image size}\,(3.5) - \text{object size}\,(3.0)}{\text{object size}\,(3.0)}$$

$$= 0.5/3.0 = 0.167 \times 100 = 16.7, \text{ or } 17\%$$

CHAPTER 12
RADIATION BIOLOGY

Concept Thinking Questions

1. LET is the transfer of energy from ionizing radiation to tissue. Highly ionizing radiation will deposit more energy in tissue as it passes through it than will a lower ionizing radiation. LET shares a direct relationship with relative biological effect (RBE); the more energy transferred to tissue, the more notable the biological effect.

2. hematologic syndrome, gastrointestinal syndrome, and central nervous syndrome

3. A stochastic effect is a random, unpredictable biological effect from radiation exposure; a response may or may not occur. A nonstochastic effect is a determined biological effect associated with a specific quantity of radiation exposure.

4. A congenital effect is a genetic anomaly present at birth.

5. The master molecule of the cell is the DNA (located within the nucleus of a cell).

6.

A *somatic cell* is a nonreprodcution cell found throughout the body. Somatic cells proliferate through the process of mitosis.

A *germ cell* is a reproductive cell, either a spermatozoa or an ova. Germ cells proliferate through the process of meiosis.

7. Possible biological effects include:

- no effect
- an indirect effect
- a direct effect

8. Radiolysis is the breakdown or destruction of water molecules within the cell as the result of ionizing radiation. This occurrence can produce free radicals within the cell, which can result in damage to the cell and even cellular death.

9.

- linear nonthreshold, which is the standard for radiographic diagnostic imaging procedures
- linear threshold
- nonlinear nonthreshold
- nonlinear threshold

10.

- embryonic stem cell
- adult stem cell

11. The $LD_{50/60}$ signifies an acute whole-body radiation dose resulting in 50% of the population dying within 60 days after exposure. The $LD_{50/60}$ for humans is approximately 320–520 rad, depending on medical treatment received.

12.

- muscle cells (myocytes)
- nerve cells (neurons)

Practice Exercises

1. prophase, metaphase, anaphase, telophase

2. germ cells (reproductive cells)

3. leukemia, genetic anomalies

4. alopecia, sterility

5. *Refer to Figure 12–3.*

6. The doubling dose refers to the quantity of radiation necessary to double the amount of genetic mutations within a population. The estimated doubling dose for the human population is 50–250 rad.

7. alpha particles and fast neurons

8. x-rays and gamma rays

9.

- **hematologic syndrome** – The hematologic syndrome, also referred to as the hematopoietic syndrome, is caused by an acute whole-body radiation dose of approximately 100–1000 rad.
- **gastrointestinal syndrome** – The gastrointestinal syndrome is caused by an acute whole-body radiation dose of approximately 1000–5000 rad.
- **central nervous syndrome** – The central nervous syndrome is caused by an acute whole-body radiation dose of approximately 5000 rad or greater.

10. The two main components of a cell are the cytoplasm and the nucleus. The semipermeable membrane is a selective membrane that only permits certain substances to enter and exit the cell.

11. Nonmembranous organelles:
- cilia
- microvilli
- centrioles
- ribosomes

Membranous organelles:
- smooth and rough endoplasmic reticulum (ER)
- golgi apparatus
- lysosome
- mitochondria
- nucleus

12. age in years (37) $\times$ 1 rem = 37 rem maximum annual cumulative dose

Matching

1. mitochondria

2. restitution

3. undifferentiated

4. radioresistant

5. OER

6. radiolysis

7. radiosensitive

8. epilation

9. gene

10. desquamation

11. mutation

12. fractionation

Retention of Material

1.

- **prodromal stage** – The prodromal stage is the first stage of acute radiation syndrome, in which the onset of symptoms occur.
- **latent stage** – The latent stage can be considered a dormant period during which no visible symptoms appear even though biological damage has occurred.
- **manifest stage** – The manifest stage is the stage in which symptoms become visibly noticeable.
- **recovery or death stage** – The recovery or death stage is dependent on the radiation dose; either the body will begin to recover (generally doses lower than 600 rad) or death will result. Death is inevitable at a whole-body radiation dose of 1000 rad or greater.

2. 10 rad or more delivered to the whole body at one time

3. The law of Bergonié and Tribondeau states that cells that are most sensitive to radiation are:

- immature (young)
- undifferentiated (not specialized in function)
- possess a high metabolic rate (divide rapidly)

This information is important in establishing thresholds for radiation exposure and biological responses. This is the premise upon which radiation therapy is based.

4.
- deoxyribose
- phosphoric acid
- 4 organic nitrogenous bases
  - purines (adenine and guanine)
  - pyrimidines (thymine and cytosine)

5. Lysomes are membranous organelles within the cell that contain enzymes to aid in the digestion or destruction of pathogens and damaged or old organelles.

6. RNA (ribonucleic acid), and DNA (deoxyribonucleic acid)

7. Rough ER contains ribosomes and aids in the production of proteins for transport out of the cell. Smooth ER contains no ribosomes and aids in the production of carbohydrates and lipids.

8.
- **anabolic** – a metabolic building process (hormone synthesis)
- **catabolic** – a metabolic breakdown process (breakdown of muscle or fat for energy)

9.
- proteins
- carbohydrates
- lipids
- nucleic acids (RNA and DNA)

10. *Refer to Table 12–2.*

CHAPTER 13
RADIATION PROTECTION

Concept Thinking Questions

1. Explain procedure to patient; provide instructions, shielding patients, obtain medical history, shield patients of child-bearing age, use optimal exposure techniques, use collimation.

2. QA (quality assurance) and QC (quality control)

3. The Joint Commission serves as a guide in providing medical facilities with compliance standards for high-quality patient care delivery.

4. 100 sievert

5. synchronous motor spin test

6. personnel monitoring devices and field survey instruments

7. concrete, gypsum, wood, steel

8. To minimize radiation exposure, reduce the time of exposure, increase the distance between the source and you, and use protective shielding whenever possible.

9. because the radiation field size is immediately reduced to the size of the IR being used

10. NCRP

Practice Exercises

1. Primary barriers are those toward which the x-ray source can be directed. Secondary barriers are those toward which the x-ray source is not directed.

2. A controlled area is any area within a medical facility where occupational workers can be found. An uncontrolled area is any area within a medical facility where the general public can be found.

3. The acceptable kVp range for a setting of 80 kVp would be 75 kVp – 85 kVp (+/− 5 kVp variation from the selected kVp setting).

4. The RSO is the person responsible either at the medical facility or the educational institution whose responsibility it is to ensure radiation safety measures are established and enforced.

5. Exposure linearity refers to various combinations of mA stations and exposure times to produce the same overall mAs without exceeding a +/− 10% variation of radiation intensity for adjacent mA stations.

6. pinhole camera, star pattern, slit camera, and line pair resolution tools

7. OSL

8. It is inexpensive and provides a permanent legal record.

9. It can only be worn for a 1-month period and cannot detect radiation levels less than 10 mrem.

10. ionzation chamber, Geiger-Muller counter, and the scintillation counter

Matching

1. TLD

2. leakage radiation

3. HVL

4. QA

5. accident

6. mA min/wk

7. beam/light congruency

8. shadow shield

9. 5 rem

10. 0.25 mm Pb

11. 5 mSv

12. primary barrier

Retention of Material

1. Use optimal exposure techniques, shield the patient, collimate on all four sides of the image (as long as it does not hinder the anatomy of interest), and provide proper instructions to the patient (e.g., hold your breath, don't move).

2. To protect the occupational worker (e.g., technologist, radiologist).

3. A patient slips and falls; a technologist sticks himself or herself with a needle.

4. distance (D), occupancy (T), use factor (U), and workload (W)

5. Radiation exposure has a cumulative effect on the body; therefore, occupational workers are provided with their report cycle reading, year-to-date reading, and cumulative reading. To calculate the cumulative effective dose limit, an occupational worker would use the following formula: age $\times$ 1 rem = cumulative effective dose limit.

6. Increasing collimation means creating a smaller radiation field size, which means less radiation to the patient.

7. no

8. Geiger-Müller counter and scintillation counter

9. contact shielding

10. $120 \times 0.15 = 18$ dots

CHAPTER 14
ORGAN SYSTEM ANATOMY

Concept Thinking Questions

1. digestive system and endocrine system

2. to provide the body with oxygenated blood and eliminate deoxygenated blood from the body

3. brain and spinal cord

4. 206 bones

5. cardia, fundus, body, and pylorus

6. duodenum

7. ileocecal valve

8. the transverse colon and the sigmoid colon

9. The kidneys lie retroperitoneal and alongside the vertebral column (approximately at the level of T12–L4). They are positioned at a 30° angle to the coronal plane with the upper poles of the kidneys more posterior than the lower poles of the kidney. The right kidney is positioned slightly lower than the left kidney due to the location and size of the liver.

10. The pelvis includes two innominate bones, the sacrum and coccyx.

11. to provide the body with an internal defense system for protection from harmful pathogens

12. five layers

Practice Exercises

1. ascending colon, transverse colon, descending colon, and the sigmoid colon

2.
   - proximal row
     - scaphoid
     - lunate
     - triquetrum
     - pisiform
   - distal row
     - trapezium
     - trapezoid
     - capitate
     - hamate

3.

- 1 frontal bone
- 2 parietal bones
- 2 temporal bones
- 1 ethmoid
- 1 sphenoid
- 1 occipital

4.

- 2 lacrimal bones
- 2 nasal bones
- 2 inferior nasal conchae
- 2 zygomatic bones
- 1 vomer
- 2 palatine bones
- 2 maxillary bones
- 1 mandible

5. The cervical vertebrae; the foramina serve as a passage way for the vertebral artery, veins, and nerves to pass through.

6.

- oral cavity
- pharynx
- esophagus
- stomach
- small intestines
- large intestines
- anus

7. three lobes: the superior lobe, the middle lobe, and the inferior lobe

8. endocrine system

9.

- skeletal muscle tissue, attached to skeletal bones
- smooth muscle tissue, located at visceral organs
- cardiac muscle tissue, located within the heart

10. An example of voluntary motion would be moving picking up a glass, which involves the central nervous system, skeletal system, and muscular system.

11. An example of involuntary motion would be the beating of the heart, which involves the muscular system (cardiac muscle tissue) along with the endocrine and nervous system affecting heart beat rate.

12. *Refer to Figure 14–17.*

Matching

1. axial

2. PNS

3. carpal bone

4. atlas

5. kidney

6. axon

7. T5

8. alveoli

9. smooth muscle tissue

10. tarsal bone

11. heart

12. larynx

Retention of Material

1. lymphatic system

2. Gas exchange occurs in the alveoli of the lungs through the process of diffusion.

3. Similarities: The cervical, thoracic, and lumbar vertebra have in common a vertebral body and a vertebral arch, vertebral foramen, transverse processes, and a spinous process.

Differences: C1 and C2 do not resemble the typical vertebra and have very unique characteristics. Different from the thoracic and lumbar vertebrae, the cervical vertebrae are smaller in size, possess transverse foramina, and have a bifid spinous process tip with overlapping vertebral bodies. C2 has an odontoid process (dens), and in C7 the spinous process (vertebra prominens) is large and palpable. The thoracic vertebrae have facets or demifacets on the vertebral body for articulating with the ribs. The lumbar vertebrae are the largest of the three vertebrae, with a large vertebral body and spinous process but rather narrow transverse processes.

4. reproductive system

5.

- from the right atrium
- through the tricuspid valve

- to the right ventricle
- to the semilunar valve
- to the main pulmonary artery
- to the left and right pulmonary arteries
- to the lungs
- from the lungs to the pulmonary veins
- to the left atrium
- through the mitral valve
- to the left ventricle
- to the aortic valve
- to the aorta
- to all parts of the body
- to the superior and inferior vena cava

6. because the liver, being a large organ, is positioned superior to it

7. sphenoid bone

8. The largest moveable facial bone is the mandible, and the largest immovable facial bone is the maxilla (right and left).

9. The epiglottis is a cartilage of the larynx, which is part of the respiratory system. It serves as a flap to cover the opening of the trachea when swallowing to prevent food particles from entering the lungs and causing aspiration.

10. liver, gallbladder, and pancreas

11. They allow the colon to expand and contract to assist with the movement of waste material toward the rectum.

12. Nephrons are the smallest functional units of the kidney and span the cortex and medulla of the kidney.

CHAPTER 15
POSITIONING TERMS, LANDMARKS, AND LINES

Concept Thinking Questions

1. stomach, splenic flexure of the colon, left kidney

2. liver for the RUQ and the stomach for the LUQ

3. umbilical region

4. L4–L5

5. duodenum

6. RLQ, hypogastric region

7. prominent rib

8. submentovertex

9. transverse plane

10. LOA

11. glabella

12. gonion

Practice Exercises

1.
- **brachycephalic** – short, broad-shaped skull with petrous ridges angled greater than 47° to the mid-sagittal plane
- **dolichocephalic** – narrow, long-shaped skull with petrous ridges angled less than 47° to the mid-sagittal plane
- **mesocephalic** – average shaped skull with petrous ridges angled 47° to the mid-sagittal plane

2. glabelloalveolar (GAL)

3. greater trochanter (femur)

4. supination

5. The seventh cervical vertebra is considered a bony landmark because it has a very large spinous process.

6. interpupillary line and the mid-sagittal plane

7. It is necessary to check for the presence of fluid within the paranasal sinuses.

8. bucky

9.
- **superior row** – right hypochondriac region (rhr), epigastric region (er), left hypochondriac region (lhr)
- **medial row** – right lumber region (rlr), umbilical region (ur), left lumbar region (llr)
- **inferior row** – right inguinal region (rir), right hypogastric (pubic) region (rhgr), left hypogastric (pubic) region (lhgr)

10. free intraperitoneal air between the liver and the lateral margin of the abdominal cavity

Matching

1. TEA

2. OML

3. vertebra prominens

4. inion

5. L2–L3

6. MML

7. ulnar deviation

8. diaphragm

9. S1–S2

10. dorsal surface

11. supination

12. posterior

Retention of Material

1. right lateral decubitus

2. The chin needs to be tilted up (extending the neck).

3. anterior and inferior to the iliac crest

4.

- ASIS
- greater trochanter
- iliac crest
- prominent rib
- symphysis pubis
- vertebra prominens
- xiphoid process

5. lateral position

6. PA projection

7. Instead of the orbits being superimposed, one orbit will appear superior to the other.

8. Instead of the orbits being superimposed, one orbit will appear anterior to the other.

9. The PA projection places the sinuses closest to the IR (increases recorded detail) and reduces radiation exposure to the patient's eyes.

10. IOML

11. Trendelenburg

12. Anatomic structures found in the RUQ include the liver, gallbladder, pyloric antrum of the stomach, hepatic flexure of the colon, proximal part of the small intestines (duodenal bulb, duodenum, ileum), head of the pancreas, right suprarenal gland, and right kidney.

Reference List

Adler, A. M., and Carlton, R. R. (2007). *Introduction to radiologic sciences and patient care* (4th ed.). St. Louis, MO: Saunders Elsevier.

American Heart Association. (2010). *2010 Guidelines for cardiopulmonary resuscitation and emergency cardiovascular care.* Dallas, TX: AHA.

American Registry of Radiologic Technologists. (2010). *Radiography: Certification handbook and application materials.* St. Paul, MN: ARRT.

American Society of Registered Technologists. (2010). *ASRT practice standards.* Albuquerque, NM: ASRT.

American Society of Registered Technologists (2010). *Code of ethics.* Albuquerque, NM: ASRT.

Association of Surgical Technologists, Inc. (2008). *Surgical technology for the surgical technologist: A positive care approach* (3rd ed.). Clifton Park, NY: Delmar Cengage Learning.

Ballinger, P. W., and Frank, E. D. (2003). *Merrill's atlas of radiographic positions and radiologic procedures* (10th ed., Vols. I–III). St. Louis, MO: Elsevier Mosby.

Beebe, R., and Funk, D. (2008). *Fundamentals of emergency care.* Clifton Park, NY: Delmar Cengage Learning.

Bontrager, K. L., and Lampignano, J. P. (2010). *Textbook of radiographic positioning and related anatomy* (7th ed.). St. Louis, MO: Elsevier Mosby.

Bushong, S. C. (2004, 2008). *Radiologic science for technologists: Physics, biology, and protection* (8th and 9th eds.). St. Louis, MO: Elsevier Mosby.

Campeau, F. E., and Fleitz, J. (2010). *Limited radiography* (3rd ed.). Clifton Park, NY: Delmar Cengage Learning.

Carlton. R. R., and Adler, A. M. (2006). *Principles of radiographic imaging: An art and a science* (4th ed.). Clifton Park, NY: Delmar Cengage Learning.

Centers for Disease Control and Prevention. (2010). *Standard precautions.* Retrieved March 14, 2011, from http://www.cdc.gov.

Daniels, R., and Nicoll, L. H. (2007). *Contemporary medical-surgical nursing* (1st ed.). Clifton Park, NY: Delmar Cengage Learning.

Dowd, S. B., and Tilson, E. R. (1999). *Practical radiation protection and applied radiobiology* (2nd ed.). Philadelphia, PA: Saunders.

Edge, R. S., and Krieger, J. L. (1998). *Legal and ethical perspectives in health care: An integrated approach.* Clifton Park, NY: Delmar Cengage Learning.

Ehrlich, R. A, McCloskey, E. D., and Daly, J. A. (2004). *Patient care in radiography: With an introduction to medical imaging* (6th ed.). St. Louis, MO: Mosby.

Forshier, S. (2009). *Essentials of radiation biology and protection* (2nd ed.). Clifton Park, NY: Delmar Cengage Learning.

Greathouse, J. S. (2006). *Radiographic positioning & procedures: A comprehensive approach.* Clifton Park, NY: Delmar Cengage Learning.

Hegner, B., Acello, B., and Caldwell, E. (2008). *Nursing assistant: A nursing process approach* (10th ed.). Clifton Park, NY: Delmar Cengage Learning.

Hoeltke, L. (2006). *The complete textbook of phlebotomy* (3rd ed.). Clifton Park, NY: Delmar Cengage Learning.

Institute for Caregiver Education (2010). *Good body mechanics/employee safety: A skills update.* Retrieved March 14, 2011, from http://www.caregivereducation.org/products/sample_inservice.pdf.

International Union of Pure and Applied Chemistry (IUPAC) (2007). *Periodic table of the elements.*

The Joint Commission. (2008, November 24). *Requirements for criminal background checks.* Retrieved June 29, 2010, from http://www.jointcommission.org/AccreditationPrograms/LongTermCare/Standards/09_FAQs/HR/requirements_vfor_criminal.htm.

Landauer, Inc. (2010). *Radiation dosimetry report.* Glenwood, IL: Landauer, Inc.

Lindh, W. Q., Pooler, M. S., and Dahl, B. M. (2010). *Delmar's comprehensive medical assisting: Administrative and clinical competencies* (4th ed.). Clifton Park, NY: Delmar Cengage Learning.

Long, B. W., Frank, E. D., and Ehrlich, R. A. (2006). *Radiography essentials for limited practice* (2nd ed.). Philadelphia, PA: Elsevier Saunders.

MedlinePlus Medical Encyclopedia. The U.S. National Library of Medicine National Institutes of Health (2/2009). *Vital signs.* Retrieved March 14, 2011, from http://www.nlm.nih.gov/medlineplus/ency/article/002341.htm.

Merck Manuals Online Medical Library (2010). *Drug names.* Retrieved March 14, 2011, from http://www.merck.com.

National Council on Radiation Protection and Measurements (NCRP) (2010). *Ionizing radiation exposure of the population of the United States* (Report No. 93). Bethesda, MD: NCRP.

National Council on Radiation Protection and Measurements (NCRP) (2010). *Limitation of exposure to ionizing radiation* (Report No. 116). Bethesda, MD: NCRP.

National Council on Radiation Protection and Measurements (NCRP) (2010). *Quality assurance for diagnostic imaging equipment* (Report No. 99). Bethesda, MD: NCRP.

Rizzo, D. C. (2010). *Fundamentals of anatomy physiology* (3rd ed.). Clifton Park, NY: Delmar Cengage Learning.

Saia, D. A. (2008). *Lange Q&A radiography examination* (7th ed.). New York, NY: McGraw Hill.

Scott, A. S., and Fong, E. (2009). *Body structures & functions* (11th ed.). Clifton Park, NY: Delmar Cengage Learning.

Seeram, E. (2011). *Digital radiography: An introduction.* Clifton Park, New York: Delmar Cengage Learning.

Seikel, J. A., King, D. W., and Drumright, D. G. (2010). *Anatomy & physiology for speech, language, and hearing.* Clifton Park, NY: Delmar Cengage Learning.

Tabers Cycopedic Medical Dictionary. (2010). *Medical abbreviations* (21st ed.). Philadelphia, PA: F. A. Davis.

Wallace, J. E. (1995). *Radiographic exposure principles & practice.* Philadelphia, PA: F. A. Davis.

Widmer, R. S., and Van Soelen, K. W. (1999). *Radiography: Study guide and registry review.* Philadelphia, PA: Saunders.

World Health Organization (2007, May). Avian influenza, including influenza A (H5N1), in humans: WHO *interim infection control guideline for health care facilities.* Retrieved March 14, 2011, from http://www.wpro.who.int/internet/resources.ashx/CSR/Publications/AI_Inf_Control_Guide_10May2007.pdf.

Index

Note: Page numbers with an italicized letter refer to the following: *b,* boxes; *f,* figures; *t,* tables.

A

A (ampere), 140
Å (angstrom), 85
A number (atomic mass number), 86, 356
a- prefix, 19
ab- prefix, 19
abbreviations
  answer key, 348–349
    concept thinking questions, 348
    matching, 348
    practice exercises, 348
    retention of material, 349
  defined, 16
  overview, 16–18
  projections and positions, 299–301
  radiographic examinations, 299
abdominal aorta, 294f
abdominal quadrants, 305f
abdominopelvic
  body quadrants, 304
  body regions, 304–305
abduction, 306, 307f
absorbed dose equivalent, 235
absorption, 85
AC (alternating current), 86, 87f, 115
Academy of Molecular Imaging, 323
Academy of Radiology Research, 323
acanthiomeatal line (AML), 316f
acanthion, 315f
acceleration, 85
accessory organs, digestive system, 267, 272
accreditation
  defined, 6, 347
  importance of, 346
Accreditation Commission for Home Care,
    Inc. (ACHC), 11t
accreditation standards, 6–7
acetic acid, 201t
ACHC (Accreditation Commission for Home
    Care, Inc.), 11t
Achilles tendon, 281f
acr/o combining form, 20
acromion process, 290t
activators, film processing, 201t
actual electron flow, 115
actual focal spot, 144

acute, 235
acute radiation dose, 235
acute radiation symptoms, 235–236, 236t
acute radiation syndrome staging, 237
ad- prefix, 19
ADC (analog-to-digital converter), 160
added filtration, 143
adduction, 306, 307f
adductor magnus, 281f
adductors of thigh, 280f
adenine, 240f
aden/o combining form, 20
adipose tissue, 285f
adrenal gland
  hormone secretions, 275t
  location of, 276f, 294f
adult stem cells, 245
advanced health care directive (AHCD), 26,
    350
AEC (automatic exposure control) devices,
    112–113, 250
AEC (automatic exposure control) selectors,
    114–115
afferent arteriole, 295f
afterglow, 206
aggravating factors, Sacred Seven patient
    care questions, 35, 350
AHCD (advanced health care directive), 26,
    350
airborne droplets, 58
airborne precautions, 47
airborne transmission, 58
air-gap technique, 181, 182f, 363
ALARA (as low as reasonably achievable)
    principle, 7, 181, 184, 249, 250, 348
-algia suffix, 22
allergic reaction, 63
alleviating factors, Sacred Seven patient care
    questions, 35, 350
alopecia, 237
alpha radiation, 93
alternating current (AC), 86, 87f, 115
alveolar duct, 288f
alveoli, 287f, 288f
ambulatory, 26
American Association for Women
    Radiologists, 323
American Board of Nuclear Medicine, 323

American Board of Radiology, 323
American College of Medical Physics, 323
American College of Nuclear Medicine, 323
American College of Radiology, 323
American heart association, 2010 guidelines
    for CPR, 333–335
American Osteopathic College of Radiology,
    323
American Radium Society, 324
American Registry of Diagnostic Medical
    Sonographers (ARDMS), 8t, 330
American Registry of Radiologic
    Technologists. *See* ARRT
American Roentgen Ray Society, 324
American Society for Therapeutic Radiation
    Oncology, 330
American Society of Emergency Radiology,
    324
American Society of Head and Neck
    Radiology, 324
American Society of Neuroradiology, 330
American Society of Radiologic
    Technologists. *See* ASRT
Americans with Disabilities Act (1990), 33
AML (acanthiomeatal line), 316f
ammeter, 116t, 122
ammonium thiosulfate, 201t
ampere (A), 140
amplitude, 85
ampule, 63, 353
ampulla of vater, 274f
amu (atomic mass unit), 86
anabolic, 237, 370
anal canal, 273f
anal opening, 285f
analog signal, 160
analog-to-digital converter (ADC), 160
anaphase, mitosis, 243
angi/o combining form, 20
angstrom (Å), 85
annihilation reaction, 95
anode, 85, 140, 166f, 167, 362
anode angle, 146
anode cooling chart, 153, 154f
anode cracking, 152
anode heel effect, 140–141, 141f, 359, 364
anode mass, 146
anode melting, 152

anode rotor, vacuum x-ray tube, 360
anode target, 141
ante- prefix, 19
anterior direction, 306
anterosuperior iliac spine (ASIS), 314
anti- prefix, 19
antibiotic, 43
antibodies, 43
antiseptic, 43
anus, 273*f*
appendicular skeleton, 286, 288–289*t*
aprons, protective, 259*t*
arcing, 153
ARDMS (American Registry of Diagnostic
    Medical Sonographers), 8*t*, 330
areola, 285*f*
Arizona State Society of Radiologic
    Technologists, 325
Arkansas Society of Radiologic Technologists,
    325
ARRT (American Registry of Radiologic
    Technologists), 346
  continuing education credits, 3
  defined, 7
  eligible candidate, 8
  examination and certifications, 8*t*
  National Certification Examination, 8–9
  rules and regulations, 9
  Rules of Ethics, 26
  standards of ethics, 9
arterial distribution, 64*f*
arterial system, 63
arteries, 63
arterioles, 63
arthr/o combining form, 20
artificially produced permanent magnets, 121*t*
as low as reasonably achievable (ALARA)
    principle, 7, 181, 184, 249, 250, 348
ascending colon, large intestine, 273*f*
asepsis, 43
ASIS (anterosuperior iliac spine), 314
ASRT (American Society of Radiologic
    Technologists), 324, 346–347
  Code of Ethics, 26
  defined, 9
  Mission Statement, 34b
  Practice Standards for Medical Imaging
      and Radiation Therapy, 26–27
  scope of practice, 331–332
assault, 37, 349
associated manifestations, Sacred Seven
    patient care questions, 35, 350
Association for Medical Imaging
    Management, 323
Association of Educators in Imaging and
    Radiological Sciences, 323
Association of Vascular and Interventional
    Radiographers, 323
atom
  defined, 85–86
  with orbital shells, 90

atomic mass number (A number), 86,
    356
atomic mass unit (amu), 86
atomic number (Z number), 356
  contrast media and, 72*t*
  defined, 86
  human tissues and, 72*t*
attenuation, 86, 181
audible (5-minute) timer, 160
auricle, 315*f*
authorization, legal, 27
autoclave, 43–44
automatic exposure control (AEC) devices,
    112–113, 250
automatic exposure control (AEC) selectors,
    114–115
automatic processor, film, 200
autonomic nervous system, 277
autonomy, 27
autotransformer, 128, 133, 357
auxiliary imaging devices, 165
average gradient, characteristic curve, 183,
    364
awards of accreditation, 6
axial projection, 311, 312*f*
axial skeleton, 286, 288–289*t*
axillary nodes, 278*f*
axillary temperature reading, 28
axon, 282*f*

B

backscatter radiation, 100
backup time, 114
bacteria, 50, 352
barium enema (BE), 269
barrel, syringe, 76, 77*f*
base plus fog density, 183, 188, 364
battery (physical harm), 37, 349
battery, electric circuit, 116*t*
battery-operated x-ray unit, 148
BD (bone densitometry), 3*t*
BE (barium enema), 269
beads of myelin, neuron, 282*f*
beam-restricting devices, 181
bearings, vacuum x-ray tube, 360
becquerel (Bq), 104, 227
beneficence, 27
beta radiation, 93
bevel, needle, 50
bi- prefix, 19
biceps brachii, 280*f*
biceps femoris, 281*f*
biennium reporting cycle, 10
binding energy, 88
biohazard, 44
biological effect, 237
biology, 237. *See also* radiation biology
biospill, 44

blood composition, 268*t*
blood pressure, 39
blood pressure rate, 349
blood pressure reading, 27
bodily fluids, 44
body
  of pancreas, 274*f*
  of stomach, 271*f*
  of uterus, 284*f*
body mechanics, 27–39
body planes, 303–304, 303*f*
body quadrants (abdominopelvic), 304
body regions (abdominopelvic), 304–305
body temperature reading, 27–29
Bohr's atomic model, 86
bolus injection, 73
bone densitometry (BD), 3*t*
bony landmarks, 314–315
Bowman's capsule, 295*f*
Bq (becquerel), 104, 227
brachy- prefix, 19
brachycephalic skull, 317*f*, 318, 373
brain, 282*f*
brain stem, 282*f*
branching of cell, cardiac muscle, 279*f*
breach of duty, 38
breast, female, 285*f*
breast sonography (BS), 3*t*
bremsstrahlung radiation, 100–101, 102*f*
brightness control, 160
British Columbia Radiological Society, 329
British Institute of Radiology, 329
broad ligament, 284*f*
bronchi, 286*t*, 288*f*
bronchiole, 287*f*, 288*f*
bronchus, 287*f*
BS (breast sonography), 3*t*
buccinator muscle, 271*f*
Bucky, Gustov, 165
bucky slot cover, 165, 259*t*
bucky tray, 165–166
building words, 16
bulbourethral gland, 285*f*
butterfly needle, 72, 73*f*

C

CAAHEP (Committee on Accreditation of
    Allied Health Education Programs), 7*t*
calcaneal tendon, 281*f*
calcaneus, 290*t*
calcium tungstate phosphors, 207
calculation for mA and distance, exposure
    maintenance formula, 219
calculation for time and distance, exposure
    maintenance formula, 219
California Society of Radiologic
    Technologists, 325
Canadian Association of Radiologists, 329

cannula, needle, 50
capacitor, electric circuit, 116*t*
capacitor discharge unit, 148–149
capillaries, 63
capillary net, 295*f*
carcinogen, 237
cardiac muscle
    cells, 279*f*
    characteristics of, 279*t*
cardiac-interventional radiography (CI), 4*t*
cardi/o combining form, 20
cardiopulmonary resuscitation. *See* CPR
cardiovascular system, 267
    American heart association 2010
        guidelines for CPR, 333–335
    blood composition, 268*t*
    heart, 268*f*
CARE Bill, 33
CARF (Commission on Accreditation of
    Rehabilitation Facilities), 11*t*
c-arm, 160–161
carpals, 290*t*
carriage, 161
cartilage ring, 288*f*
cassette-loaded spot-film, 166
catabolic, 237, 370
cathartic, 63
cathode, 86, 141
cathode ray tube (CRT), 161, 162*f*
cauda equina, 283*f*
caudal, 307
causation, 38
CCAC (Continuing Care Accreditation
    Commission), 11*t*
CDC (Centers for Disease Control and
    Prevention), 42–43
CE (continuing education), 9–10
cecum, large intestine, 273*f*
cell
    components and functions, 239*t*
    defined, 237
    overview, 238*f*
cell body, 282*f*
cell membrane, 239*t*
Centers for Disease Control and Prevention
    (CDC), 42–43
central nervous syndrome, 236, 369
central ray, 181–182
central venous catheter, 63–65
central venous (cv) line, 63
centrally located nucleus, cardiac muscle,
    279*f*
centrioles, 238*f*, 239*t*
cephalic, 307
cerebellum, 282*f*
cerebr/o combining form, 20
cerebrum, 282*f*
certification, ARRT, 9, 346, 347
cervical nodes, 278*f*
cervical spinal nerves, 283*f*
cervical vertebrae, 290*t*, 292*f*
cervix of uterus, 284*f*
chambers, AEC, 114

CHAP (Community Health Accreditation
    Program), 11*t*
characteristic curve, 182–183, 363–364
characteristic radiation, 101
charge-coupled device, 161
charting, 35
chemical energy, 88
chemical name, drug, 69
Chicago Radiological Society, 326
choke coil, 115, 358
chol/e combining form, 20
chondr/o combining form, 20
chromosome, 237–238
chronic, 238
chronic radiation dose, 238
chronology, Sacred Seven patient care
    questions, 35, 350
chyme, 267
CI (cardiac-interventional) radiography, 4*t*
Ci (curie), 104, 195*t*, 227
cilia, 239*t*
cinefluorography, 166
circuit breakers, 115, 133
circuitry
    AEC devices, 112–113
    AEC selectors, 114–115
    answer key, 356–359
        concept thinking questions, 356–357
        matching, 356
        practice exercises, 357–358
        retention of material, 358–359
    choke coil, 115
    circuit breaker, 115
    conductor, 115
    coulomb, 115
    current, 115
    current types, 115
    electric circuit, 117
    electric circuit symbols, 117
    electrical circuit wiring, 115–117
    electrical grounding, 117
    electrification, 117
    electrodynamics, 117
    electromagnet, 117
    electromagnetic induction, 118
    electromagnetism, 118–120
    electrostatic field, 120
    EMF, 120
    generator, 120
    helix, 120
    hertz, 120–121
    horsepower, 121
    insulator, 121
    inverter circuit, 121
    magnet, 121
    magnetism, 122
    meter, 122
    motor, 122
    ohm, 122
    Ohm's law, 122–123
    overview, 111–112
    power, 123
    power loss, 123

    rectification, 123–125
    rectification formula, 125–126
    rectifier, 126
    resistance, 126–127
    resistor, 127
    rheostat, 127
    rpm, 127
    solenoid, 127
    TR, 131
    transformer, 128–130
    transformer laws, 130–131
    transformer power loss, 131
    volt, voltage, 131
    voltage ripple, 131–132
    watt, 132
    x-ray circuit, 132–135
    x-ray tube, 135
circular muscle layer, stomach, 271*f*
classical scattering, 94
clavicle, 290*t*
clearing agent, film processing, 201*t*
closed switch, electric circuit, 116*t*
closed-core transformer, 128, 129*f*
coccyx, 290*t*, 292*f*
coccyx spinal nerve, 283*f*
code of ethics, 322
coherent scattering, 94
collaboration between school-based
    practitioners and psychologists in other
    settings, 1
collimation, 183–184
Colorado Society of Radiologic Technologists,
    325
combining forms, 16, 20–21
Commission on Accreditation of
    Rehabilitation Facilities (CARF), 11*t*
Committee on Accreditation of Allied Health
    Education Programs (CAAHEP), 7*t*
common bile duct, 274*f*
common hepatic duct, 274*f*
communicable disease, 44
communication, 29–30
Community Health Accreditation Program
    (CHAP), 11*t*
compassion, 30
compensating filters, 142
competence, 30
compliance, 30
compression, 184
compton scattering, 95
computed radiography (CR), 161–163, 181,
    184–185, 185*t*
computed tomography (CT), 4*t*
conducting material, 126
conduction, 146
conductor, 115, 357
confidentiality, 33
congenital effect, 238, 368
Connecticut Society of Radiologic
    Technologists, 325
contact precautions, 46
contact shields, 259*t*
contamination, 44

Continuing Care Accreditation Commission (CCAC), 11*t*
continuing education (CE), 9–10
continuous quality improvement (CQI), 259
contrast, 186–187
contrast contraindications, 65, 67*t*
contrast media. *See also* pharmacology
   allergic reaction, 63
   ampule, 63
   answer key, 353–355
      concept thinking questions, 353
      matching, 354
      practice exercises, 354
      retention of material, 354–355
   arterial system, 63
   cathartic or laxative, 63
   central venous catheter, 63–65
   contrast contraindications, 65, 67*t*
   contrast reactions, 66–67
   defined, 66
   related atomic number and, 72*t*
   venipuncture, 342–343
contrast reactions, 66–67
contrast resolution, 163
control console components, 132
controlled area, 258, 370
controlling factors
   contrast, 186*t*
   defined, 187
   distortion, 193*t*
   radiographic density, 188, 189*t*
   recorded detail, 211*t*
conus medullaris, 283*f*
convection, 146
conventional current, 115
conventional units, 262*t*
conviction, 30
Coolidge, William D., 152
Coolidge tube, 152
Cooper's ligament, 285*f*
copper loss, 131
copy film, 199
coronal plane, 303
coronal suture, 291*f*
cortex
   hormone secretions, 275*t*
   kidney, 294*f*
cosmic radiation, 104
cost/o combining form, 20
Coulomb, Charles-Augustin de, 88, 217
Coulomb unit, 115
Coulomb's law, 88, 217
CPR (cardiopulmonary resuscitation), 29, 333–335
   delivery rescue breaths, 335
   establish airway, 334–335
   initiate chest compressions, 333–334
CQI (continuous quality improvement), 259
CR (computed radiography), 161–163, 181, 184–185, 185*t*
crash cart, 67–68
credentials, ARRT, 10
criminal background check, 30

Crookes, William, 152
Crookes' tube, 152
cross-hatch grid, 202
crossover, 187
crosstalk, 187
CRT (cathode ray tube), 161, 162*f*
CT (computed tomography), 4*t*
cultural diversity, 30
cumulative exposure, 238
curie (Ci), 104, 195*t*, 227
current, 86, 115, 142, 223, 358
Cutie Pie, 112, 113*f*, 250, 252*t*
cv (central venous) line, 63
cyan/o combining form, 20
cycle of infection, 45
cystic duct, 274*f*
cyt/o combining form, 21
cytoplasm, 239*t*
cytosine, 240*f*
cytosol, 239*t*

D

D (distance), 258
D log E curve, 182–183
damage, 38
DC (direct current), 86, 87*f*, 115
dead-man foot pedal, 163
dead-man switch, 142
death stage, acute radiation syndrome, 237, 369
decubitus, 301
defamation, 37
defendant, 30
defibrillator, 68*f*, 69
deltoid, 280*f*, 281*f*
dendrites, neuron, 282*f*
densitometer, 187, 190*f*, 364
density, 114, 187–190, 217
density maintenance formula, 197, 218–219, 365, 367
deoxyribonucleic acid (DNA), 239, 240*f*
dependent, 30
dermis, 276
derm/o combining form, 21
descending colon, large intestine, 273*f*
desquamation, 238
detent position, 142
deterministic effect, 245
developers, film processing, 201*t*
deviation, 307
DF (digital fluoroscopy), 163
diagnosis, 30, 351
diagnostic imaging equipment, 260*t*
diagnostic x-ray range, 86–87, 191
diameter of conductor, 126–127
diaphragm, 287*f*
diastolic blood pressure, 27, 39
dielectric oil, 142
diencephalon, 282*f*
differentiated cell, 238–239

digestive system
   defined, 267, 269
   duodenum, 274*f*
   esophagus, 269*b*
   gallbladder, 273*t*, 274*f*
   large intestine, 269–270*t*, 273*f*
   liver, 273*t*, 274*f*
   overview, 270*f*
   pancreas, 273*t*, 274*f*
   pharynx, 269*b*
   salivary glands, 271*f*
   small intestine, 269–270*t*, 272*f*
   stomach, 269–270*t*, 271*f*
digital fluoroscopy (DF), 163
digital image acquisition, 191–192
digital pixel size, 368
digital radiography (DR), 181, 185*t*
diode/rectifier, electric circuit, 116*t*
-dipsia suffix, 22
direct acquisition, 185*t*
direct amorphous selenium, 185*t*
direct contact transmission, 58
direct current (DC), 86, 87*f*, 115
direct digital radiography, 163–164, 192
direct effect, ionizing radiation, 246
direct square law, 197, 218–219, 365, 367
direct-exposure film, 198
directional terms, 306–311
directional x-ray tube terms, 311–314
disease, 44
disinfectant, 44
distal, 307
distal convoluted tubule, 295*f*
distance (D), 258
distortion, 192–195
diuretic, 69
D-max, characteristic curve, 183, 364
DNA (deoxyribonucleic acid), 239, 240*f*
DNR (do not resuscitate) code, 31
doctrine, 31
dolichocephalic skull, 317*f*, 318, 373
dorsoplantar projection, 299, 301*f*
dose-effect relationships, 240
dose-response curves, 240
dosimeters, 250–252*t*
dosimetry report, 345
double-emulsion film, 199
doubling density, 190*t*
doubling dose, 240, 369
DR (digital radiography), 181, 185*t*
drip infusion, 69
droplets, 48
drug
   defined, 69
   screening/testing, 31
dual-field image intensifier tube, 171
dual-focus tube, 142
duodenum of small intestine, 271*f*, 272*f*, 274*f*
duplicating film, 199
dura mater, 283*f*
duty, 38
dynamic image, 164

dynamic image recording, 171*t*
dynamometer, 122
dys- prefix, 19

E

EAM (external acoustic meatus), 316*f*
EAM (external auditory meatus), 291*f*, 315*f*
ecto- prefix, 19
-ectomy suffix, 22
eddy current loss, 131
Edison, Thomas A., 164
effective dose limit recommendations, 252–253
effective focal spot, 144
effects of radiation, 240–241
efferent arteriole, 295*f*
EI (exposure index) number, 196–197
ejaculatory duct, 285*f*
elective booking, 36
electric circuit
    defined, 117
    symbols, 116*t*, 117
    wiring, 115–117
electrical energy, 90
electrical grounding, 117
electrification, 87, 117
electrodynamics, 87, 117
electromagnetic energy, 90
electromagnetic induction, 118
electromagnetic radiation, 91–92
electromagnetic spectrum, 87
electromagnetic stators, vacuum x-ray tube, 360
electromagnetism, 118–120
electromagnets, 117, 121*t*, 356–357
electromotive force (EMF), 120
electronic timers, 133
electrons, 87, 166*f*, 167
electrostatic field, 87*f*, 120
electrostatic focusing lenses, 166*f*, 167, 362
electrostatics, 87–88
element, 88
elongation, 192, 193, 363
embryonic stem cells, 245
EMF (electromotive force), 120
empathy, 31
endo- prefix, 19
endocrine system
    defined, 272
    location of glands, 276*f*
    organs and glands, 275*t*
endometrium, 284*f*
endoplasmic reticulum (ER), 239*t*
endotracheal tube, 69
energy, 88–90
enteral feeding routes, 74*f*
enter/o combining form, 21
entrance skin exposure (ESE)
    calculating, 243
    defined, 241

for fluoroscopic procedures, 253
envelope, vacuum x-ray tube, 360
epi- prefix, 19
epidermis, 276
epididymis, 285*f*
epiglottis, 287*f*, 373
epilation, 241
ER (endoplasmic reticulum), 239*t*
erect, 301
erthyocytes, 245
erythema, 241
erythr/o combining form, 21
ESE. *See* entrance skin exposure
esophagram, 269
esophagus, 269*b*, 270*f*, 287*f*
ethics, 31, 350
ethmoid bone, 291*f*
European Society of Radiology, 329
eversion, 308
excitation, 94
exit radiation, 100
exposure, 195
exposure factors/technique, 195–196
exposure index (EI) number, 196–197
exposure linearity, 253–255, 370
exposure maintenance formula, 197, 218–219, 365, 367
exposure reproducibility, 255
exposure switch. *See* exposure timer circuit
exposure timer
    accuracy, 255
    test tools, 219–220, 255–256
exposure timer circuit
    defined, 133
    electronic timers, 133
    mAs, timers, 134
    synchronous, timers, 134–135
extension, 307*f*
extensors, hand and fingers, 280*f*, 281*f*
external acoustic meatus (EAM), 316*f*
external anal sphincter, large intestine, 273*f*
external auditory meatus (EAM), 291*f*, 315*f*
external naris, 287*f*
external oblique, 280*f*
external os, 284*f*
extrafocal radiation, 100
extravasation, 69
eyeglasses/goggles, 259*t*

F

face, sagittal section, 287*f*
face shield, 51*f*
facemask, 51
falciform ligament, 274*f*
false imprisonment, 37
Faraday's laws, 118
fat-soluble iodinated contrast media, 66
FDA (Food and Drug Administration), 52
felony, 31–32, 349
female gonads, 275*t*

female reproductive organs, 284*f*, 284*t*
femur, 290*t*
fetal personnel monitoring device, 257
FG (flux gain), 169–170, 221, 362
fibula, 290*t*
fidelity, 31
field of view (FOV), 164, 191
field size, x-ray tube, 142
field survey instruments, 252*t*
fifteen percent (15%) rule, 197–198, 220
filament, vacuum x-ray tube, 142–143, 360
filament saturation, 149
filament transformer (FT), 116*t*, 128, 134, 357
filament vaporization, 143
film
    defined, 198
    types of, 198–200
film badge dosimeter, 251*t*, 254*f*
film cassette, 200
film contrast, 200
film cubic lattice, 199*f*
film processing, 200, 201*t*
film speed, 182, 200–201
film-screen combination, 164, 200
filtration, 143–144, 201
fimbriae, 284*f*
first digit, hand, 290*t*
"five rights," drug administration, 70
5-minute timer, 160
fixed fluoroscopic units, 174
fixers, film processing, 201*t*
flat contact shield, 256
Fleischner Society, 324
Fleming, John Ambrose, 119
Fleming's hand rules, 119, 359
flexion, 307*f*, 308
flexors, hand and fingers, 280*f*
flight-or-fight response, 32
Florida Patient's Bill of Rights and Responsibilities (381.026), 336–340
    overview, 336
    responsibilities of patients, 338–340
    rights of patients, 336–338
        access to health care, 338
        experimental research, 338
        financial information and disclosure, 338
        individual dignity, 336–337
        information, 337–338
        patient's knowledge of rights and responsibilities, 338
Florida Radiological Society, 325
Florida Society of Radiologic Technologists, 325
fluorescence, 91, 206
fluoro curtain/drape, 259*t*
fluoroscope, 164
fluoroscopic image, 164
fluoroscopic mA range, 164
fluoroscopic system, 164–169
fluoroscopic unit, 146
fluoroscopic x-ray tube, 168
fluoroscopy
    ADC, 160

analog signal, 160
answer key, 361–363
  concept thinking questions, 361
  matching, 362
  practice exercises, 361–362
  retention of material, 362–363
audible (5-minute) timer, 160
brightness control, 160
c-arm, 160–161
carriage, 161
charge-coupled device, 161
computed radiography, 161–163
contrast resolution, 163
CRT, 161
dead-man foot pedal, 163
defined, 169
DF, 163
direct digital radiography, 163–164
dynamic image, 164
film-screen combination, 164
fluoroscope, 164
fluoroscopic image, 164
fluoroscopic mA range, 164
fluoroscopic system, 164–169
flux gain, 169–170
focal point, 170
FOV, 164
illumination, 170
image recording, 170
magnification, 170
minification gain, 170
multifield image intensification, 170–171
overview, 159–160
patient dose, 171
photoemission, 172
photopic vision, 172
quantum mottle, 172
raster pattern, 172
recording system, 172
remote fluoroscopic system, 172–173
scotopic vision, 173
spatial resolution, 173
spot imaging, 173
static image, 173
tabletop exposure rate, 173
total brightness gain, 173
TV camera tube, 173
vignetting, 173–174
x-ray source to patient distance, 174
flushing, 71
flux gain (FG), 169–170, 221, 362
focal point, 170
focal spot, 144–145
focal spot selector, 134
focal spot testing, 256
focal track, 145
focused nonlinear grid, 202, 203f
focusing cup, 145
fog, 202
Foley catheter, 71
fomite, 59
Food and Drug Administration (FDA), 52
foreshortening, 192, 193, 363

foreskin, 285f
fornix, 284f
four prime factors, 202
four radiographic properties, 202
fourth digit, hand, 290t
FOV (field of view), 164, 191
Fowler's position, 301
fractional-focus tube, 145
fractionation, 241
fraud, 32
free radical, 241
frequency, 91
friction, 87
frontal bone, 290t, 291f
frontalis, 280f
FT (filament transformer), 116t, 128, 134, 357
fulcrum, x-ray tube, 360
full-wave rectification, 124, 131–132
fundamental particles, 91
fundus
  stomach, 271f
  uterus, 284f
fungi, 50, 352

G

GAL (glabelloalveolar line), 316f
gallbladder, 270f, 273t, 274f
galvanometer, 122
gamma rays, 92, 93f
gastr/o combining form, 21
gastrocnemius, 280f, 281f
gastrointestinal syndrome, 236, 369
Geiger-Muller counter, 252t
gene, 241
generator, 120
generic name, drug, 69
genetic effect, radiation exposure, 241
genetic significant dose (GSD), 241–242
genetics, 241
geometric blur, 173, 202, 208–209
geometric properties, 202
Georgia Society of Radiologic Technologists, 325
germ cell, 242, 245, 368
glabella, 315f
glabelloalveolar line (GAL), 316f
glabellomeatal line (GML), 316f
glandular tissue, 285f
glass envelope, 166f, 167, 361
glomerular capsule, 295f
glomerulus, 295f
gloves, 52, 259t
glucagon, 71
glucophage, 71
glutaraldehyde, 201t
gluteus maximus, 281f
GML (glabellomeatal line), 316f
goggles, 52
golgi apparatus, 238f, 239t
gonadal shield, 256

gonads, 242, 275t
gonion, 315f
good body mechanics
  best practice rules, 28t
  defined, 27
Good Samaritan Law, 33–34, 351
gowns, protective, 52
gracilis, 281f
-gram/-graphy suffix, 22
great toe, 290t
greater trochanter, 314
grid, 202–204
grid cut-off, 202–203
grid frequency, 204, 204f
grid radius, 204
grid ratio, 204, 220, 221t
grid ratio/mAs formula, 220
grid-controlled tube, 152
Groshong catheter, 64, 355
GSD (genetic significant dose), 241–242
guanine, 240f

H

H&D curve, 182
HAI (health care-associated infection), 45
hair cap, 52
half-life, 91
half-value layer (HVL), 145, 204, 209, 256
half-wave rectification, 124, 132
halving density, 190t
hamstrings, 281f
hand washing, 44
hard palate, 287f
hardeners, film processing, 201t
Hawaii Society of Radiologic Technologists, 325
head-tilt/chin-lift method, CPR, 334
health care, 32
health care accreditation, 10
health care power of attorney, 27
health care proxy decision maker, 26
health care team, 32
health care-associated infection (HAI), 45
Health Insurance Portability and Accountability Act (HIPAA) 1996, 33, 349
health organizations, 44
heart
  hormone secretions, 275t
  physiology of, 268f
heat, 145
heat dissipation, 145–146
heat transfer, 146
heat unit (HU), 146–147, 220–221
Heimlich maneuver, 32
helix, 120, 358
hemat/o combining form, 21
hematologic syndrome, 235, 369
hematopoietic syndrome, 235, 369
hemi- prefix, 19

hem/o combining form, 21
HEPA (high-efficiency particulate air) filter, 47
hepatic ducts, 274f
hepatic flexure, large intestine, 273f
hepat/o combining form, 21
heredity, 242
hertz, 91, 120–121
heter/o combining form, 21
heterogeneous beam, 147
Hickman catheter, 64
high osmolarity, 75
high-efficiency particulate air (HEPA) filter, 47
high-frequency rectification, 124–125, 132
high-osmolality contrast agent, 354
high-speed film, 200-201
high-tension transformer (HTT), 116t, 128–129, 134, 357
high-voltage section components, 133
HIPAA (Health Insurance Portability and Accountability Act) 1996, 33, 349
hist/o combining form, 21
histogram, 204–205, 205f
homeo combining form, 21
horizontal beam, 311
horizontal plane, 304
horsepower (hp), 121, 221
hospice, 33
host, 45
housing cooling chart, 153
hp (horsepower), 121, 221
HTT (high-tension transformer), 116t, 128–129, 134, 357
HU (heat unit), 146–147, 220–221
hub, needle, 50
human tissue
    contrast media and, 71–72
    effective atomic number and, 72t
humerus, 290t
HVL (half-value layer), 145, 204, 209, 256
hydr/o combining form, 21
hydroquinone, 201t
hyoid bone, 287f
hyper- prefix, 19
hyperextension, 308
hyperflexion, 309
hypo- prefix, 19
hypodermic needle, 72–73
hypothalamus, 275t, 282f
hysteresis loss, 131
hyster/o combining form, 21

I

-ia suffix, 22
iatrogenic infection, 45
ICRU (International Commission on Radiologic Units), 104, 261
Idaho Society of Radiologic Technologists, 326
idiopathic, 45

ileocecal valve, large intestine, 273f
ileum
    large intestine, 273f
    small intestine, 272f
iliac crest, 314
iliotibial tract, 281f
ilium, 290t
Illinois State Society of Radiologic Technologists, 326
illumination, 170
illuminator device, 217
IM (intramuscular) injection, 76f, 354
image blur, 173, 202, 208–209
image forming radiation, 100
image intensifier mathematical equations, 221–222
image intensifier tube, 166
image magnification, 205, 222
image production
    air-gap technique, 181
    ALARA principle, 181
    answer key, 363–366
        concept thinking questions, 363–364
        matching, 364–365
        practice exercises, 364
        retention of material, 365–366
    attenuation, 181
    beam-restricting devices, 181
    central ray, 181–182
    characteristic curve, 182–183
    collimation, 183–184
    compression, 184
    contrast, 186–187
    controlling factors, 187
    CR, 184–185
    crossover, crosstalk, 187
    densitometer, 187
    density, 187–190
    density maintenance formula, 190
    diagnostic x-ray range, 191
    digital image acquisition, 191–192
    direct digital radiography, 192
    direct square law, 192
    distortion, 192–195
    EI number, 196–197
    exposure, 195
    exposure factors/technique, 195–196
    exposure maintenance formula, 197
    fifteen percent (15%) rule, 197–198
    filament, 198
    film, 198
    film cassette, 200
    film contrast, 200
    film processor, 200
    film speed, 200–201
    film type, 198–200
    film/screen combination, 200
    filtration, 201
    fog, 202
    four prime factors, 202
    four radiographic properties, 202
    geometric blur, 202
    geometric properties, 202

grid, 202–204
grid frequency, 204
grid radius, 204
grid ratio, 204
histogram, 204–205
HVL, 204
image magnification, 205
image stitching, 206
influencing factors, 206
intensifying screen, 206
intensifying screen phosphors, 207
intensity, 207
inverse square law, 207
IR, 206
isotropic, 207–208
latent image, 208
manifest image, 208
moiré pattern, 208
non-screen film, 208
OID, 208
overview, 180
PACS, 209
parallax, 208
penetrometer, 208
penumbra, 208–209
photographic properties, 209
quality, 209
quantity, 209
quantum mottle, 209
radiolucent, 209
radio-opaque, 209
reciprocity law, 209–210
recorded detail, 210
resolution, 210
scatter, 210
sensitometer, 210–211
SOD, 211
step wedge, 211
subject contrast, 211
tube angulation, 211–212
umbra, 212
window level, 212
window width, 212
image receptor (IR), 206
image recording, 170
image stitching, 206
imaging modalities, 2–12
    accreditation, 6
    accreditation standards, 6–7
    ALARA principle, 7
    answer key, 346–348
        concept thinking questions, 346
        matching, 347
        practice exercises, 346–347
        retention of material, 347–348
    ARRT, 7–8
        eligible candidate, 8
        National Certification Examination, 8–9
        rules and regulations, 9
        Standards of Ethics, 9
    ASRT, 9
    CE, 9–10
    certification, 9

credentials, 10
health care accreditation, 10
licensure, 10
organizations, 329–330
overview, 2–5
radiologic technologist/radiographer, 10–11
radiologic technology, 11
radiologist, 11
radiologist assistant, 11–12
registry, 12
imaging plates (IPs), 184
imaging principles
answer key, 366–368
concept thinking questions, 366
matching, 367
practice exercises, 366–367
retention of material, 367–368
immobilization methods, 37–38
immunity, 45
immunization, 45
immunization record, 45
incident electron, 91
incident report, 33, 256–257, 344
incorrect tube angulation, 203
Indiana Society of Radiologic Technologists, 326
indirect acquisition, 185t
indirect amorphous silicon, 185t
indirect contact transmission, 58
indirect effect, ionizing radiation, 246
induction, 87
induction motor, 122, 147
infection control, 42–59
answer key, 351–353
concept thinking questions, 351–352
matching, 352–353
practice exercises, 352
retention of material, 353
antibiotic, 43
antibodies, 43
antiseptic, 43
asepsis, 43
autoclave, 43–44
biohazard, 44
biospill, 44
bodily fluids, 44
communicable disease, 44
contamination, 44
disease, 44
disinfectant, 44
hand washing, 44
health organizations, 44
host, 45
idiopathic, 45
immune, immunity, 45
immunization, 45
immunization record, 45
infection, 45
inoculation, 45
isolation, 45–49
microorganism, 49
MSDS sheet, 49

needle, 49–50
needle recapping, 50
needleless devices, 50
needlestick injury, 50
overview, 42–43
parasite, 50
pathogen, 50–51
PPE, 51–55
proliferate, 56
skin prep kit, 56
standard precautions, 56
sterile, 56
sterile field, 56
sterile technique, 56–57
superbug, 58
surgical scrub, 58
toxin, 58
transmission mode, 58–59
vaccination, 59
vaccine, 59
inferior vena cava, 294f, 309
infiltrate, 73
influencing factors
contrast, 186t
defined, 206
distortion, 193t
radiographic density, 188, 189t
recorded detail, 211t
informed consent, 73, 341, 354
infra- prefix, 19
infraorbital foramen, 291f
infraorbital margin, 315f
infraorbitalmeatal line (IOML) positioning, 313f, 316f
infraspinatus, 281f
infundibulum, 284f
infusion port (Port-a-Cath), 355
inguinal nodes, 278f
inherent filtration, 143
injections, 73
inner canthus, 315f
inoculation, 45
input phosphor, 166f, 167, 361
insulator, 121, 357
integumentary system, 272
intensifying screen, 206
intensifying screen phosphors, 207
intensity, 207
intentional misconduct, 38, 349
inter- prefix, 19
intercalated disc, cardiac muscle, 279f
internal anal sphincter, large intestine, 273f
internal os, 284f
internal rotation, 309
International Commission on Non-Ionizing Radiation Protection, 329
International Commission on Radiologic Units (ICRU), 104, 261, 329
international organizations, 328–329
International Society for Magnetic Resonance in Medicine, 329
International Society of Radiology, 324
interphase, somatic cellular cycle, 243

interpupillary line, 316f
intestinal crypt cells, 245
intra- prefix, 19
intramuscular (IM) injection, 76f, 354
intrathecal injection, 73, 355
intravascular injection, 73
intravenous (IV) injection, 76f, 354, 355
intravenous urogram (IVU) compression device, 184f
intubation, 69
inverse square law, 207, 222, 365, 366, 367
inversion, 309
inverter circuit, 121
IOML (infraorbitalmeatal line) positioning, 313f, 316f
ion, 91
ionic contrast media, 66, 353, 354
ionization, 91, 92f
ionization chamber, 112, 113f, 250, 252t, 358
ionizing radiation, 91–93, 104, 227, 261–262
Iowa Society of Radiologic Technologists, 326
IPs (imaging plates), 184
IR (image receptor), 206
irritant laxatives, 63
ischium, 290t
-ism suffix, 22
iso- prefix, 19
isobar, 93
isolation, 45–49
isolation mask, 51
isomer, 93
isotone, 93
isotope, 93, 355
isotropic, 94, 147, 207–208
isthmus, 276f
-itis suffix, 22
IV (intravenous) injection, 76f, 354, 355
IV push, 73
IVU (intravenous urogram) compression device, 184f

J

jaw thrust, CPR, 334
JCAHO (Joint Commission on Accreditation of Healthcare Organizations), 259
jejunum, small intestine, 272f
Joint Commission on Accreditation of Healthcare Organizations (JCAHO), 259
joint movements, 307f
Joint Review Committee on Education in Diagnostic Medical Sonography (JRC-DMS), 7t
Joint Review Committee on Education in Radiologic Technology (JRCERT), 7t
Joint Review Committee on Educational Programs in Nuclear Medicine Technology (JRCNMT), 7t
JRC-DMS (Joint Review Committee on Education in Diagnostic Medical Sonography), 7t

JRCERT (Joint Review Committee on Education in Radiologic Technology), 7*t*
JRCNMT (Joint Review Committee on Educational Programs in Nuclear Medicine Technology), 7*t*

K

"K" shell, 98
Kansas Society of Radiologic Technologists, 326
khU (kilovolt heat unit), 223
kidney, 294*f*
kilovolt (kV), 131, 147, 196, 222
kilovolt heat unit (khU), 223
kilovoltage peak (kVp), 147, 196
kinetic energy, 90, 223
kV (kilovolt), 131, 147, 196, 222
kVp (kilovoltage peak), 147, 196

L

lacrimal bone, 291*f*
lactiferous duct, 285*f*
lambda (λ), 94
landmarks, bony
    answer key, 373–374
        concept thinking questions, 373
        matching, 373–374
        practice exercises, 373
        retention of material, 374
    overview, 314–315
large intestine, 269–270*t*, 272*f*, 273*f*
laryngopharynx, 287*f*
larynx, 286*t*, 287*f*, 288*f*
laser film, 199
latent image, 208
latent stage, acute radiation syndrome, 237, 369
lateral, 309
lateral decentering, 203
lateral position, 302
lateral rotation, 310, 311*f*
latex-free gloves, 52
latissimus dorsi, 281*f*
law, 33–34
law of Bergonié and Tribondeau, 242
law of conservation of energy, 88
laws of electromagnets, 118
laws of electrostatics, 88
laxatives, 63
LD$_{100}$, 242
LD$_{50/60}$, 242, 368–369
lead gloves, 52
leakage radiation, 102, 103*f*, 257
left brachiocephalic vein, 278*f*
left hepatic duct, 274*f*
left internal jugular vein, 278*f*
left lower quadrant (LLQ), 304, 305*f*
left renal artery, 294*f*
left subclavian vein, 278*f*

left upper quadrant (LUQ), 304, 305*f*
left-hand rule, 119–120
left-hand thumb rule, 120
legal guardian, 27
legal terms. *See* medical and legal terms
legislature, 34
length of conductor, 127
LET (linear energy transfer), 242
lethal, 242
leuk/o combining form, 21
licensure, 10
line focus principle, 147–148
line monitor, 133
line voltage compensator, 133
linea alba, 280*f*
linear energy transfer (LET), 242
linear grid, 203, 311
linear tomography, 150–151
linear-nonthreshold relationship, 240
linear-threshold relationship, 240
lip/o combining form, 21
lipsmeatal line (LML) positioning, 316*f*
lith/o combining form, 21
lithotomy, 302
liver, 270*f*, 273*t*, 274*f*
LLQ (left lower quadrant), 304, 305*f*
LML (lipsmeatal line) positioning, 316*f*
lobes, 285*f*
localization, Sacred Seven patient care questions, 35, 350
long scale of contrast, 186
longitudinal muscle layer, stomach, 271*f*
look-up table (LUT), 205
loop of Henle, 295*f*
Los Angeles Radiological Society, 325
Louisiana Society of Radiologic Technologists, 326
lower gastrointestinal series, 269
low-osmolality contrast agent, 75, 354
lumbar spinal nerves, 283*f*
lumbar vertebrae, 292*f*
luminescence, 94
lungs, 286*t*, 287*f*
LUQ (left upper quadrant), 304, 305*f*
LUT (look-up table), 205
lymphatic system, 276–277, 278*f*
lymph/o combining form, 21
lymphocytes, 245
lysosome, 238*f*, 239*t*, 370

M

mA (milliampere), 148, 197
mA meter, 134
mA selector, 135
macro- prefix, 19
magnet, 121
magnetic resonance (MR) imaging, 4*t*, 329
magnetism, 122
magnification, 170, 194
main pancreatic duct, 274*f*

main power switch, 133
major calyces, kidney, 294*f*
major kVp selector, 133
male gonads, 275*t*
male reproductive organs, 284*t*, 285*f*
malice, 34, 350
malpractice, 38
mammography, 4*t*
mandible, 290*t*, 291*f*, 373
manifest image, 208
manifest stage, acute radiation syndrome, 237, 369
manual spin top test, 219, 255
Maryland Society of Radiologic Technologists, 326
mAs (milliamperes), 148, 196, 223
mAs timers, 134
mass, 94
Massachusetts Society of Radiologic Technologists, 326
masseter, 280*f*
masseter muscle, 271*f*
mastoid process, 291*f*
Material Safety Data Sheet (MSDS), 49, 353
mathematical equations, 216–228
    answer key, 366–368
        concept thinking questions, 366
        matching, 367
        practice exercises, 366–367
        retention of material, 367–368
    Coulomb's law, 217
    density, 217
    direct square law, 217
    exposure maintenance formula, 218–219
    exposure timer test tools, 219–220
    fifteen percent (15%) rule, 220
    grid ratio, 220
    grid ratio/mAs formula, 220
    hp, 221
    HU, 220–221
    image intensifier mathematical equations, 221–222
    image magnification, 222
    inverse square law, 222
    khU, 223
    kV, 222
    mAs, 223
    mechanical energy, 223
    ohm, 223
    Ohm's law, 223
    OID, 223
    orbital shell formula, 223
    overview, 216–217
    patient dose, 223–224
    penumbra formula, 224
    pixel size formula, 224
    Planck's constant, 224
    power, 225
    power loss formula, 225
    reciprocity law, 225
    rectification formula, 225
    RSV, 225
    transformer current law, 225–226

transformer voltage law, 226
tube angulation, 226–227
units to measure ionizing radiation, 227
units to measure radioactivity, 227
velocity, 227–228
watt, 228
weight, 228
work, 228
mathematical triangle
  manual spin top test, 255*f*
  synchronous motor spin test, 256*f*
matrix, 191, 192*f*
matter, 94
matter interaction, 94–98
maxilla, 290*t*, 291*f*, 373
mean marrow dose, 242
means of transmission, 45
mechanical energy, 90, 223
medial, 309
medial rotation, 310, 311*f*
median plane, 304, 316*f*
medical and legal terms
  AHCD, 26
  ambulatory, 26
  answer key, 349–351
    concept thinking questions, 349–350
    matching, 351
    practice exercises, 350–351
    retention of material, 351
  ARRT Rules of Ethics, 26
  ASRT
    Code of Ethics, 26, 322
    Practice Standards for Medical Imaging
      and Radiation Therapy, 26–27, 331
  authorization, 27
  autonomy, 27
  beneficence, 27
  blood pressure reading, 27
  body mechanics, 27–39
  body temperature reading, 27–29
  communication, 29–30
  compassion, 30
  competence, 30
  compliance, 30
  conviction, 30
  CPR, 29
  criminal background check, 30
  cultural diversity, 30
  defendant, 30
  dependent, 30
  diagnosis, 30
  DNR code, 31
  doctrine, 31
  drug screening/testing, 31
  empathy, 31
  ethics, ethical, 31
  felony, 31–32
  fidelity, 31
  flight-or-fight response, 32
  fraud, 32
  health care, 32
  health care team, 32
  Heimlich maneuver, 32

HIPAA, 33
hospice, 33
incident report, 33
law, 33–34
malice, 34
medical record, 34
misdemeanor, 34
mission statement, 34
morals/morality, 34
overview, 25–26
patient assessment data collection, 34
patient chart, 34–35
patient history, 35–36
patient type, 36
plaintiff, 36
pregnancy, 36–37
prognosis, 37
reprimand, 37
sanction, 37
state regulations, 37
tort, 37–38
values, 38
veracity, 38
vital signs, 38–39
vulnerable, 39
medical asepsis, 43, 352
medical record, 34
medulla, 275*t*
medulla oblongata, 282*f*
-megaly suffix, 22
meiosis, 242–243
membranous organelles, 239*t*
mental foramen, 291*f*
mentomeatal line (MML), 316*f*
mentum, 315*f*
mesocephalic skull, 318*f*, 373
mesovarium, 284*f*
metacarpals, 290*t*
metaphase, mitosis, 243
metatarsals, 290*t*
meter, electric circuit, 116*t*, 122
MG (minification gain), 170, 221–222, 362
Michigan Society of Radiologic
  Technologists, 326
micro- prefix, 19
microorganism, 49
microvilli, 239*t*
midbrain, 282*f*
mid-coronal plane, 303
Middle States Association of Colleges and
  Schools, 6
midlateral orbital margin, 315*f*
mid-sagittal plane, 304, 316*f*
mild reactions, contrast agents, 67
milliampere (mA), 148, 196, 197, 223
minification gain (MG), 170, 221–222, 362
minimum reaction time, AEC, 114
Minnesota Society of Radiologic
  Technologists, 327
minor calyces, kidney, 294*f*
minor calyx, kidney, 294*f*
minor kVp selector, 133
miscibility, 73

misdemeanor, 34, 349
mission statement, 34, 351
Missouri Society of Radiologic Technologists,
  327
mitochondria, 238*f*, 239*t*
mitosis, 243
MML (mentomeatal line), 316*f*
mobile fluoroscopic units, 174
mobile x-ray unit, 148–149
moderate reactions, contrast agents, 67
moiré pattern, 208
molecule, 98, 243
morals/morality, 34, 350
motor, 122
mouth, 270*f*
MR (magnetic resonance) imaging, 4*t*
MSDS (Material Safety Data Sheet), 49, 353
multifield image intensification, 170–171
muscle tissue
  cardiac
    cells, 279*f*
    characteristics of, 279*t*
  overview, 279*t*
  skeletal
    anterior view, 280*f*
    cells, 279*f*
    characteristics of, 279*t*
    posterior view, 281*f*
  smooth
    cells, 279*f*
    characteristics of, 279*t*
muscular system, 277
mutation, 243
mutual induction, 118, 357
myel/o combining form, 21
myofibrils, 279*f*
myometrium, 284*f*

N

N (nuclear medicine technology), 4*t*, 330
N95 respirator, 52
nasal bone, 291*f*
nasal cavity, 287*f*
nasion, 315*f*
nasoenteric tube (NE tube), 73–74
nasogastric tube (NG tube), 74
nasopharynx, 287*f*
The National Association for Proton Therapy,
  329
National Council on Radiation Protection
  and Measurements (NCRP), 238, 252,
  253*t*, 257
National Institute for Occupational Safety
  and Health (NIOSH), 52
National Institutional Accrediting Agencies, 6
national organizations, 328–329
natural magnets, 121*t*
NCRP (National Council on Radiation
  Protection and Measurements),
  160, 174, 238, 252, 253*t*, 257

NE tube (nasoenteric tube), 73–74
Nebraska Society of Radiologic Technologists, 327
neck, sagittal section, 287*f*
necr/o combining form, 21
needle, 49–50
needle recapping, 50
needleless devices, 50
needlestick injury, 50
negative contrast agent, 66, 354
negative pressure room, 47
negligence, 38
negligence doctrines, 38
nephr/o combining form, 21
nephron, 295*f*, 373
nervous system, 277
neur/o combining form, 21
neuron, 282*f*
neuron soma (cell body), 282*f*
neutral, 309
neutron, 98
New England Association of Schools and Colleges, 6
New Mexico Society of Radiologic Technologists, 327
New York State Society of Radiologic Sciences, Inc., 327
New York State Society of Radiologic Technologists, 327
NG tube (nasogastric tube), 74
NIOSH (National Institute for Occupational Safety and Health), 52
nipple, 285*f*
nitroglycerin, 77, 354
NMTCB (Nuclear Medicine Technology Certification Board), 8*t*
noise, 171
nomogram, 241, 243, 244*f*
nonionic contrast media, 66, 353
nonionizing radiation, 98
nonlinear-nonthreshold relationship, 240
nonlinear-threshold relationship, 240, 241
nonmembranous organelles, cell, 239*t*, 369
non-screen film, 198, 208
nonstochastic effect, 245
North American Society for Cardiac Imaging, 330
North Carolina Society of Radiologic Technologists, 327
North Central Association of Colleges and Schools, 6
Northwest Commission on Colleges and Universities, 6
nosocomial infection, 45
NRC (Nuclear Regulatory Commission), 257
nuclear arrangements, 93*t*
Nuclear Council on Radiation Protection (NCRP), 160, 174
nuclear energy, 90
Nuclear Medicine Technology Certification Board (NMTCB), 8*t*
nuclear medicine technology (N), 4*t*, 330
Nuclear Regulatory Commission (NRC), 257

nucleolus, 238*f*
nucleons, 98
nucleus
  cell, 238*f*, 239*t*
  neuron, 282*f*
  skeletal muscle, 279*f*
  smooth muscle, 279*f*
numbered stroke surgical scrub method, 58, 352

O

objective data, 34, 349
object-to-image distance (OID), 195*f*, 208, 223
oblique muscle layer, stomach, 271*f*
oblique position, 302, 309
occipital bone, 290*t*, 291*f*
occipitalis, 281*f*
occlusal plane, 303
occupancy (T), 258
octet rule, 98
OD (optical density), 188, 217
OER (oxygen enhancement ratio), 243–244
Oersted, hans Christian, 119
Oersted experiment, 119
off -centering, 203
off-focus radiation, 100, 101*f*, 203
off-level grid, 203
Ohio Society of Radiologic Technologists, 327
ohm (W), 122, 223
Ohm's law, 122–123, 223, 367
OID (object-to-image distance), 195*f*, 208, 223
Oklahoma Society of Radiologic Technologists, 327
olecranon process, 290*t*
olig- prefix, 19
-ologist suffix, 22
-ology suffix, 22
-oma suffix, 22
OML (orbitalmeatal line), 316*f*
onset, Sacred Seven patient care questions, 35, 350
open switch, electric circuit, 116*t*
optical density (OD), 188, 217
optically stimulated luminescence dosimeter (OSL), 251*t*, 254*f*
oral route, drug administration, 77*t*
oral temperature reading, 28
orbicularis oculi, 280*f*
orbicularis oris, 280*f*
orbital shell
  corresponding electrons, 99*t*
  with corresponding electrons, 224*t*
  defined, 98
orbital shell formula, 98, 223
orbitalmeatal line (OML), 316*f*
Oregon Society of Radiologic Technologists, 328

organ systems
  answer key, 371–373
    concept thinking questions, 371
    matching, 372
    practice exercises, 371–372
    retention of material, 372–373
  autonomic nervous system, 277
  cardiovascular system, 267
  digestive system, 267–272
  endocrine system, 272, 275*t*
  integumentary system, 272
  lymphatic system, 276–277, 278*f*
  muscular system, 277
  nervous system, 277
  overview, 266–267
  peripheral nervous system (PNS), 277
  reproductive system, 280
  respiratory system, 281, 283, 286*t*
  skeletal system, 286, 288*t*
  thoracic duct entering venous system, 278*f*
  urinary system
    anatomy of, 293*t*
    defined, 286
    structures of, 294*f*
organelles, 239*t*
oropharynx, 287*f*
-osis suffix, 22
OSL (optically stimulated luminescence dosimeter), 251*t*, 254*f*
osmolarity, 75
osmosis, 75
oste/o combining form, 21
-ostomy suffix, 22
-otomy suffix, 22
outer canthus, 315*f*
output phosphor, 166*f*, 167, 362
ovarian ligament, 284*f*
ovary, 276*f*, 284*f*
overexposure, 181
overhead x-ray tube, 168–169
over-the-needle catheter, 72, 73*f*
overview, 180
oxygen administration, 75
oxygen enhancement ratio (OER), 243–244

P

PACS (picture-archiving communication systems), 209
pair production, 95
palatine tonsils, 287*f*
palmar, 309, 310*f*
pancreas
  anatomy of, 273*t*
  duodenum and, 274*f*
  hormone secretions, 275*t*
  location of, 276*f*
  overview, 270*f*
panoramic tomography, 151
parallax, 187, 208
parallel circuit wiring, 115–117

parallel grid, 203, 311
parasite, 50
parathyroid gland
    hormone secretions, 275*t*
    location of, 276*f*
parenteral route, drug administration, 77*t*
parietal bone, 290*t*, 291*f*
parotid duct, 271*f*
parotid gland, 271*f*
particulate radiation, 92
particulate respirator, 52, 56*f*
patella, 280*f*, 290*t*
patellar ligament, 280*f*
path/o combining form, 21
pathogen, 50–51, 352
pathogenic organism, 45
patient assessment data collection, 34
patient chart, 34–35
patient dose, 171, 223–224
patient history, 35–36, 75
patient type, 36
patients, responsibilities of (Florida), 338
patients, rights of (Florida), 336–338
    access to health care, 338
    experimental research, 338
    financial information and disclosure, 338
    individual dignity, 336–337
    information, 337–338
    patient's knowledge of rights and
        responsibilities, 338
Patient's Bill of Rights, 29
PBL (positive beam limitation), 183–184, 257
PCF (phase conversion factor), 125–126, 225
pectoralis major muscle, 280*f*, 285*f*
penetrability, 149
penetrometer, 208, 211
-penia suffix, 22
penis, 285*f*
penumbra, 173, 202, 208–209
penumbra formula, 224
peri- prefix, 19
perimetrium, 284*f*
periodic table of elements, 89*f*
peripheral nervous system (PNS), 277
peripherally inserted central catheter (PICC)
        line, 65, 355
peroneus brevis, 281*f*
peroneus longus, 280*f*, 281*f*
perpendicular, 312
perpendicular plate of ethmoid bone, 291*f*
personal protective equipment (PPE), 51–55
personnel monitoring devices, 250–251
PFCs, 226*t*
-phagia suffix, 22
phalanges, 290*t*
pharmaceutical, 75
pharmacology
    answer key, 353–355
        concept thinking questions, 353
        matching, 354
        practice exercises, 354
        retention of material, 354–355
    crash cart, 67–68

defibrillator, 69
diuretic, 69
drip infusion, 69
drug, 69
endotracheal tube, 69
extravasation, 69
"five rights" of drug administration, 70
flushing, 71
Foley catheter, 71
glucagon, 71
glucophage, 71
human tissue, 71–72
hypodermic needle, 72–73
infiltrate, 73
informed consent, 73
injections, 73
IV push, 73
miscibility, 73
NE tube, 73–74
NG tube, 74
osmolarity, 75
osmosis, 75
overview, 62–63
oxygen administration, 75
patient history, 75
pharmaceutical, 75
prescription, 76
radiolucent, 76
radio-opaque, 76
routes of drug administration, 76
syringe, 76
tourniquet, 76–77
vasoconstrictor, 77
vasodilator, 77
venipuncture, 78
venous system, 78
vial, 79
viscosity, 79
pharynx, 269, 287*f*
phase conversion factor (PCF), 125–126, 225
-phasia suffix, 22
phenidone, 201*t*
phleb combining form, 21
phosphorescence, 206
photocathode, 166*f*, 167, 361
photocells, 114
photodisintegration, 96
photoelectric absorption, 96–97, 97*f*
photoemission, 172, 362
photographic properties, 209
photomultiplier tube, 113, 250, 358
photon, 98–99
photopic vision, 166, 172
photospot camera, 167, 362
photostimuable phosphors (PSP), 184
phototime, AEC, 114
physics terminology
    absorption, 85
    acceleration, 85
    amplitude, 85
    amu, 86
    angstrom (Å), 85
    anode, 85

answer key, 355–356
    concept thinking questions, 355
    matching, 356
    practice exercises, 356
    retention of material, 356
atom, 85–86
atomic mass number, 86
atomic number, 86
attenuation, 86
Bohr's atomic model, 86
cathode, 86
current, 86
diagnostic x-ray range, 86–87
electrification, 87
electrodynamics, 87
electromagnetic spectrum, 87
electron, 87
electrostatics, 87–88
element, 88
energy, 88–90
fluorescence, 91
frequency, 91
fundamental particles, 91
half-life, 91
hertz, 91
incident electron, 91
ion, 91
ionization, 91
ionizing radiation, 91–93
isobar, 93
isomer, 93
isotone, 93
isotope, 93
isotropic, 94
lambda, 94
luminescence, 94
mass, 94
matter, 94
matter interaction, 94–98
molecule, 98
neutron, 98
nonionizing radiation, 98
nucleons, 98
orbital shell, 98
orbital shell formula, 98
overview, 84–85
photon, 98–99
Planck's constant, 99
polyenergetic, 99
proton, 99
quanta/quantum, 99
quarks, 99
radiation
    human-made, 99–104
    natural, 104
radioactivity, 104
sinusoidal wave, 104
speed of light, 104
units of ionizing radiation, 104
velocity, 104–105
wavelength, 105
wave-particle duality, 105
weight, 105

work, 105
  x-ray circuit, x-ray unit, 105
  x-ray production, 106
  x-ray properties, 106
PICC (peripherally inserted central catheter)
    line, 65, 355
picture-archiving communication systems
    (PACS), 209
pineal gland
  hormone secretions, 275t
  location of, 276f
pitting, 153
pituitary gland
  hormone secretions, 275t
  location of, 276f
pixel size formula, 224
pixels, 191, 192f
plaintiff, 36
Planck's constant, 99, 224
plantodorsal projection, 299, 302f
plasma membrane, 238f
-plegia suffix, 22
plumbicon, 173
plunger, syringe, 76, 77f
pluridirectional tomography, 151
-pnea suffix, 22
pneum/o combining form, 21
PNS (peripheral nervous system), 277
pocket dosimeter, 251t
poly- prefix, 19
polyenergetic, 99
pons, 282f
portable fluoroscopic units, 174
Port-a-Cath port, 65
positioning
  abbreviations
    projections and positions, 299–301
    radiographic examinations, 299
  answer key, 373–374
    concept thinking questions, 373
    matching, 373–374
    practice exercises, 373
    retention of material, 374
  body quadrants (abdominopelvic),
    304
  body regions (abdominopelvic),
    304–305
  bony landmarks, 314–315
  directional terms, 306–311
  directional x-ray tube terms, 311–314
  overview, 298–299
  skull morphology, 318
  skull positioning lines, 316–318
  skull topography, 315–316
  vocabulary terms, 301–304
positive beam limitation (PBL), 183–184,
    257
positive contrast agent, 66, 354
positive ion, 356
post- prefix, 20
posterior direction, 309
postprimary pathway, ARRT, 9
potassium alum, 201t

potassium bromide, 201t
potential energy, 90, 223
powdered gloves, 52
power, 123, 225
power loss, 123
power loss formula, 123, 225
PPE (personal protective equipment), 51–55
Practice Standards, 25–26
pre- prefix, 20
prefixes, 16, 19–20
pregnancy, 36–37
pregnant radiographer/trainee, 257
prepuce, 285f
prereading kVp meter, 133
prescription, 76
preservatives, film processing, 201t
primary bronchus, 288f
primary pathway, ARRT, 9
primary protective barrier, 258, 370
primary radiation, 100
privacy, 33
prodromal stage, acute radiation syndrome,
    237, 369
professional organizations, 323–330. *See also*
    imaging modalities
  answer key, 346–348
    concept thinking questions, 346
    matching, 347
    practice exercises, 346–347
    retention of material, 347–348
  imaging modalities, 329–330
  national and international organizations,
    328–329
  radiology associations, 323
  radiology societies, 324
  state organizations, 325–328
prognosis, 37, 351
projections
  abbreviations, 299–301
  axial, 311, 312f
  dorsoplantar, 299, 301f
  plantodorsal, 299, 302f
  SMV, 300f
  VSM, 301f
proliferate, 56, 244
prominent rib, 314
pronation, 309, 310f
prone, 302
prophase, mitosis, 243
prostate gland, 285f, 294f
protective barrier, 257–259
protective curtain, 167
protective devices, 258–259
protective housing, 149
protective shielding, 250
protective/reverse isolation, 49
proton, 99
protozoan parasites, 50, 352
proximal, 309
proximal convoluted tubule, 295f
PSP (photostimuable phosphors), 184
pubic bone, 285f, 314
pubis, 290t

pulse rate, 39, 349
pyel/o combining form, 21
pyloric sphincter, stomach, 271f

Q

QA (quality assurance), 259, 260t
QC (quality control), 83, 260
QM (quality management), 4t, 259–261
quadriceps tendon, 280f
quality
  defined, 350
  HVL, 209
  Sacred Seven patient care questions, 36
quality assurance (QA), 259, 260t
quality control (QC), 83, 260
quality factor. *See* radiation-weighting factor
    (WR)
quality management (QM), 4t, 259–261
quanta/quantum, 99
quantity, 209
quantum mottle (quantum noise), 172, 209
quarks, 99

R

R (radiography), 4t, 332
RA (radiologist assistant), 5t, 11–12
Raaf catheter, 65
radial deviation, 310
radiation
  human-made, 99–104
  natural, 104
radiation biology
  absorbed dose equivalent, 235
  acute, 235
  acute radiation dose, 235
  acute radiation symptoms, 235
  acute radiation syndrome, 235–236
  acute radiation syndrome staging, 237
  alopecia, 237
  anabolic, 237
  answer key, 368–370
    concept thinking questions, 368–369
    matching, 369
    practice exercises, 369
    retention of material, 369–370
  biological effect, 237
  biology, 237
  carcinogen, 237
  catabolic, 237
  cell, 237
  chromosome, 237–238
  chronic, 238
  chronic radiation dose, 238
  congenital effect, 238
  cumulative exposure, 238
  desquamation, 238
  differentiated cell, 238–239